clinical
an architecture of variation with repetition

Maria Hurtado de Mendoza
estudio.entresitio

Clinical means "relating to a clinic", but also "based on observation of an individual". It also means "analytical". This book is a clinical study of a trilogy of health-care centers built by estudio.entresitio in Madrid, Spain. A trilogy of three individuals, three case studies that share the same formal configuration and yet are perceived as different.

Books, as projects, have an initial stage of explosion in which many directions and possibilities are opened at once. Then comes a quieter stage, in which ideas are reorganized, distilled and rounded out. For this book, the detonator is drawing. A collection of analytical representations of the clinics are the foundation for an exploration of a number of questions in the project, in the search for their best translation. It is an iterative process in which words are a second step: they emphasize what the drawings may be already explaining and also provide an additional layer of information, structure and even room for debate.

Ideas regarding difference and repetition, ordering systems, materiality, program strategies and formal structure are unfolded in a sequential collection that talks about entresitio's strategies in the conception of architectural space – the transfer from the world of ideas to physical realization.

Maria Hurtado de Mendoza is an architect and an educator, founding partner at estudio.entresitio. She is an Associate Professor of Architecture at the New Jersey Institute of Technology. Prior to NJIT, she taught at Madrid's Polytechnic University ETSAM (her alma mater) for 15 years and at Cornell University as a visiting critic. She was also a resident scholar at the Spanish Academy in Rome.

estudio.entresitio is a Madrid-NY based practice that is invested in the material actualization of the architectural concept. The practice has extensive building experience with an emphasis on public work that utilizes novel solutions for what is functional and necessary without sacrificing creativity or exploration. A large number of international awards and recognitions for projects, and especially for built work, speak to the attention that estudio.entresitio's work gives to spatial thinking and tectonics.

In recent years, the public has begun to recognize the estudio.entresitio name before the names of its different members. That's how it should be. As a registered trademark it represents a joint effort and, in addition, entresitio has become part of us. I like to think of entresitio as an alias – a pseudonym that, curiously, various people share.

In that sense, this book belongs as much to entresitio, to which it owes an obvious debt, as is does to me. Especially to César Jiménez de Tejada: a classmate and colleague throughout my career, a constant source of support and indisputable friend; his ideas are all over – in fact, I can no longer distinguish them from my own.

And to my brother Pepe (José María) Hurtado de Mendoza, who always has the clearest sight; to follow the clinical metaphor, he usually makes the best diagnostic, the one that is truly useful. But entresitio is a lot of people: Alvar Ruiz, our associate, has been working with us for so many years that I can't remember what the firm was like without him – a tireless draftsman, he never gives up on trying "all" the options on a design, some of which are included here; and María Urigoitia, an extraordinary former student of mine and an even better collaborator, she is responsible for many of the other drawings and her patience and level-headedness were key to putting each detail in its place. I would also like to thank Ruben Petrela, a student in the Master's program at NJIT for his smart suggestions during the initial phases of the book, and which put it on the path to what it is now.

Over the years in which we developed the design and construction of the S,U,V trilogy many collaborators have come through estudio.entresitio. Some of them were more directly tied to the projects (I hope I haven't left anyone out) and I would like to thank them for their efforts: Jorge Martínez, Laura Frutos, Vicent Rodríguez, Fabrice Quemeneur, Felipe Minderico, Clara Rodríguez, Marco Plazzogna and Miguel Crespo, architects; Geasyt S.A. (Francisco Sánchez and Felipe Fernández) and María José Camporro, consultants; Juan Carlos Corona and David Gil, quantity surveyors, and Copredije S.A. for security.

I would like to make special mention of the photographers Roland Halbe and Raul Belinchón, whose work is a fundamental part of this book. Roland began photographing our work when we finished the San Blas project. Since then he has accompanied us on that special day, perhaps the only time our work belongs solely to us.

This book is about the health care centers San Blas, Usera and Villaverde which belong to Madrid Salud, an independent body under the Madrid City Council. When our design won the competition, the director of Madrid Salud was Jose Manuel Torrecilla, and his right hand was Pilar Felip. They are, most certainly, the best client we have ever had. We owe them a debt of thanks for their sincere professional respect and their intelligence. The construction of the clinics involved a long list of manufacturers and contractors, and the help of Madrid Salud, especially from Victor Martín.

Professor Val Warke, from Cornell University, who showed so much generosity in writing the foreword to this book, was the first person who encouraged me to look at 3x1 as a dissertation, and I am still grateful for the challenge. His words stuck with me somehow, and they became important again a few years later when I started working on a monographic about ideas that interest us at entresitio.

Thanks to professor Keith Krumwiede for talking with me until I had understood the book I wanted to write, and for his love of architectural drawings; and thank you to professor Karen Frank for her ability to structure and order concepts that helped me so much in the initial stages. Both are teachers and my colleagues at the School of Architecture at the New Jersey Institute of Technology, where I have taught since 2013. Support from the institute has been essential in making this book possible.

I grew as an architect with books published by Actar publishers on my desk, and I couldn't be more delighted that they are publishing this monograph. Thank you to Ramón Prat and Ricardo Devesa for leading me here.

Why are there so many paintings of women with parrots?

It doesn't seem to be a natural or obvious association. At first, in the fifteenth century, it was apparently mostly portraits of the Madonna that included parrots, with the bird having some sort of allegorical relationship to Immaculate Conception, since parrots had already been considered in classical circles as some sort of intermediary between the heavens and earth. But the *woman with parrot* theme lingered among the arts for centuries; and largely with no feasible association with virginity, or purity, or any of the other traits associated with Mary — so slippery are symbols. One thinks of Tiepolo (or was that a macaw?), Delacroix (his subject quite a distance from the Virgin Mary), Courbet (further still), Manet, Renoir, Bonnard, Cézanne, Kahlo (with many parrots), Dali, and even Botero, among many others.

The return to the theme of woman and parrot — in countless prints, paintings, and pin-ups — seems to be more than a show of technical virtuosity in incorporating bright colors in a composition or in being able to convincingly depict the texture of feathers, but also as a recurrent litmus of an artist's relation to contemporary social and political milieux. And because of the sheer number of "women with parrots," there is an inevitable intra-artistic dialogue that is opened up, with a complex network of quotations, confrontations, homages, and challenges.

This same concept of theme and variation seems to be even more ubiquitous in music. There is a fascinating paradox at the center of every musical theme with variations: while it is usually the persistence of the theme's melodic refrain that unifies and propels the composition, it is the variations of rhythm, harmony, key, range, instrumentation, and so on that drive the composition into uncharted territories. The listener's familiarity and expectation becomes jolted by the evolution of unfamiliar variants. The familiar is suddenly unfamiliar; the habitual is suddenly invigorated. Most importantly, themes with variations serve a larger purpose: in suppressing the dominance of melody, they elevate an awareness of the techniques of music-ness, or of what makes music music. (Incidentally, in our current context, it's perhaps not surprising that two of the more prevalent musical variation forms, the chaconne and the passacaglia seem to have their origins in Spain.)

It is into this context that we might place the clinics of estudio.entresitio.

Despite their assertions to the contrary, I believe it's very propitious that there are three clinics, rather than the originally planned two. When there are two similar things, one tends to understand them simply as dichotomous: lighter/darker, rougher/smoother, more opaque/more transparent, and so on. With three things, one tends to see them in an ongoing conversation, as individual utterances that are continuously elaborating and enriching each other — S to U, U to V, V to S — all the while altering our understanding and experience of the triad. And the conversation can go on.

Perhaps most importantly, with three things there is a condition of "unfinalizability": a capacity to expand understandings beyond the boundaries of the three works, and to resist closure. Two clinics would be a pair; each refers to the other. Three clinics, however, are loosened from a dialectic *pas de deux*; they oppose definitive boundaries of interpretation. Instead, an evolution is proposed; a trajectory is established. The perceptive observer begins to fantasize about possible clinics A, M, T, and so on, speculating on further permutations of the material/spatial vocabulary, designing clinics of the mind that would never have otherwise been imaginable.

The differences in material allow us to momentarily 'bracket' planimetric distinctions and to then investigate the more phenomenal realms of material distinction. In other words, the clinics of estudio.entresitio seem to establish a very tangible link between material and perception.

The typology of the mat with multiple courtyards allows the various clinics to exploit an internal autonomy that separates them from the vagaries of multiple and uncontrollable external contexts. These courtyards — "patios," in their original, Spanish incarnations — in their erasure of the immediate urban fabric, engender a sense of privacy within the community of the clinic itself, of calmness, and of refuge from daily realities.

At the same time, these glazed courts play upon all of the traits of glass: sometimes transparent, sometimes reflective, sometimes opaque. The material treatment of these courtyards poses a fascinating dichotomy: on the one hand, they provide a grand openness to the interior; on the other hand, they also seem to propose a sense of displacement, as in a labyrinthine house of mirrors.

But that is to speak of the common themes of these clinics. As is the case of the theme with variations, what is most important with these clinics — and especially with this presentation of this project — is that their variations make us extraordinarily aware of the "architectureness" of the whole endeavor. And this text represents those variations with a thrilling precision.

Rafael Moneo once pointed out that the publication of *Five Architects* had a major affect on the teaching of architecture around the world, especially in Europe and in Spain in particular. While many people superficially read the text as advocating a specific strain of architecture, Moneo and others read the text as suggestive of an intertwined network of potential pedagogies, of making a speculative architecture teachable.[1]

With this perhaps in the back of my mind, immediately after having heard Maria Hurtado de Mendoza lecture on these clinics, I sent an (uncharacteristic) email that said, among other things:

Maria--

I loved your lecture. It was one of the best I've seen in recent years .... The 3 clinics are a curriculum in themselves.

Thank you.

I still believe this.

So, as this book illustrates, there is a clear, transferrable logic to the work of estudio.entresitio, a strategy of development that explains the pedagogical and didactic values such work can have.

Similarly, there is an assertive, didactic value established by the presentation of these clinics. While this might seem contradictory, the chapters provide a logical recitation of architecture's most powerful antinomies. There are presentations of the tools at an architect's disposal; of strategies of organizing (and disorganizing) a program; of numerous field conditions that include type and fragmentation, geometry as a metaphor, and anti-gravity as spatiality; of concepts of difference through repetition; of what one might understand as the devices of producing the "scarless merger"; of resisting standardization (although not necessarily repetition); and, finally, of the palette of techniques with which the architect can rigorously "confront the inexact."

1. Rafael Moneo, lecture in session "Five Architects and After: From Structure to Performativity," part of *The '70s: The Formation of Contemporary Architectural Discourse*, conference at Cornell and Harvard, Feb. 6, 2001.

One finds also, as with many of the painterly themes and variations, another form of internal discourse within this text. Just as Manet's *Young Lady [with parrot] in 1866* refers to his earlier works of *Olympia* and *Luncheon on the Grass* by using the same model (though this time fully clothed and with a demure expression; quite probably as a critique of Courbet's more languid *Woman with a Parrot*), estudio.entresitio presents us with potential future variations on their clinic theme, showing their original "model" on a hilly site, and with a sixth façade.

Most valuable is that this is not a rigid catechism of design methodology. It is an embrasure of architecture's variabilities, its dichotomies, its humanness, and a projection of its possibilities.

One would be remiss to point out that there is also a poignancy to the fact that, due to the recent economic situation in Spain, these clinics represent some of the relatively rare recent works of Spanish architects building in Spain. And that, in another variation on a theme — a reciprocal to *Five Architects'* migration into numerous Spanish academies — many of Spain's most talented architects have turned to settling abroad, and to teaching in schools around the world, and in the United States in particular. But this is not simply a matter of economic flight. One might argue that there is a deep appreciation for the insights and sensibilities of these architects, especially with their talents for the teaching of architects.

While, on the one hand, one finds in these teachings a reverence for the clarity of the diagram; on the other, this clarity is modified by the diagram's alternative capacity to suggest sites of ambiguity, overlap, and distortion. We see in this text a dissertation on the plan's capacity for variation, and on the necessity for intelligent self-critique. It is, in its way, a suite of "Women with Parrots."

And in the end, given the effect that works like this should have on the way we think of architecture, and of the considerable affect these architects have on the teaching of architecture around the world, we might all become Spanish architects. This could be a very good thing.

Conciliation of Opposites
Introducing the clinic as the case study for this clinical book on architectural design. Through analytical drawings, it explores a polarized relationship between an interior and exterior that are, however, two sides of the same coin. This clinic, which – when considered as an archetype – has been called "3x1", is a placeless building with formal autonomy in which light comes only from above.

Programmatic Bars
An explanation of the generic clinical program's chain-like configurations and their spatial and formal structure. The relationship between circulation and program (circulation serves program) is informed by the waiting areas and the desire for natural light and ventilation. The layout of programmatic bars around and through exterior spaces introduces the logics of the clinical grain.

Field Condition
When the programmatic bars are placed alongside one another to become an extended field and the façade is no longer an option for lighting the entire floor plan, new rules apply. 3x1 is a mathematical field condition with a characteristic rhythm that establishes the relationship between order, space and structure.

Difference and Repetition
Building the same building three times becomes a learning process in itself: what is the same but different, how different can the spatial translations of one plan be, what is the consequence of the material physicality of what is built, are some of the questions that arise. The question of the one and the many, across scales and components.

The Scarless Merger
However many different components or parts a project may have, we tend to erase their independency in favor of the whole. It is like the hand to arm continuity, where there is no clear division between one and the other. Like a typical condition in human skin, when we build the idea is to cut and join things in parts so that they look complete once the parts are put together.

Towards the Nonstandard
The nonstandard appears when varying from the usual. It is about questioning the given status quo and, from there, the role of the discipline-based creativity of architectural design. It involves the consideration of certain ordering systems and their specific way of addressing gravity, scale, and the width and depth of what is being built.

Conciliation of Opposites

Introducing the clinic as the case study for this clinical book on architectural design. Through analytical drawings, it explores a polarized relationship between an interior and exterior that are, however, two sides of the same coin. This clinic, which – when considered as an archetype – has been called “3x1”, is a placeless building with formal autonomy in which light comes only from above.

The idea of the conciliation of opposites is well represented by Le Corbusier's drawing the Sun and Medusa: a hybrid between two realities, meaning that opposites can reach a certain point where they are no longer one thing or another but both things at the same time. A certain estrangement (the uncanny) comes with these ambiguous pairings; it is presented as something easy to understand and yet hard to convey.

In this dialectical opposition, opposites are not in confrontation; instead they work in reciprocal advantage and help us understand dichotomies not as the need for choosing between things but as the possibility of exploring what is in between.

It also becomes a special kind of freedom for the mind that does not need to take a strong position; black or white, open or closed, order or disorder, false or true… rather, it can embrace “this and that” (the power of and!).

It can be understood here as the aim for synthetic thinking as well, when in the translation of abstract conceptual ideas into physical space, one same solution is posited for all the different questions – including the aesthetic ones.

Very closely related to these questions is the idea of harmony as the equilibrium of proportions between the different parts (aspects) of a whole – especially from the perspective of ancient Greek thinking (Heraclitus), where harmony is understood not only as a mathematical and static consequence but as the dynamic balance of opposing forces which does not allow one to exceed the other, and the disappearance of one will lead to the disappearance of its opposite (the bow and the lyre).

3x1 is a trilogy of healthcare clinics that estudio.entresitio built in Madrid, Spain.
Why there were three may not be relevant anymore. It all started with an unusual competition to build two clinics for the same client (Madrid's city council) with the same budget, the same functional program, and on two different sites.
Our answer to those initial conditions was to work with the idea of a "placeless building" as a strategy to insert a cohesive whole into irrelevant environments. A great sense of autonomy was required in formal, functional and even conceptual terms to allow the building to exist no matter where. This so-called placeless building takes on the opposition between hermetic and open as a conceptual framework and initiator for the project.
The third clinic came along later in the game as an expanded possibility for variation on the initial scheme.

S- San Blas, U- Usera, V- Villaverde are the three neighborhoods in the eastern and southern outskirts of Madrid, where the clinics are located.

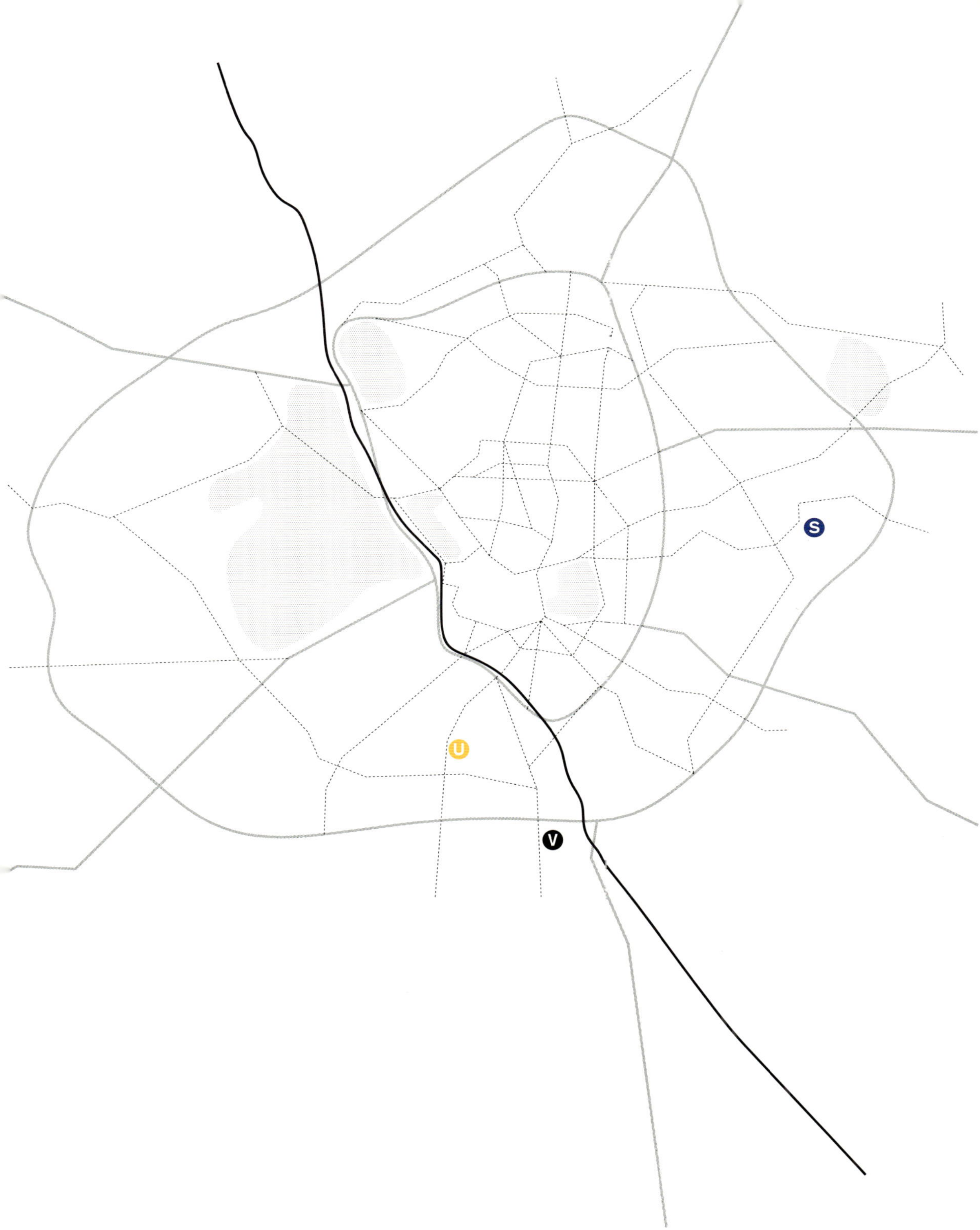

S
U
V

Placeless becomes different than siteless; "the site is not the place" is something Enric Miralles used to say when talking about the work of the exact disposition of a building on a site.
The two words may be synonyms, but they do have different nuances:
- site (situs) as a portion of space, real or imagined, in which something is located.
- place (locus) as a portion of space that fulfills a certain condition (in mathematics, equation).
Although we are used to saying "this building is placed on this site", potentially 3x1 can be sited on any/every place. As a placeless building, 3x1 is, thus, interiority; it is not oriented (the light comes from above). The fact that it gets light from above as the only requirement and main reason for its autonomy, and the lack of almost any other kind of relationship with the context, allows this "box" to suit all possible urban conditions.
However, in the work of its exact disposition on each site, it addresses the urban context with a desire for frontality. No matter how large the site is, the building is related to the street in a direct and frontal way, as if the rest didn't matter.

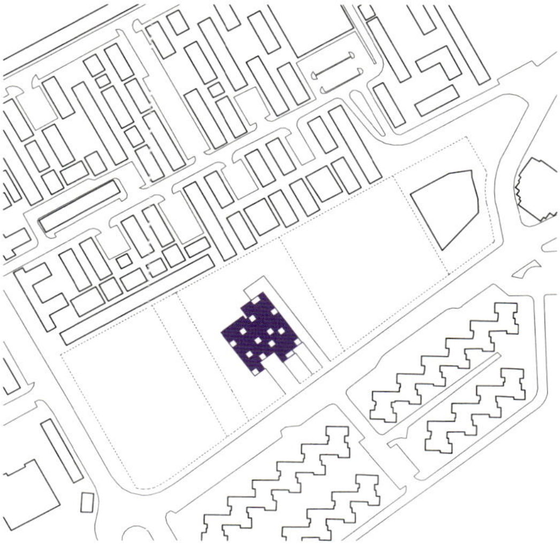

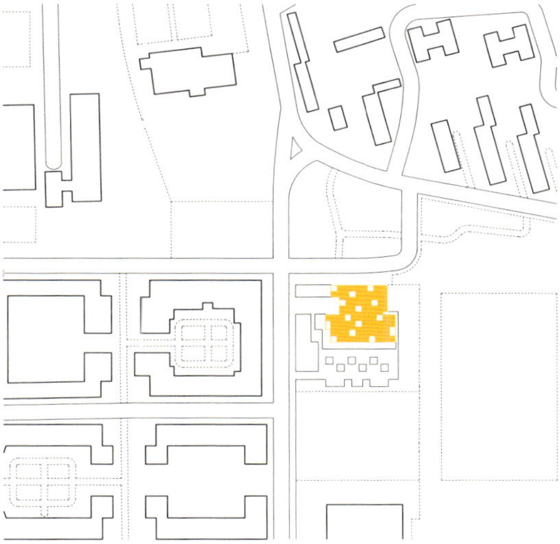

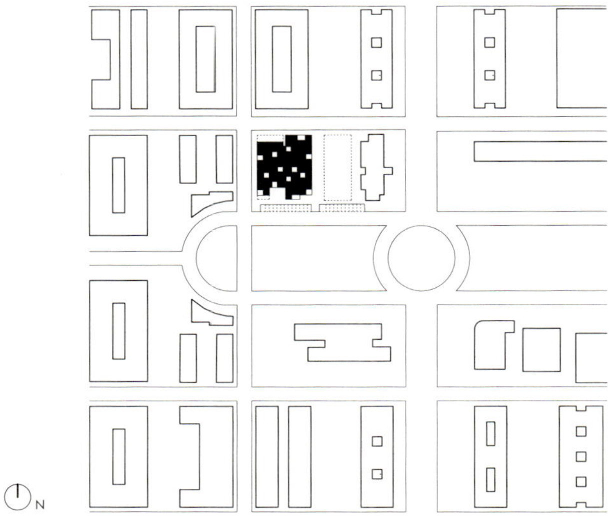
N

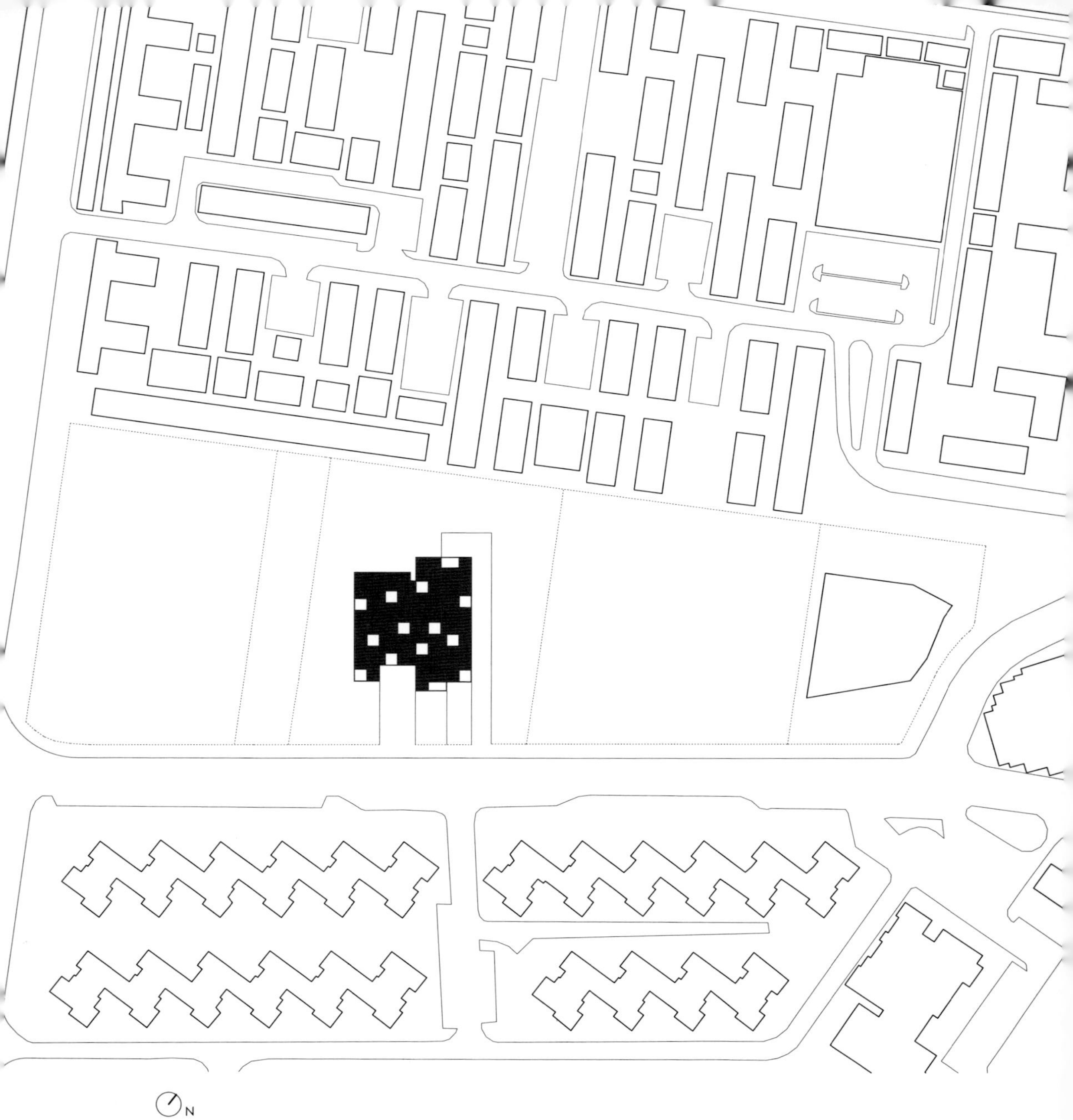

N

Looking closer into the relationship of the building to each specific site, in the case of S there are four "degrees of freedom". Front, back, right and left are open questions as the free-standing building becomes a kind of pavilion in the park. Parking is hidden underground which abounds in the free-standing condition.
The frontality of the entrance prioritizes the relationship of the built volume to the street over the surrounding social housing complex and its different alignments. However, as a reverse consequence, the roof becomes a real fifth façade exposed to the neighboring buildings' attention.

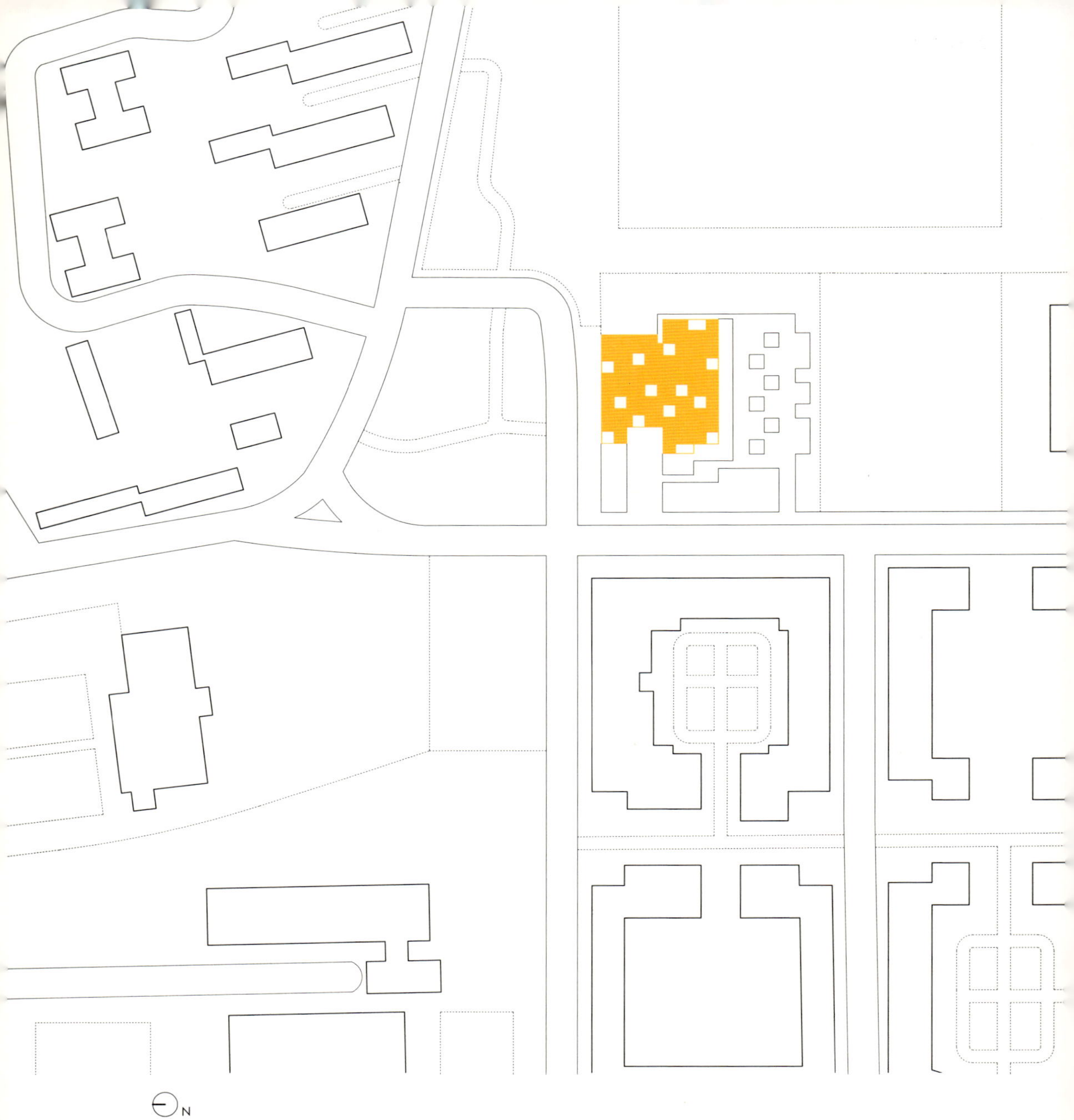
N

The U case works with one street alignment that is however not the frontal one. Therefore, three degrees of freedom allow the building to again establish that umbilical cord from the entrance, leaving the above-ground parking area to the right. The link between the street and the building door tenses this site in a similar manner that we saw in S. The corner condition of the site plays an equivalent role in presenting a free-standing shell, maybe foreign but yet precisely sited on the unqualified given platform. "The object on the tray" is perhaps a closer description of how the building is perceived in this environment.

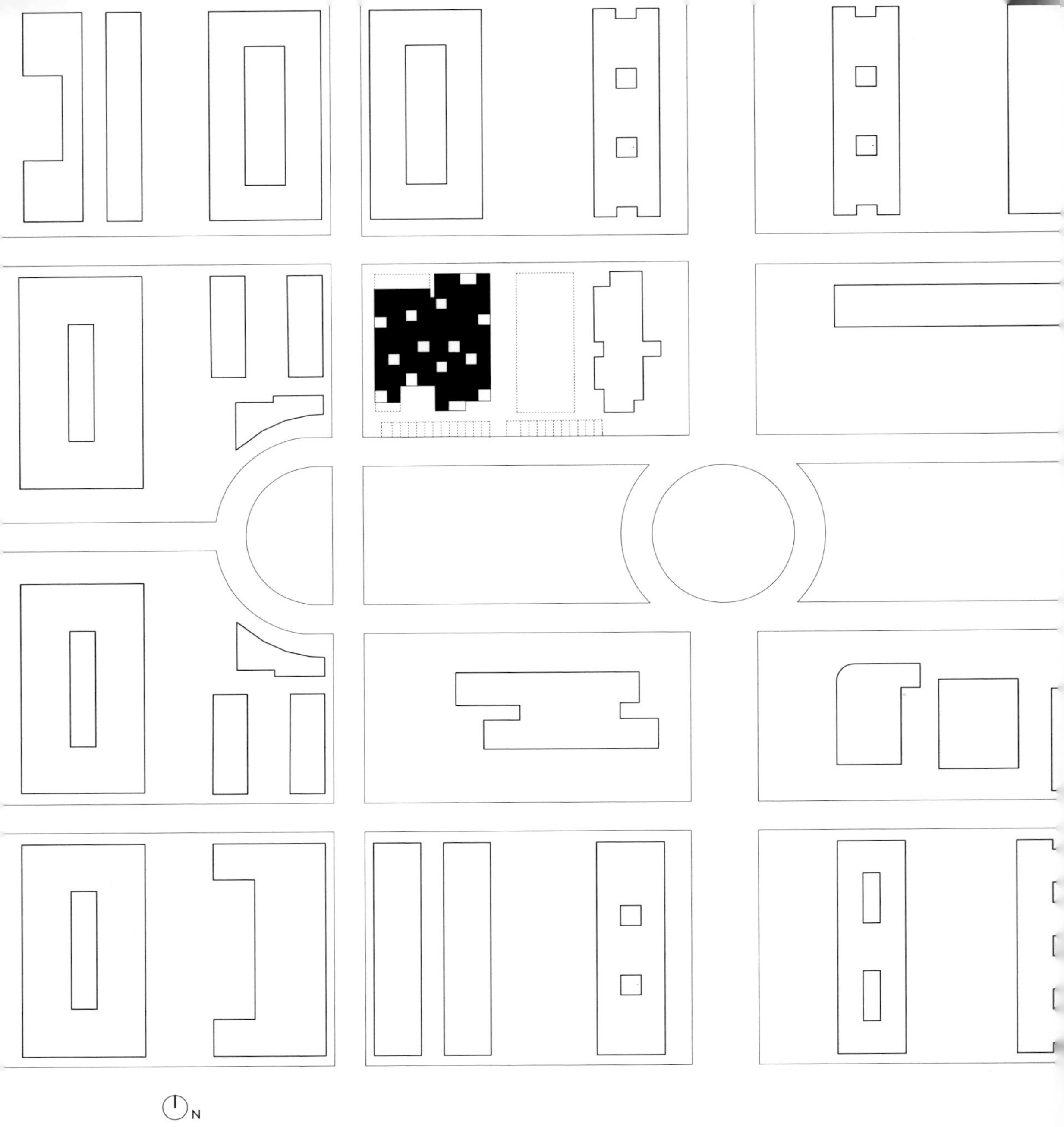
N

When a second competition was launched by the client for a third clinic, the 3x1 clinic prototype fit the given site perfectly, like it belonged there.
V case is, by chance, street aligned on three sides and set back from the neighboring wall to the right for access to the underground parking area. This time the building, almost an urban block, is much closer to the street, to the point of qualifying the urban context; however, the free-standing condition prevails. It is also much closer to the neighboring buildings and the roof plane as the fifth façade gains more relevance, like urban façades do when vertical.

parts (p. 24_25)

The three clinics have the exact same configuration; the program is disposed extensively on a single ground floor in an isotropic disposition that takes the light from above through fourteen patios.
Three main conditions arise from that disposition (from top to bottom)
- Voids and volumes in the shell.
- The "interior" public space _in orange.
- Perimeter of the outer shell _in green.

In the archetypical condition of 3x1 we can think of those characteristics as the underlying structure of three different individuals to come. The shell is a hermetic image to the exterior, which encloses the open and bright space of the interior, to emphasize its value.

Page 24:
Each of these conditions can be expressed as entities (right column) in dialectical opposition with the most relevant "parts" in isolation (left column):

- voids; subtracted / added
- public space; space possessed / space perceived (appropriated)
- program; content/continent (outer skin)

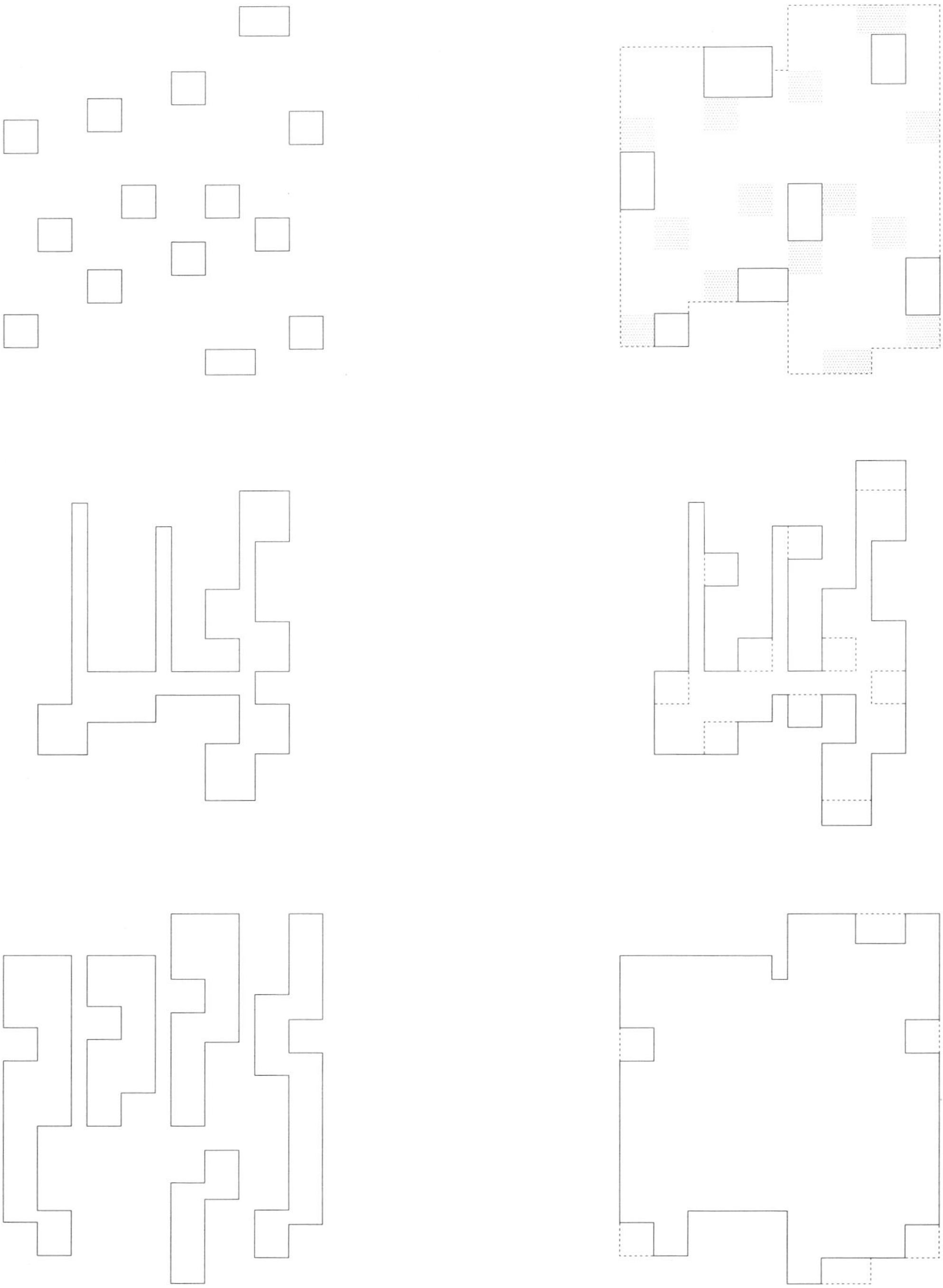

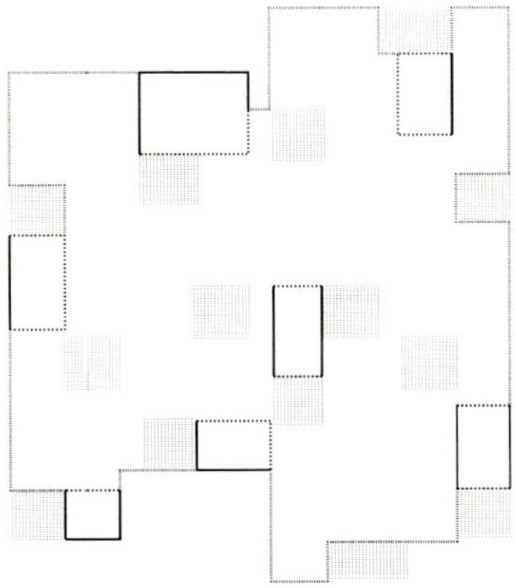

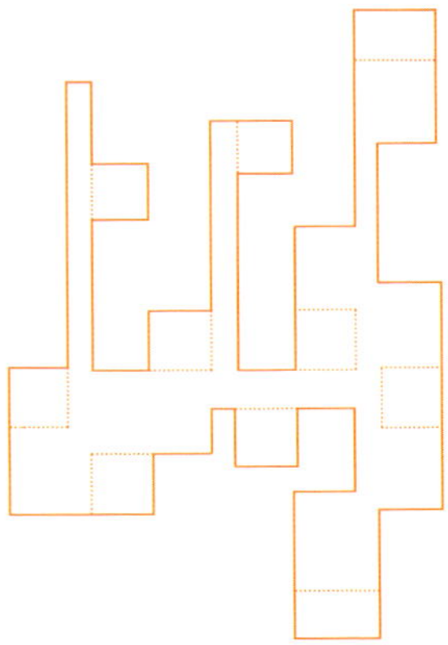

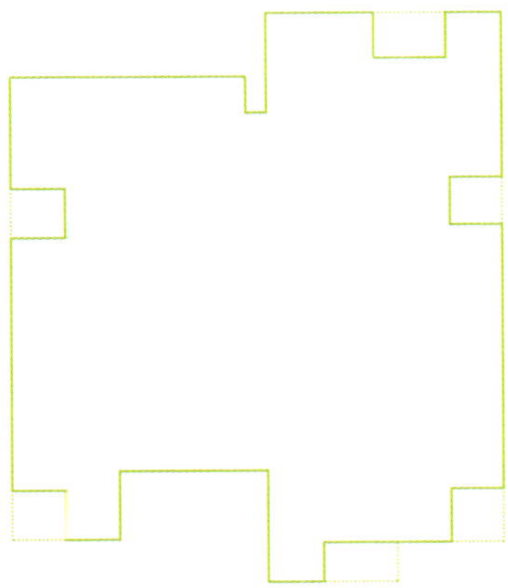

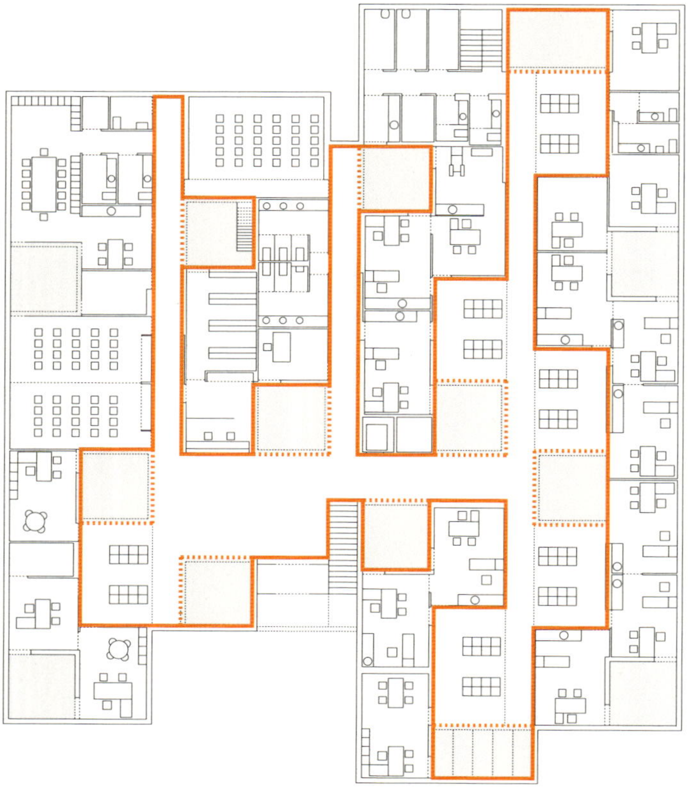

There is a non-stop visual continuity across interiors and patios that provides space enlargement; what you see inside is larger than what you can actually walk through.
The public space is extensive and non-hierarchical. The different rooms of the program are organized on a loose irregular orthogonal grid, where the patios are arranged in a zigzag pattern between the public and private rooms along three parallel (non)-corridors. The corridor vanishes to an extent; it is no longer the traditional tensed linear connecting structure, because the alternating arrangement of the empty spaces of patios and public waiting areas has a counterbalance effect between front and side.

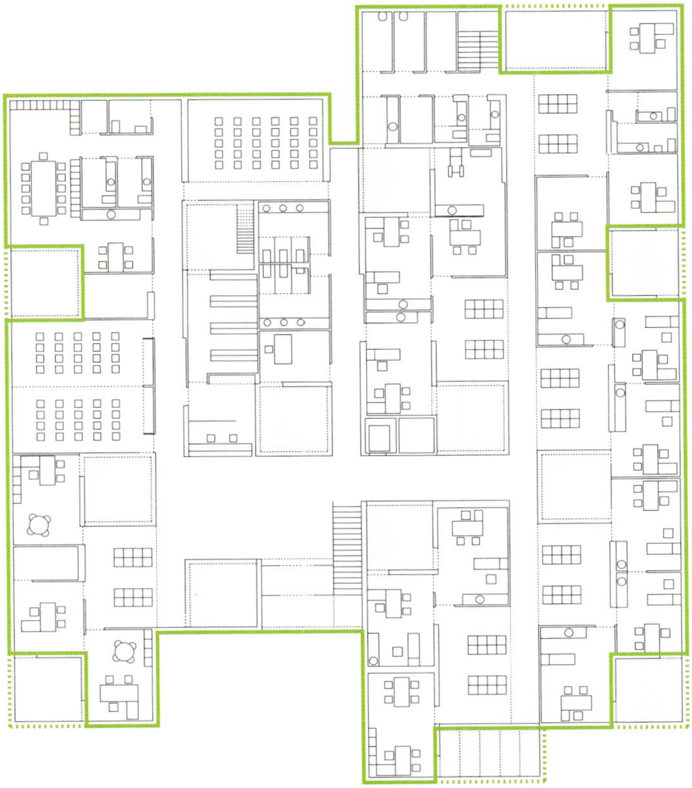

In this compact geometry, common in multi-cellular clusters, the perimeter shape is not really what matters since a different perimeter would not have made any difference. What matters are the connections between pieces: a bottom-up configuration in which "the plan" (understood as strategy) proceeds from within to without.

These two realities or conditions explained here as separate questions – interiorness and exteriorness – are apparently opposites to be reconciled: space and its qualities of enclosure and infiniteness. On the one hand, a very particular relationship with the exterior occurs within the expanded interior public space. And, on the other hand, the hermetism of the outer shell contains, provokes and preserves that condition as a vessel.

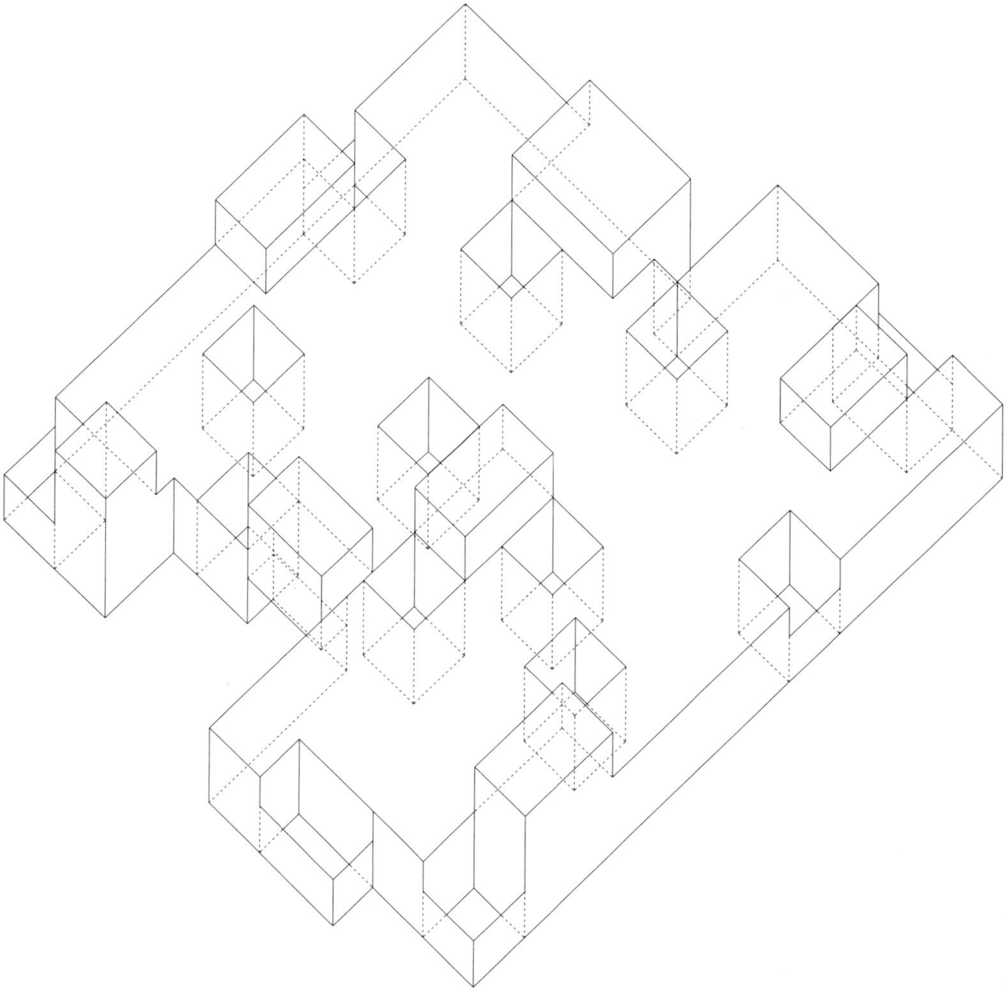

In addition to being described as an equilibrium of opposing forces, the building can be also described as a box, but a very specific one. The roof plane behaves as a sensitive membrane and actually becomes the fifth (and only) façade, allowing the building to breathe, where volumes containing double heights or services rooms emerge channeling light into the interior.
These volumes (both added and subtracted) are not exactly consequences of formal decisions; they are part of "one among many" possible results of playing by the rules. The rules regarding program and structure (spatial and load-bearing) provide certain surprises in the 3D that are as well-received as they are unexpected.

patios (p. 30_31)

The absence of hollows in the vertical walls of the exterior enclosure causes the relationship between the interior and exterior of the building to occur vertically, almost with the sky above. Courtyards bring the light inside the building and help to create a spacious and luminous interior, blurring the boundaries between inside and outside, a dissolution of the built limit. The transparency and mirroring qualities of the glass surfaces also create multiple visions, presences and absences, by reflected symmetry.

Page 30:
Patios as vertical enclosure
Materialization of light spaces
Relationship between program and (vertical) enclosure

Page 31:
Patios as relationship between ground and sky
Openings as horizontal window like cuts on the fifth façade (90° rotation from the typical)
Relationship between program and ceiling (roof)

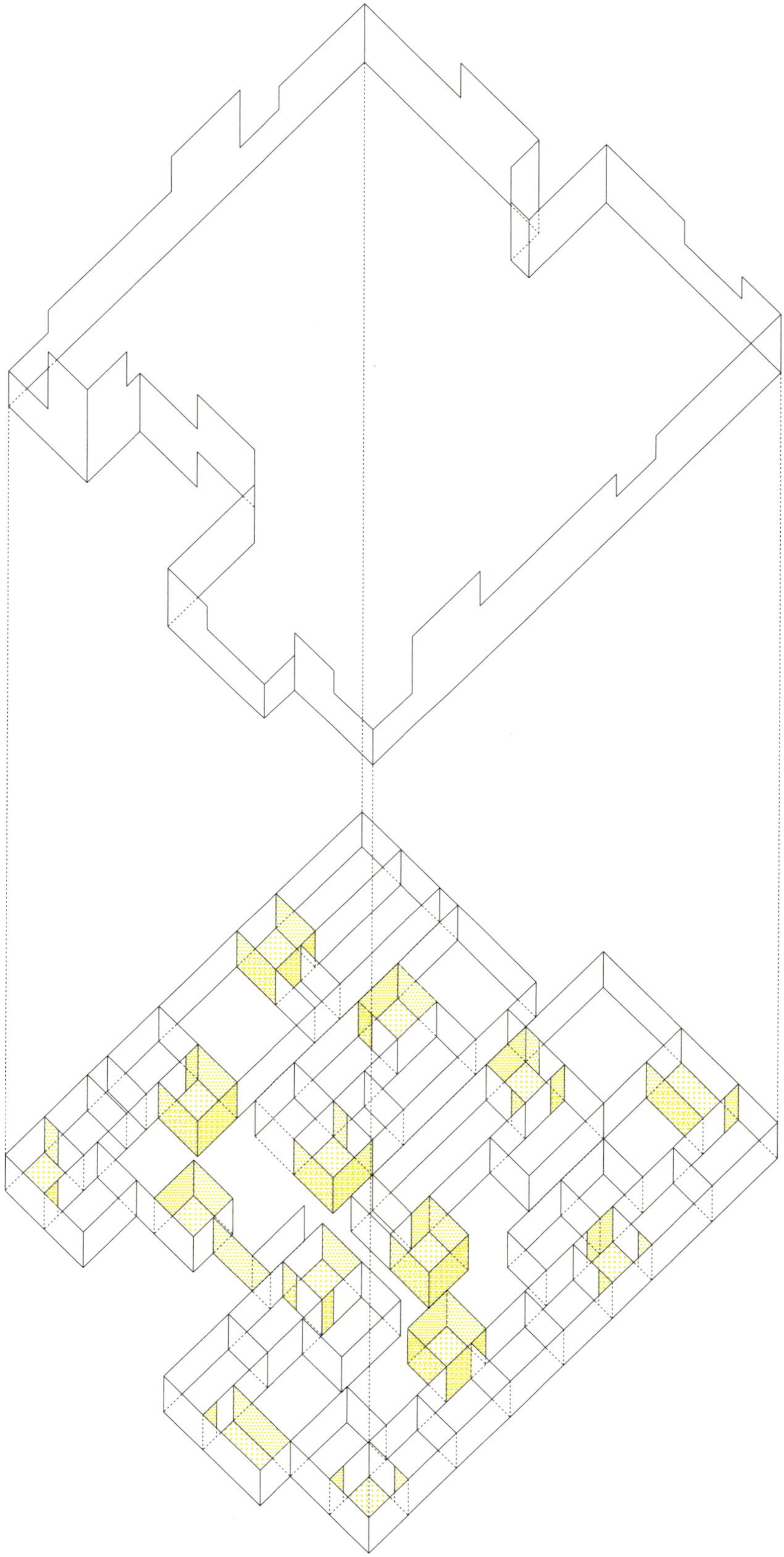

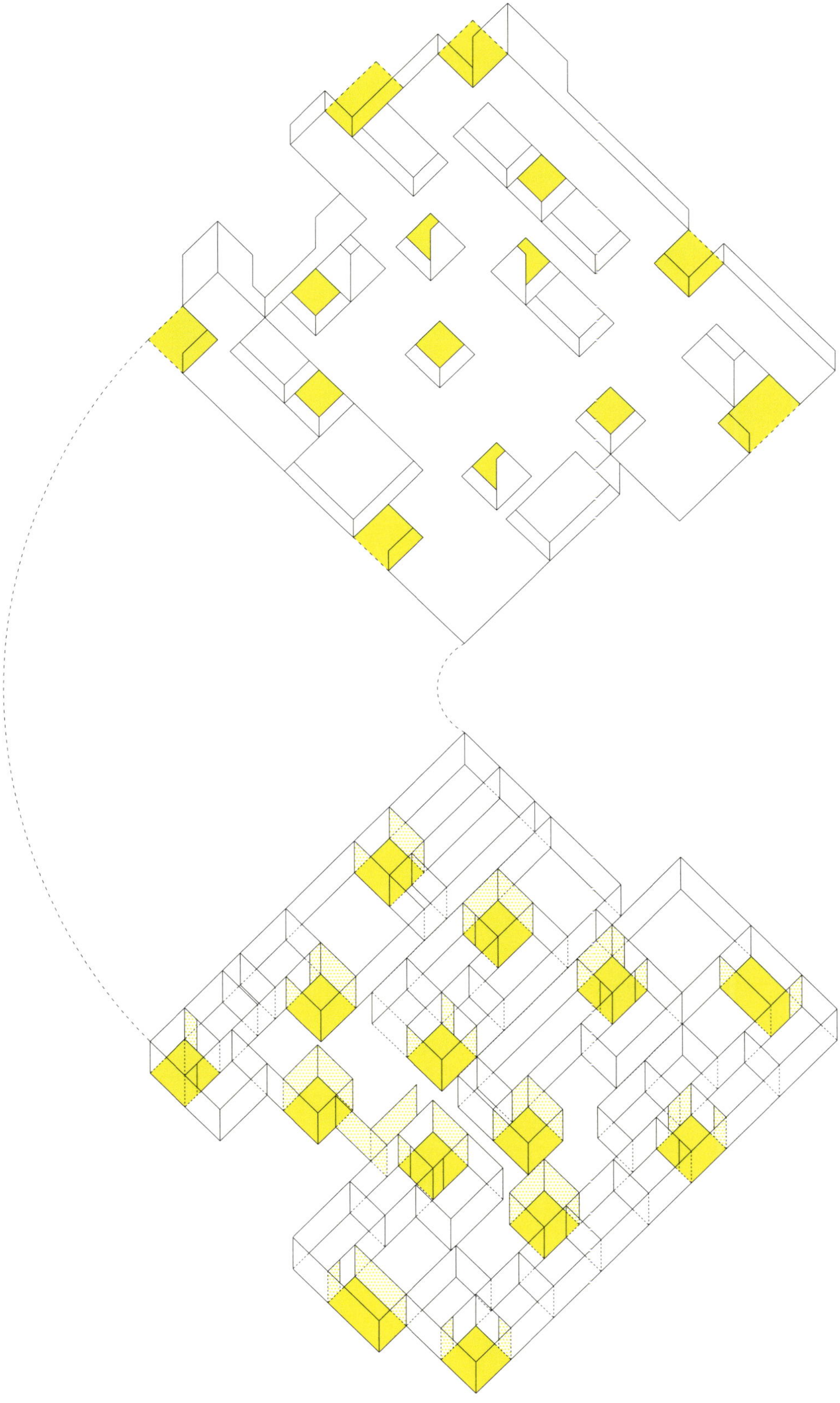

When architecture must respond to a demanding functional program, we understand that simply solving the program is not the solution, yet the solution does undoubtedly begin with solving the program. From the generic understanding to the most specific aspects of each unit, the various parts of the program are translated into spatial conditions that incorporate their own system of order with the aim of arriving at a floor plan efficiency that bypasses the obvious. Rooms (cells), although similar in size and specifications, have a certain encoded information that qualifies the connections between them (doctor-nurse contiguity, blood test in-out queuing, infants distant from pregnant women, etc.)

Rules for the spatial conditions work at different stances: (from top to bottom)

- Private-public; administration rooms – exam rooms: binuclear plan disposition
- Programmatic bars; offices and educational – public area – primary care – specialists: "Double-double" loaded corridors transversally connected
- Programmatic specialization (rooms as cells); main programs – support areas – waiting rooms: We can talk about programmatic atomization rather than sectorization; non-hierarchical atomization

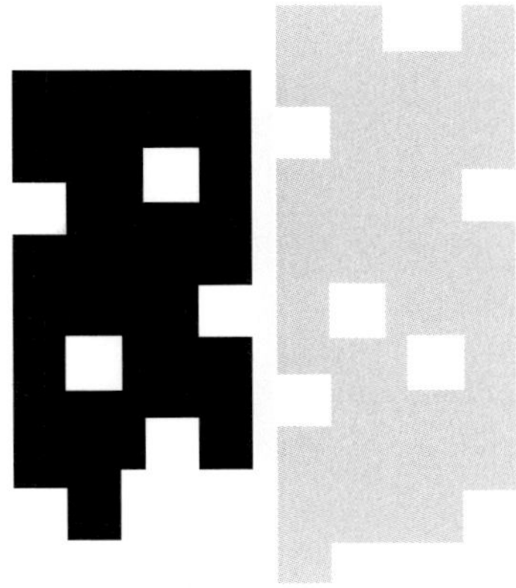

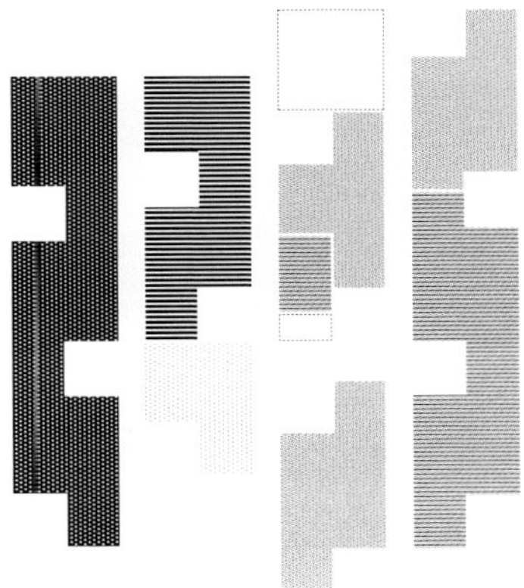

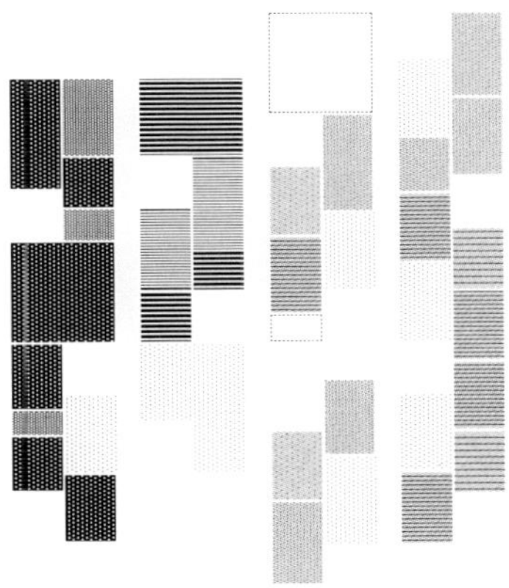

Structural rules become an input for decision making and form, a consequence of concrete dimensions. Regulate, arrange, seriate, are all actions in search of that primary rhythm Le Corbusier talked about in *Towards an Architecture* (1931, Dover Publications, Inc. New York, 1986, pg.50.):

". . . The plan bears within itself a primary and pre-determined rhythm . . . Rhythm is a state of equilibrium, is an equation; equalization (symmetry and repetition); compensation (movement of contrary parts); modulation (the development of and original plastic invention)."

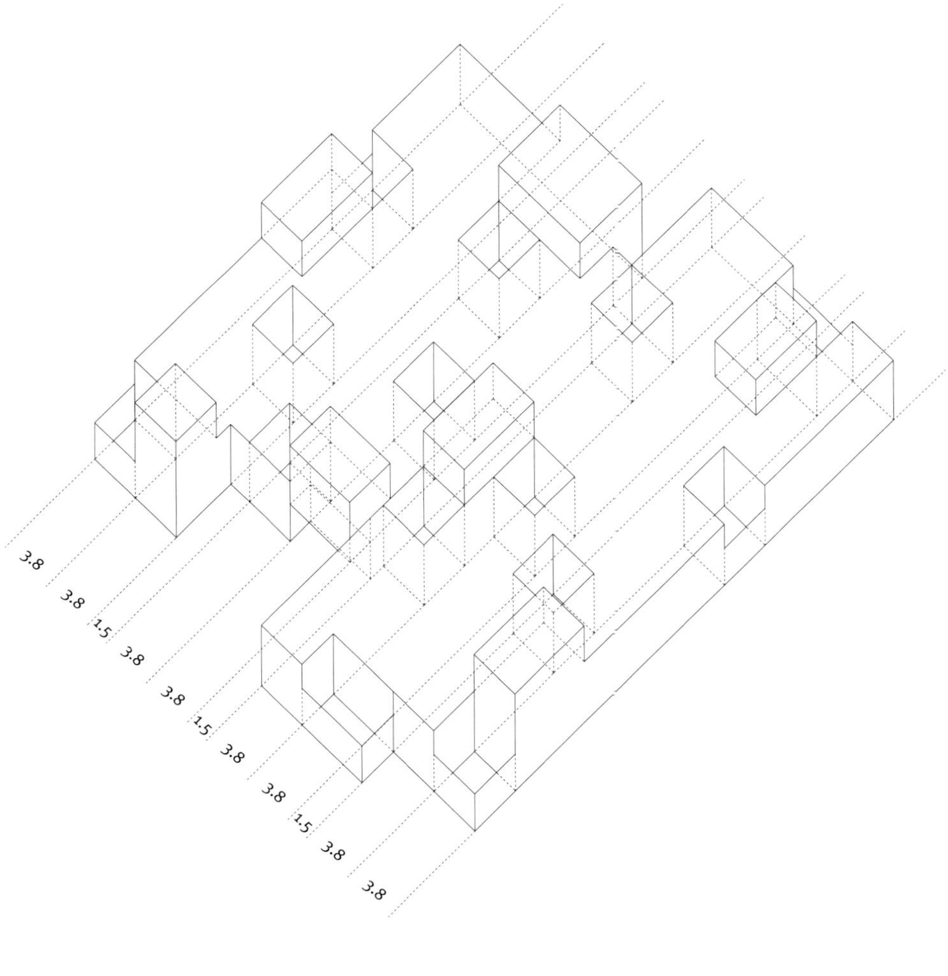
3.8
3.8
1.5
3.8
3.8
1.5
3.8
3.8
1.5
3.8
3.8

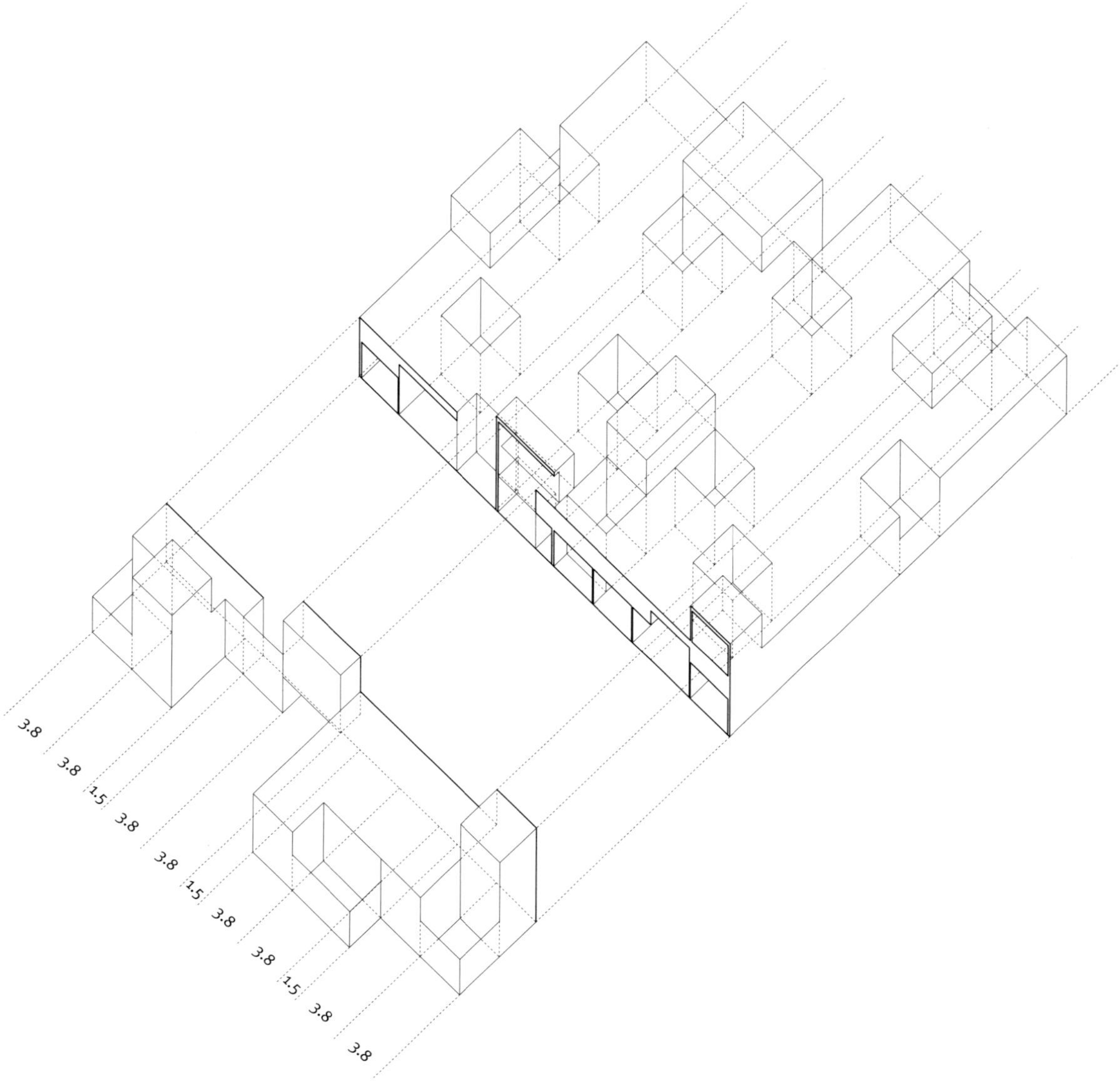

Further interpreting Le Corbusier's words, the plan is presented as an intention, a systematic modus operandi that is set before an action in order to direct and channel it. In that sense, the plan is three-dimensional; it is a spatial strategy that transcends the floor plan and incorporates sectional thinking as well (the treasures of section).

Transverse section
Spatial compression and expansion sequence;
entrance, circulation, sky, waiting area, room, sky, service

Page 37: Longitudinal section
Spatial compression and expansion sequence;
circulation, sky, waiting area, room, sky

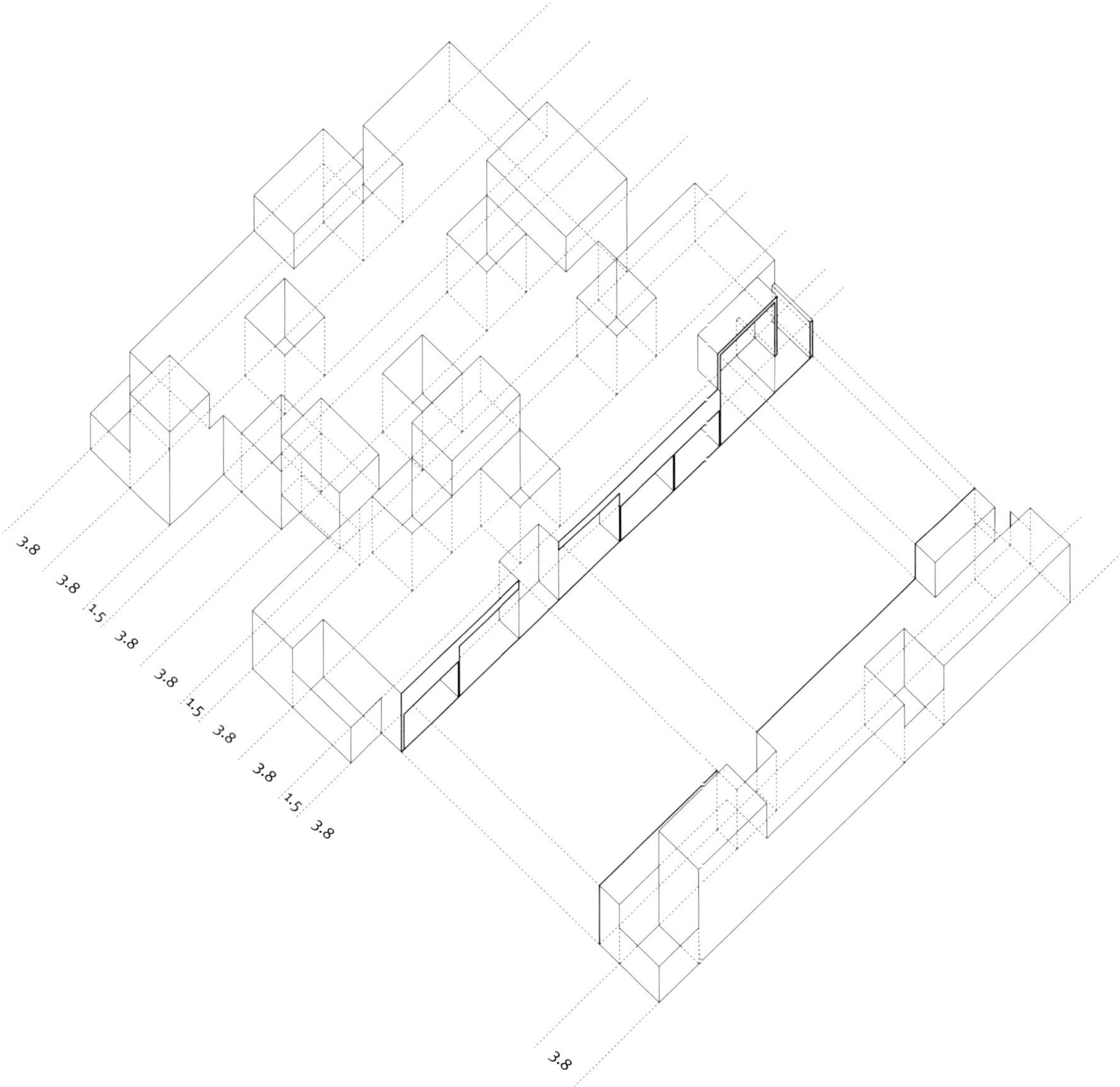
3.8
3.8
1.5
3.8
3.8
1.5
3.8
3.8
1.5
3.8
3.8

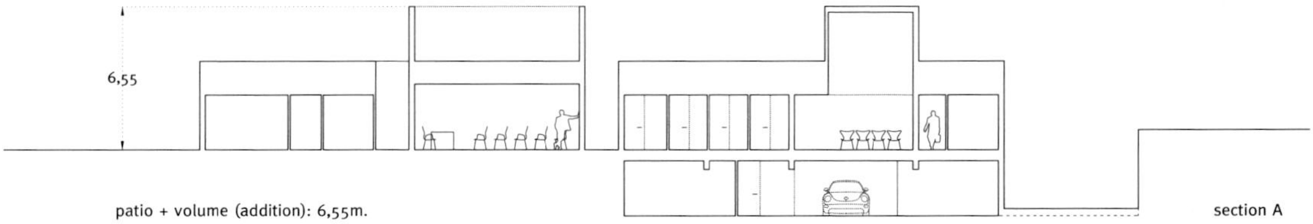

patio + volume (addition): 6,55m.

section A

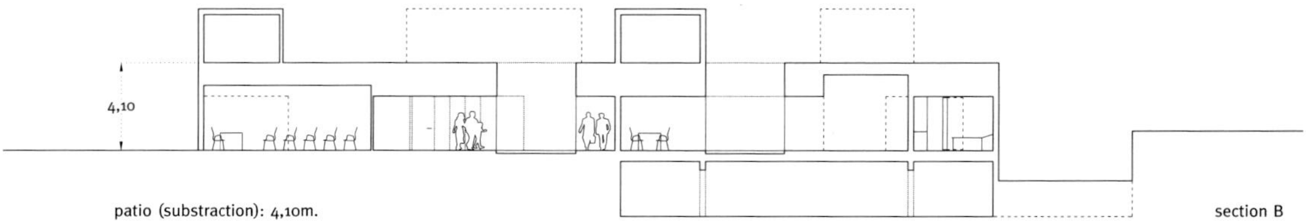

patio (substraction): 4,10m.

section B

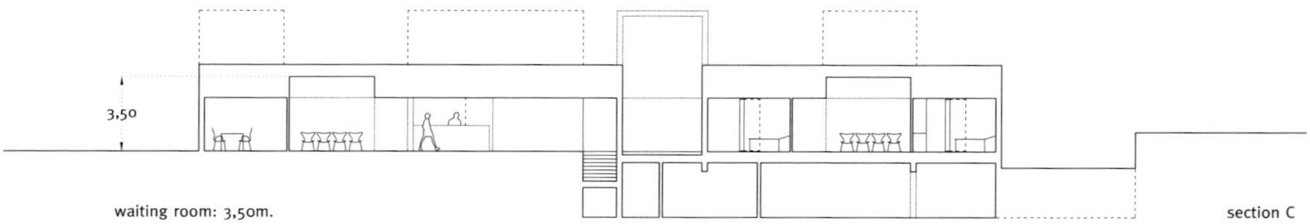

waiting room: 3,50m.

section C

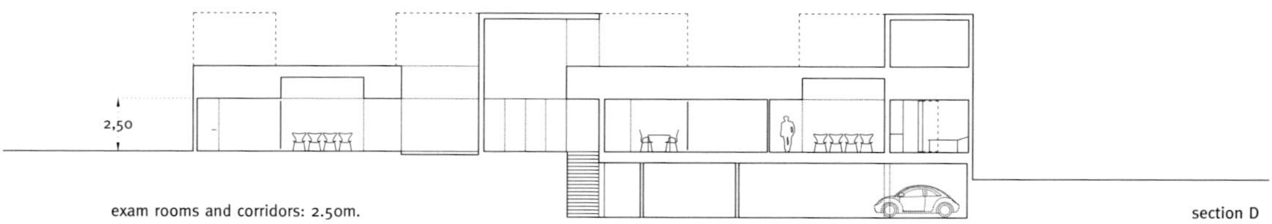

exam rooms and corridors: 2.50m.

section D

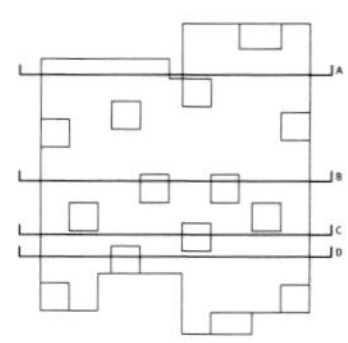

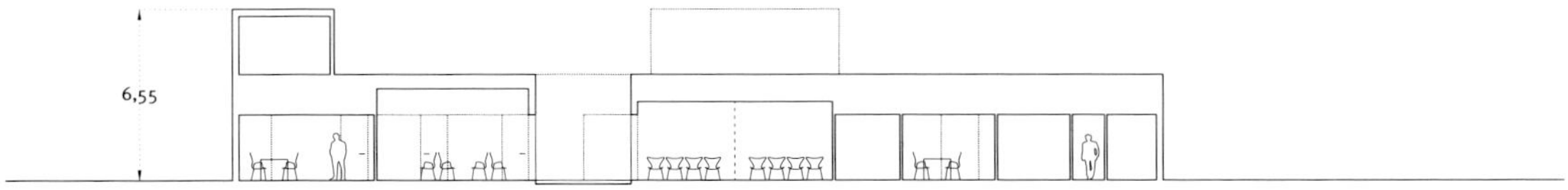

section 1

patio + volume (addition): 6,55m.

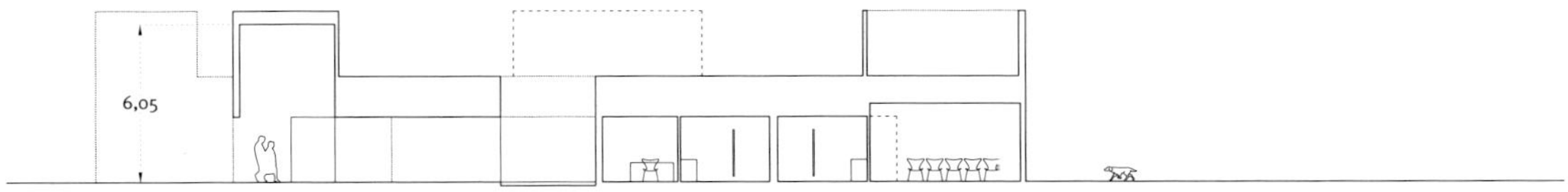

section 2

entrance: 6,05m.

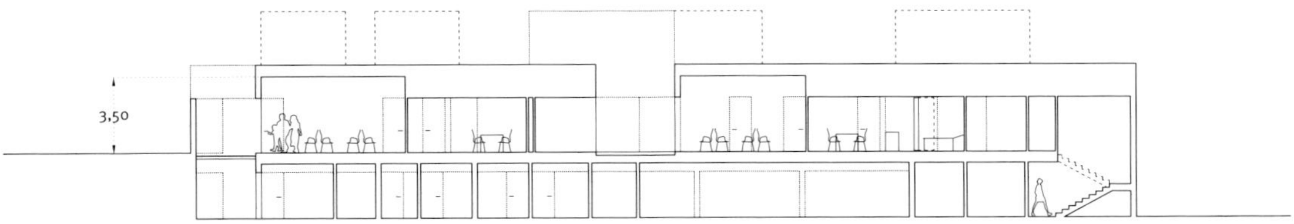

waiting room: 3,50m.

section 3

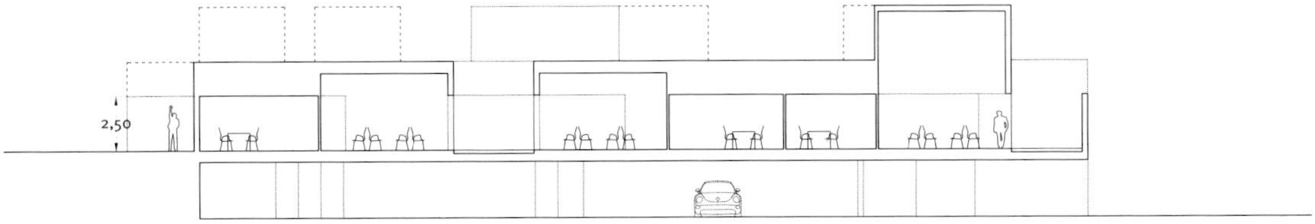

exam rooms and corridors: 2.50m.

section 4

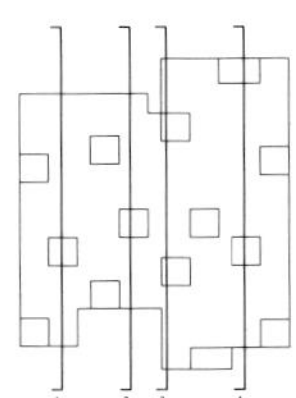

Programmatic Bars

An explanation of the generic clinical program's chain-like configurations and their spatial and formal structure. The relationship between circulation and program (circulation serves program) is informed by the waiting areas and the desire for natural light and ventilation. The layout of programmatic bars around and through exterior spaces introduces the logics of the clinical grain.

When considering program, the first thing for us involves making the conversion from individual items on a list into programmatic conditions; once the specific requirements are understood and assimilated, program becomes a collection of components with certain spatial attributes (dimension, proportion, light, ventilation, privacy).

In the case of a highly demanding program like health care, we introduce the concept of "programmatic bars" which are strips of program – chain-like configurations of different but similar elements (exam rooms, offices, waiting rooms, etc.) following the logics of aggregation rather than the subdivision of a pre-established whole.

These chains incorporate flexibility and versatility as a potential: a collection of many concatenated small pieces that can be reordered, shortened or extended as needed. This capacity of being easy to rearrange without modifying the organizational principle or structure is, at this point, still a strategy that belongs to the design process. Later there is another kind of flexibility, throughout the life of the building, when rooms need to be repurposed.

Looking closely at these examples of fragments of programmatic bars and bearing in mind the need for natural light for a good clinical environment, we can look at the evolution of our approach from top to bottom as centered on these recursive questions:
– relationship between program and circulation (circulation serves the program)
– relationship between program and enclosure (light and ventilation)
– relationship between circulation and enclosure (light)

1. one generic bay structure where the waiting area is simply the enlargement of the circulation, and exam rooms sit by adjacent to one another along the opposite façade. Public space is homogeneous. Light horizontal (lateral)
2. same with focal tension, the idea of beginning and end, an oriented bar, oriented public space
3. waiting areas are a specialized part of circulation due to the rooms' configuration, also one bay structure that needs two parallel façades. Alternating horizontal compression-expansion of public space
4. patios as rooms in a pattern, which bring light to each of the adjacent spaces regardless of function, with no required façade condition. Extensive and expansive public space. Vertical light.

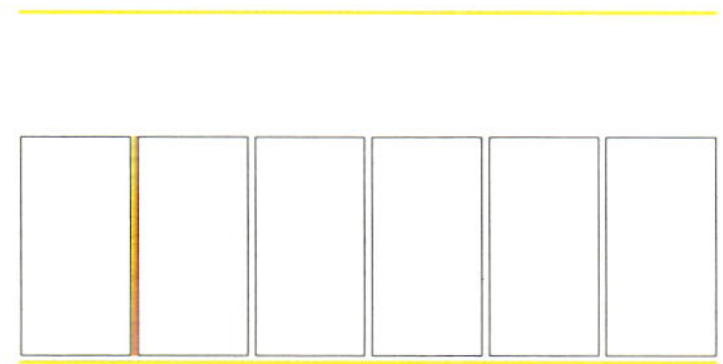

1

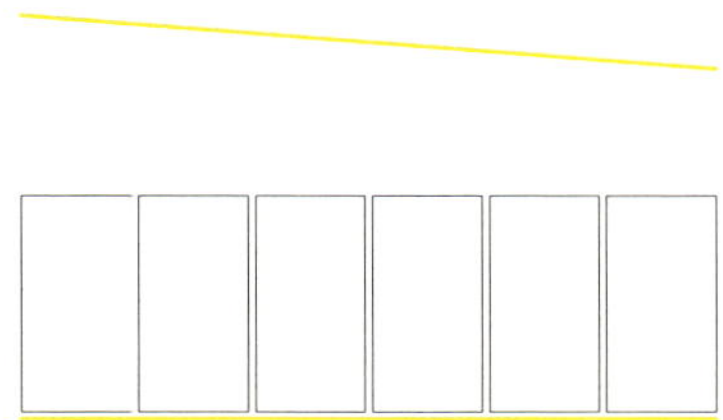

2

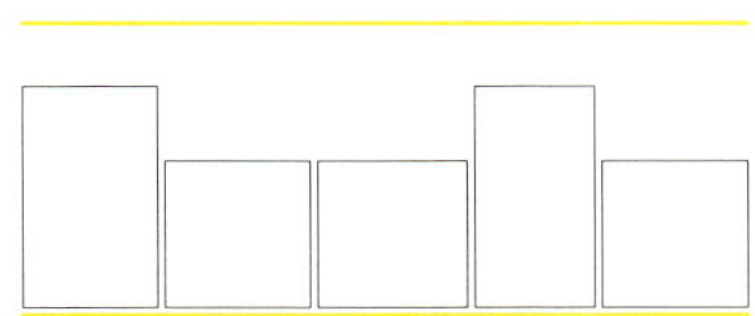

3

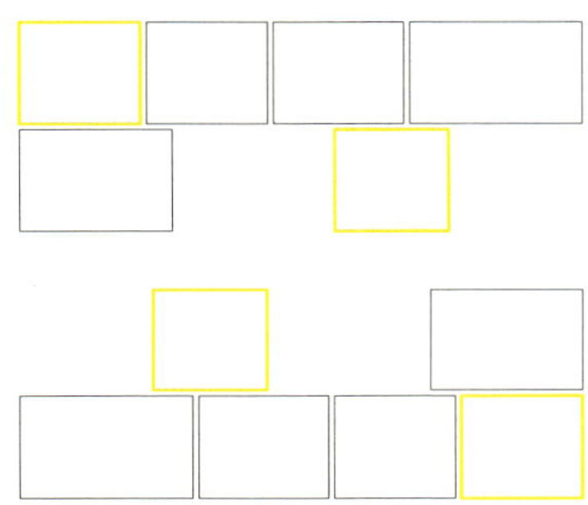

4

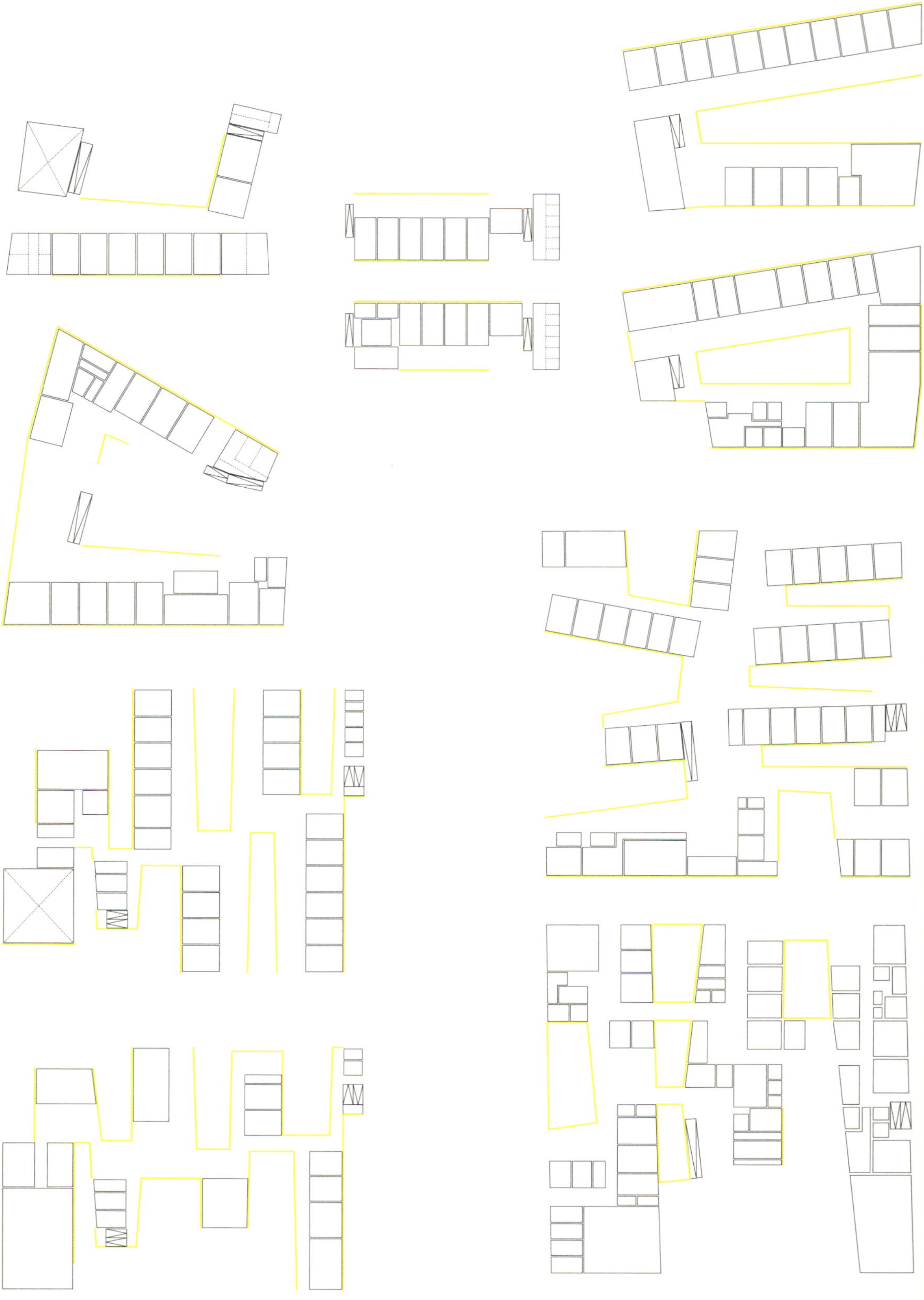

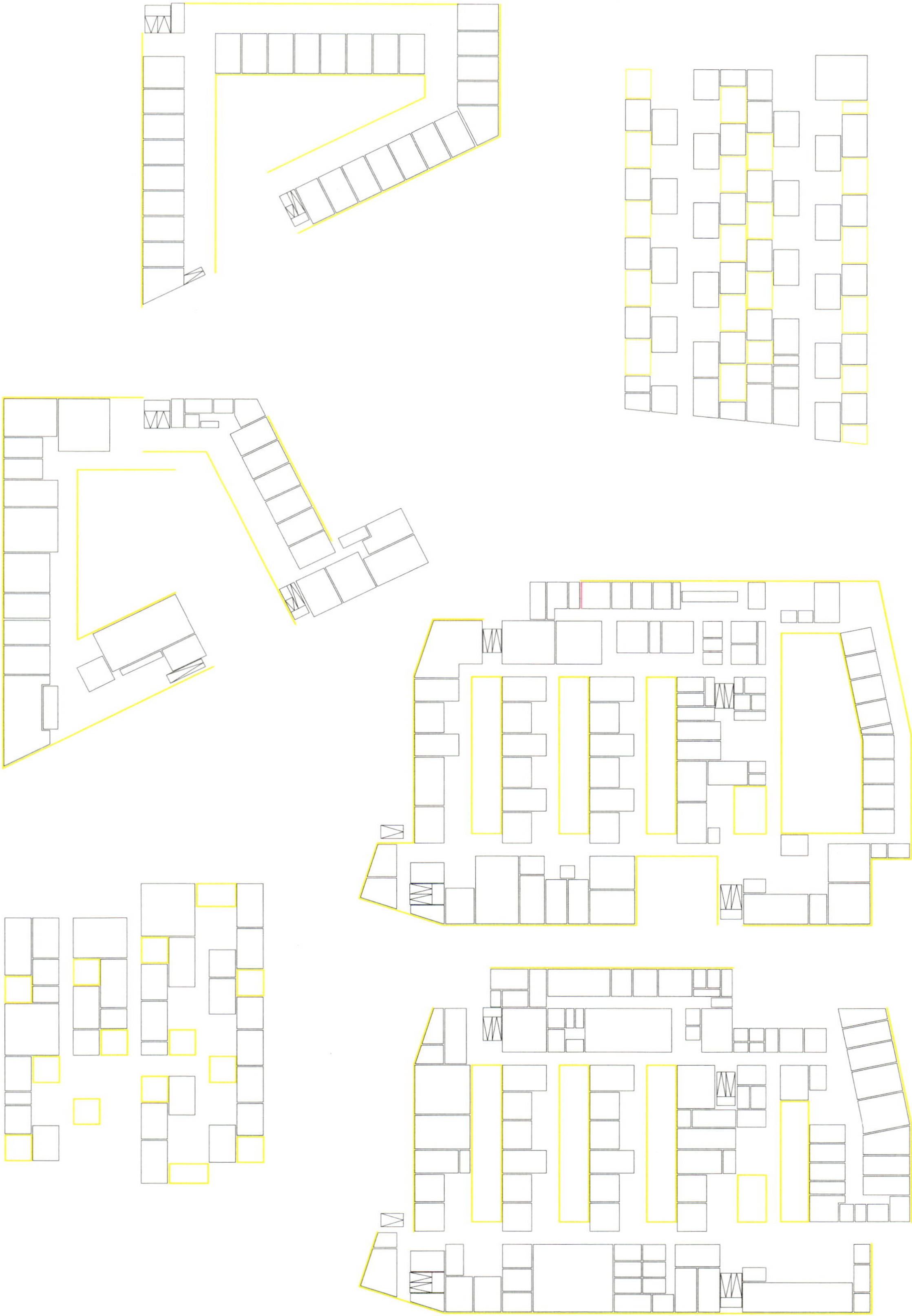

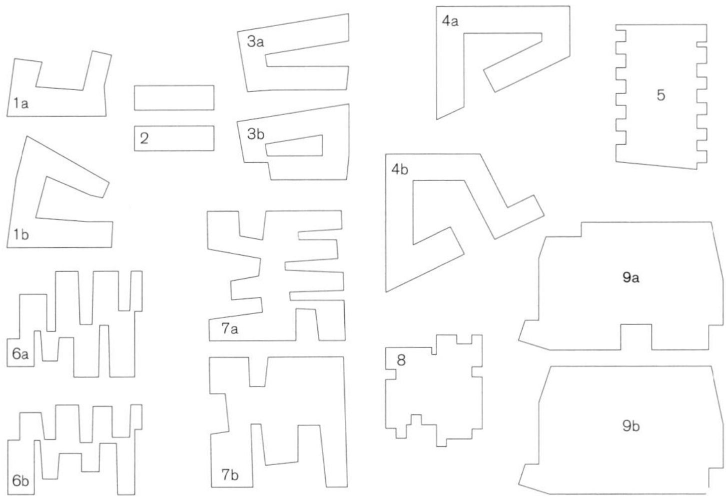

1a. Minglanilla (second floor)
1b. Minglanilla (first floor)
2. Puentenansa
3a. Marchamalo
3b. Marchamalo
4a. Camarena, Madrid
4b. Camarena, Madrid
5. Ocaña
6a. El Zurguén, Salamanca
6b. El Zurguén, Salamanca
7a. Manzanares
7b. Manzanares
8. 3x1
9a. Daimiel
9b. Daimiel

(p. 44_45)

One question is how to build the bars, another is how to put the bars together.
This is a sample of health-care building floor plans we have worked on, all on the same scale. There are cases where an inner courtyard is the form generator; other times it is the cell of the system and its logic of aggregation; yet other times it is the negotiation between the system (type of organization) and an external constraint (boundary conditions) that rules the formal decisions.
If giving form has to do with how to organize things, these diagrams are indeed organizational. Diagram drawings here serve as an analytical tool for understanding form as the dialogue between program, circulation, light, enclosure and space (in/out, open/closed, private/public). It is a typological question in which the different solutions for each type arise in relation to something concrete. In that sense, 3x1 (8) is presented as an alternative type, that of the "unlimited extension", in place of other more common types: the simple bar, the linear structure that bends, wraps, and twists with more or less deformations, the fish spine, the grid, etc.

The expression "form plays function" has been presented as a counter version of the exhausted "form follows function", providing a richer meaning (move, perform, act, interpret).
These diagrams aim to fall conceptually somewhere between Wittkower's analysis on the Palladian Villas as variations on a single theme, Franco Purini's study of architectural elements as a hypothesis of architectural spatial organizations as a form of notation and the relationship between morphology and typology (form and type), and the Texas Rangers use of "parti" (parti pris) as the "big idea" or chief organizing thought or decision behind an architect's mind presented as a simple statement (the fried egg, the snake, etc.). All of these are influential in our approach to developing a project.

(p. 48_49)

Within the spectrum from purely servant circulation (that of housing for example) on one end, and other cases where circulation occurs through the program (as in a museum) on the other, a clinic is somewhere in the middle.
If we compare it to the architecture of collective housing – where the cell or part is always very similar, if not identical, and circulation is something external to it, which runs by program – health-care program (understood as a collection of rooms) deals with a cell or base element of the organization that has a higher level of embedded information (it is for a physician, or nurse, or pediatrics, or a midwife). Parts are arranged rather than repeated, and circulation is partially programmed as well (waiting areas); it connects rooms but also specializes them.

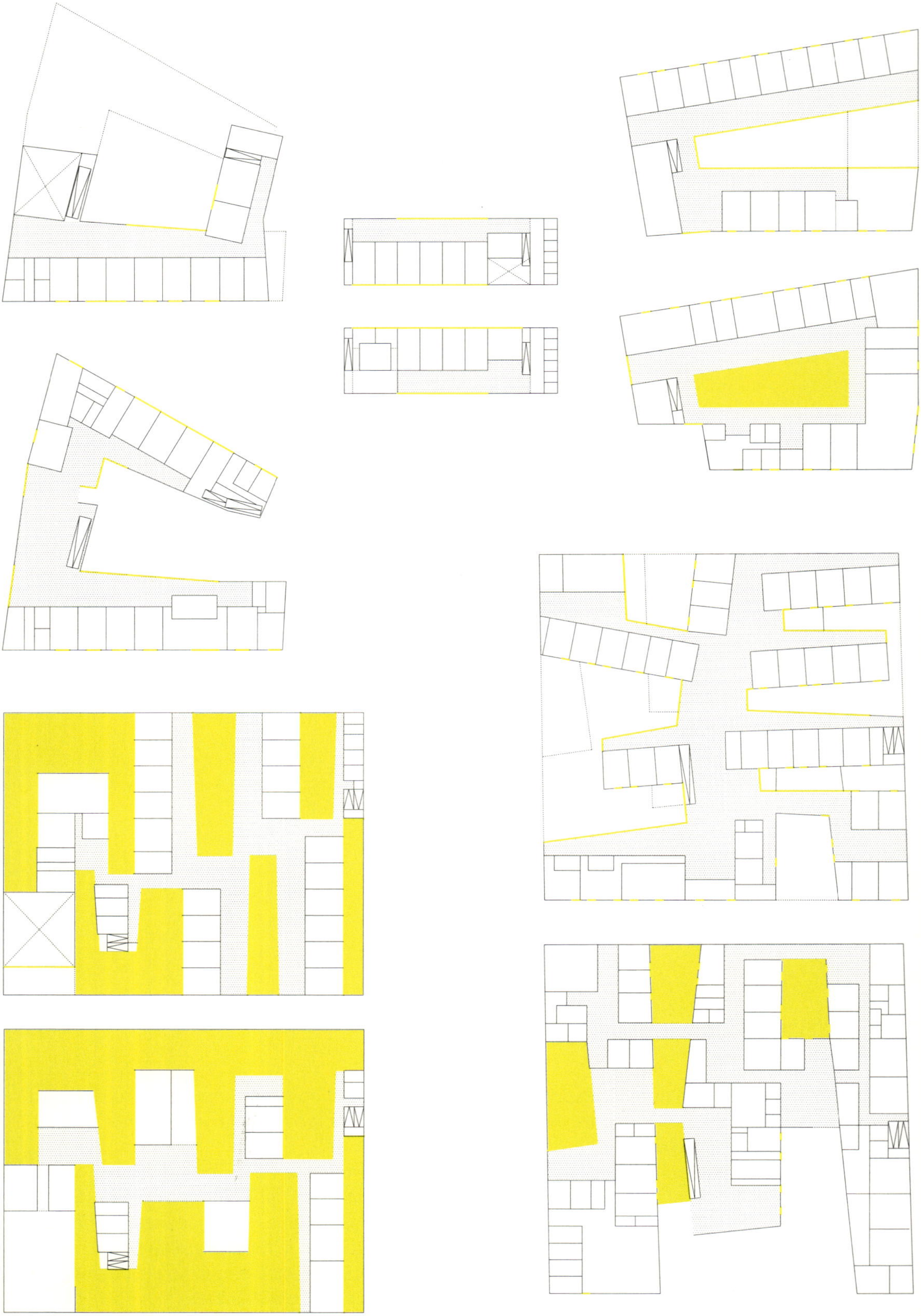

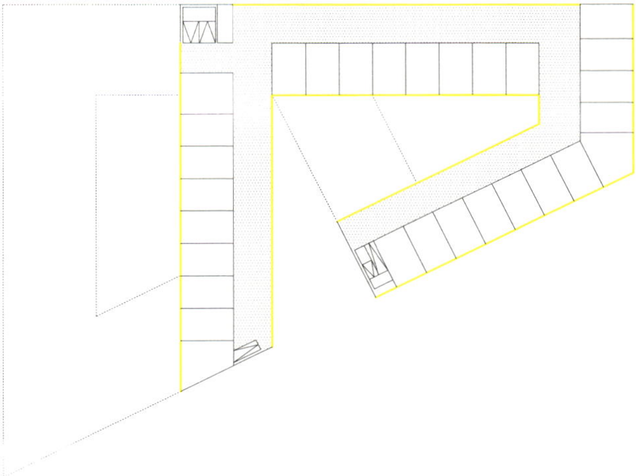
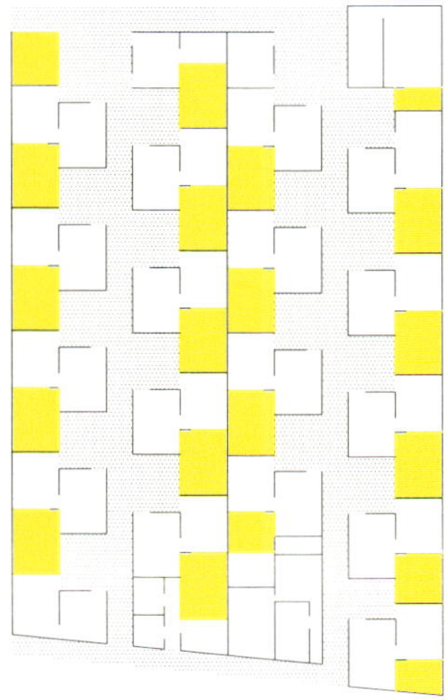
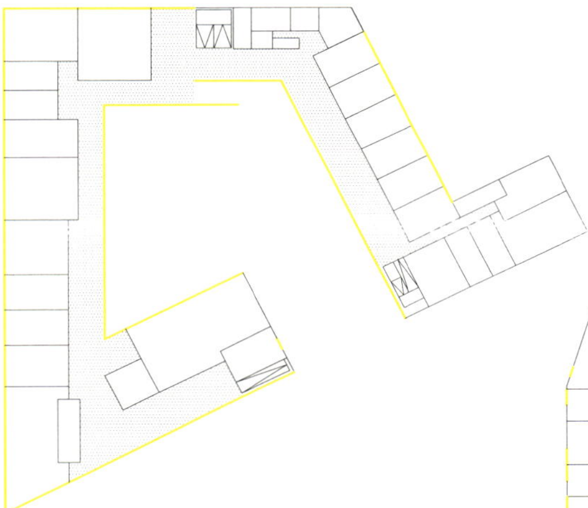
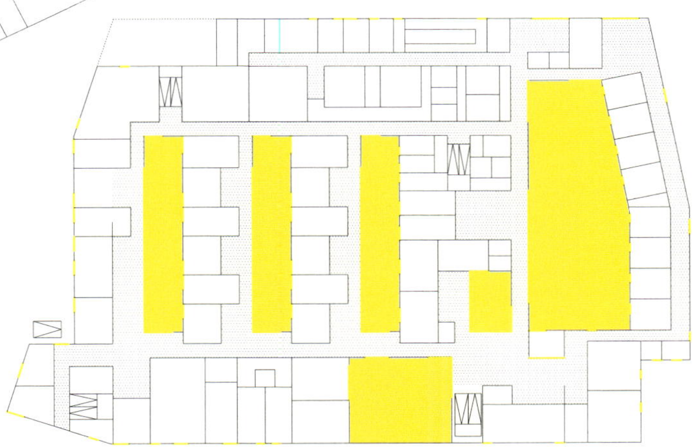
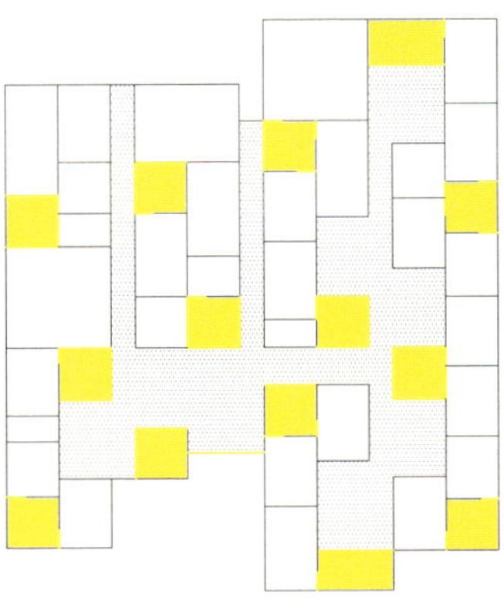
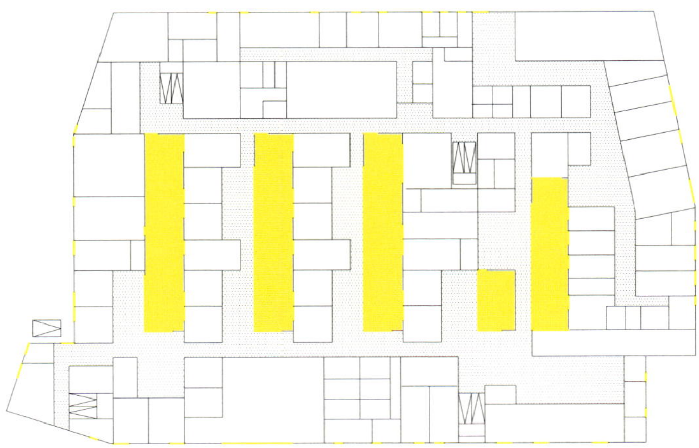

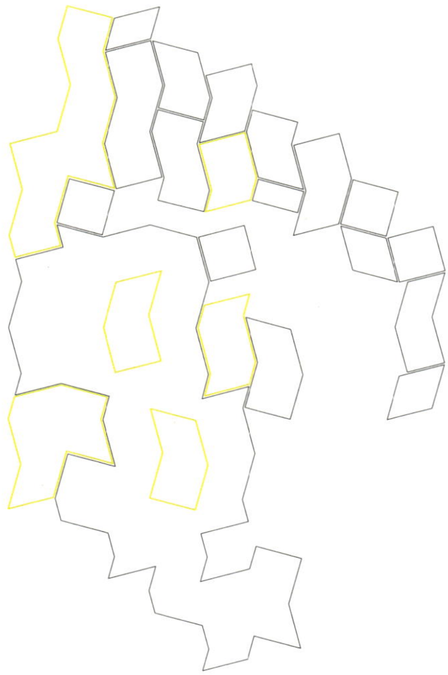

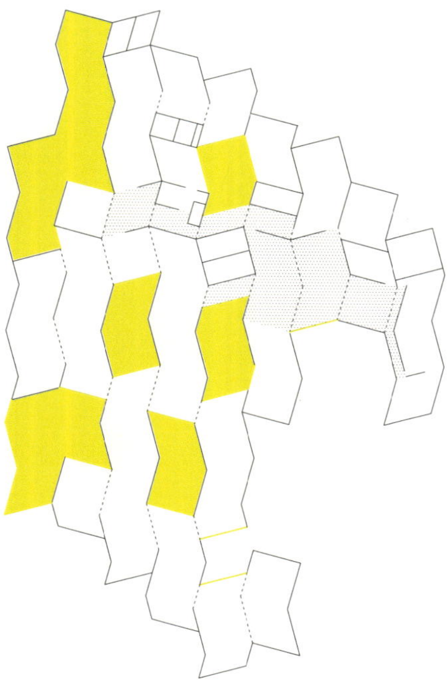

As an explicit form of citation, although in a graphic manner here, it is only fair to attribute ideas that influenced our work to their authors.
In the case of Musac (Museo de Arte Contemporaneo de León, Spain) by Mansilla-Tuñón, we paid special attention to the idea of irregular perimeter. Any perimeter shape built upon the geometrical strategy of the project would have been as plausible, although some amount of control can be identified in restraining the floor plan development inscribed with in a parallelogram. Operations of cutting or emptying a corner create an outdoor entrance space in concavity (the kind of overall shape that, in mathematics, is called a non-convex set).

Musac's floor plan is analyzed comparatively here using the same abstraction technique through diagrams.
Top: Cell diagram identifies both program enclosures and outdoor space with the emphasis on the dimensional relationships and relative position; families of similar enclosures, large versus small, how they fit next to each other, on the one hand, and relative position of outdoor spaces (included in, at the side of, amid), on the other.
Bottom: Diagram of circulation-program-light, with emphasis on the connection between rooms and between them and the light.

dissolution (p. 52_53)

Another graphic quote is a tribute to Almere by Sanaa (Cultural Centre and Theatre) and the idea of dissolution of hierarchy.
Following on the notion of diagram, Sejima's architecture was phrased as "diagram architecture" by Toyo Ito, in reference to the strength derived from the extreme reduction of the building to a special kind of diagram, where what is built acquires the abstract characteristics of its own representation.
These drawings, dual diagrams on program-circulation-enclosure-light relations like previous ones in this book, show both the competition entry floor plan (left) and the floor plan for the final project (right) on the same scale. They help to clarify the evolution of the main ideas behind the project: the patio-room insertion (patios as cells) as one type of cell among others in a system and the dissolution of hierarchy, both spatial and structural. These questions read more clearly in the competition proposal than in the final project, although they are present in both.
This is a good example of the everlasting fight that characterizes the translation process from conceptual to built architecture.

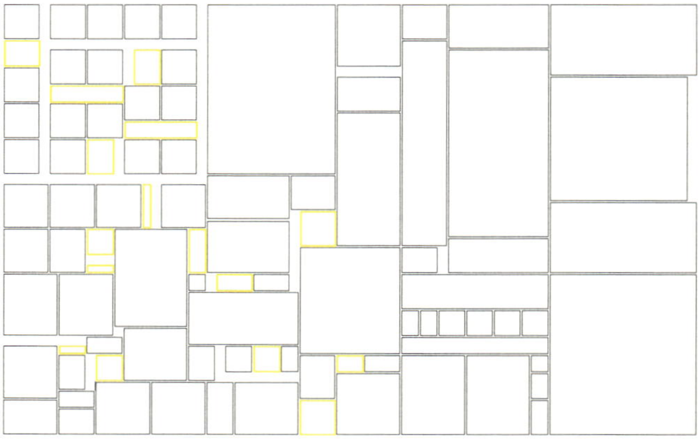

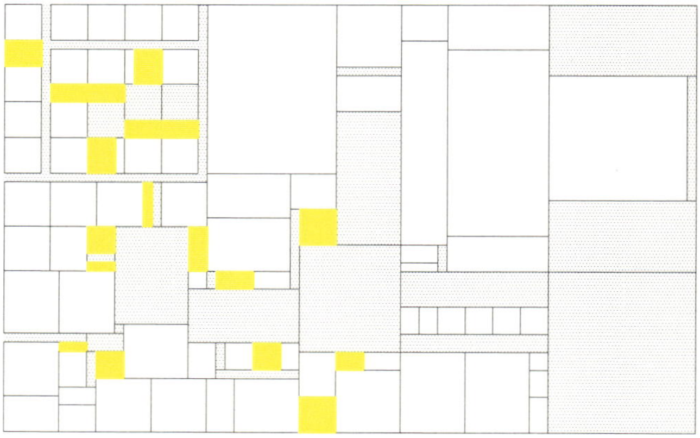

Almere Competition by Sanaa (Cultural Centre and Theatre)
The main strategy is to populate the grid, a battleship-like kind of game that is played with no distinction between “x” and ”y” coordinates.
Cells are either small and many or large and few, but they are clustered by adjacency leaving no gaps in between (accumulation). Some of these cells are also circulation but are presented like any other enclosure. There is no distinction between the servant and the served, as movement happens in a multi-path way from cell to cell, regardless of programmatic attributes.
Although it behaves as a bottom-up configuration, it takes up the strictness of the rectangular boundary as restriction and support. An undeniable spatial disorientation arises from this labyrinth disposition in which every corner is the same.

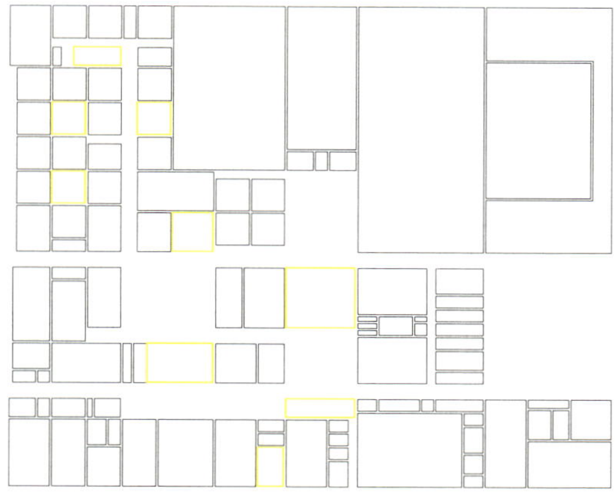

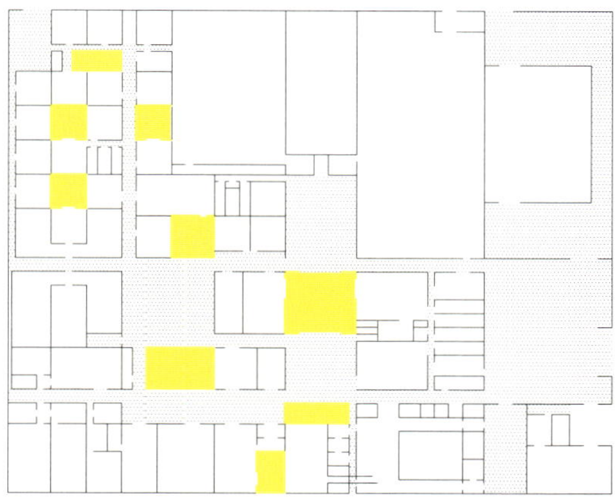

Almere Final project by Sanaa (Cultural Centre and Theatre)
The project is smaller in footprint, therefore it has fewer cells to organize. What was extremely generic before becomes more specific, if only because of its singularity.
Corridors are introduced between cells and larger gaps are now to be considered more like the absence of cells rather than a different type of cell. With corridors as "the other condition", a secondary system of order introduces the idea of threaded one-way structural bays that were not revealed in the competition and, with them, slightly greater hierarchy and less disorientation.

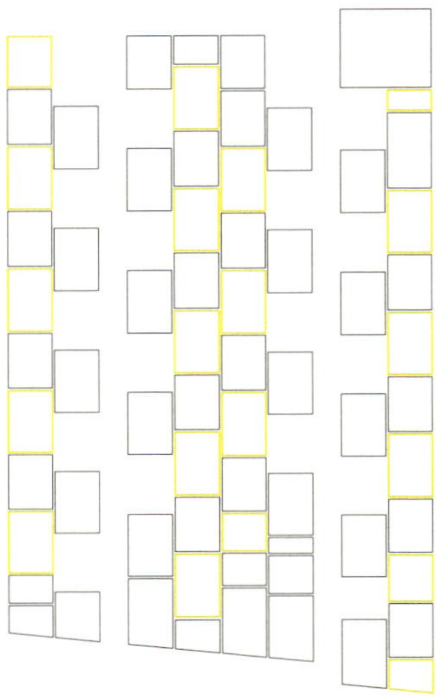

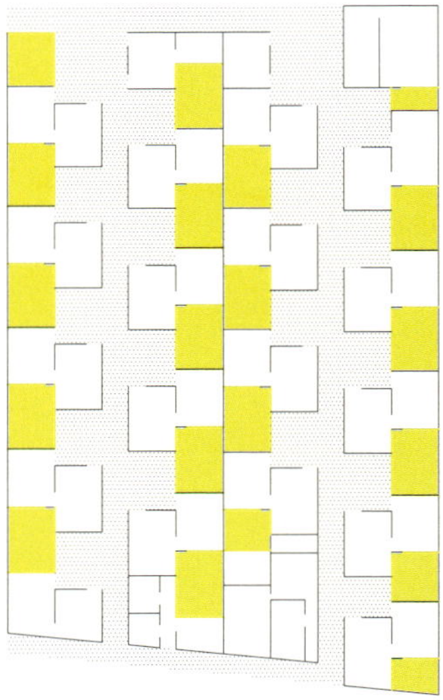

Cedt Ocaña by estudio.entresitio (primary and specialized health-care center).
Acting as a precedent for the "3x1" clinic, this project is a non-wining competition entry that represents a turning point in our spatial research. Based on the Almere's cell-to-cell strategy and the use of patio-rooms, for the first time in our work it proposes questions of a potential endless expansion of the floor plan.
One could say it is a one-way (unidirectional) interpretation of Almere's scheme, although there is a transverse or, more precisely, oblique direction that combs the floor plan in visual continuity through waiting areas and patios. It still inherits some conditions of a linear structure head-and-tail configuration in which the negotiation with the site's boundary imposition is non-existent, as it simply adopts it without any further consideration.

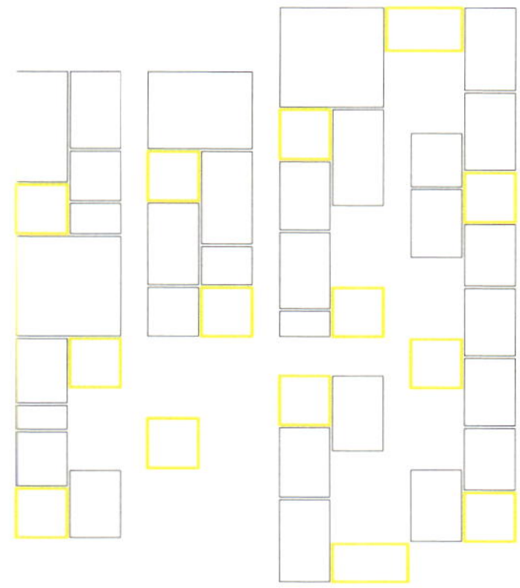

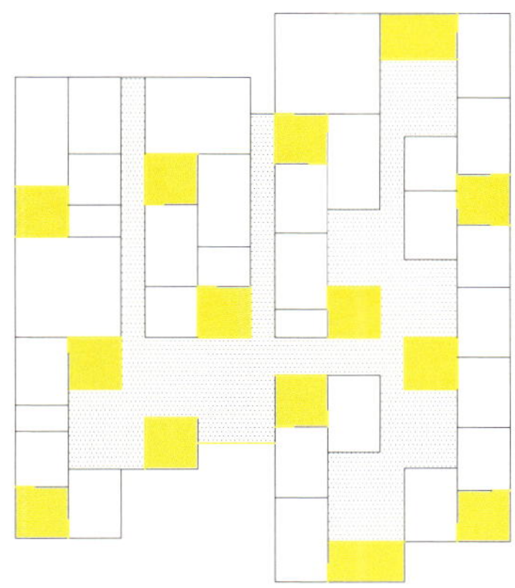

3x1.
In comparison with Ocaña's linearity, this disposition has a higher degree of complexity. There are more rules involved in the solution and the so-called programmatic bars get dissolved, enunciating the idea of a field condition.
When solving the floor plan we look to ensure that exceptions are always consistent with the system, or even emerge from it. We aim to "play" the system as the opposite of giving value to "the exception that proves the rule". This means that the system rules have to be flexible in their ability to accommodate possibility; perhaps it is our own intellectual position that needs to be flexible to admit unanticipated results as a solution in the development of a certain system logic (a serendipitous encounter).
To cite Jacques Monod, we might say that the order of a system is equal to the amount of information necessary for the description of a system; this dithering, although seemingly random, has a more complex order, which from the perspective of complexity, is a higher degree of order than the one a checkerboard may have. There are hidden variables that prevent us from understanding it up front. Thus, as a complex system, it has more information than what each part provides independently, and describing it requires understanding not only the performance of the parts but their relationship to each other.

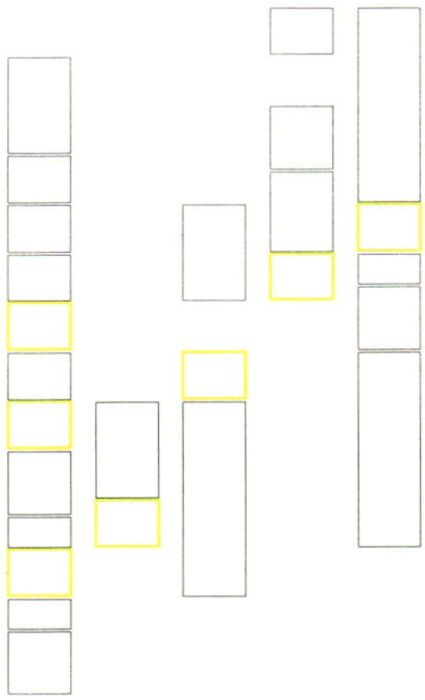

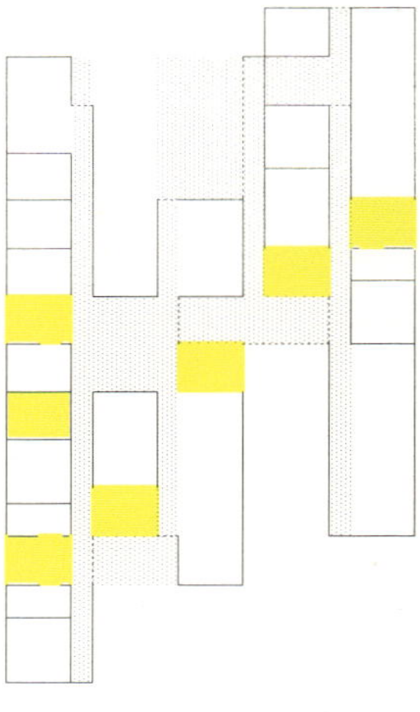

To return to the idea of a graphic citation, this project by entresitio may be understood as self-referential. Some of the findings that we encountered as we designed the clinics saw a later transposition into our work. For example, an afterthought on the dissolution of the corridor is developed in this project for a single family house in Medellín, Colombia. Following on Carlos Martí's opinion from his book *Las variaciones de la identidad* (2014), where he presents an idea of the evolution of the species that could mean a decline in the natural world, but an enrichment in the cultural world, we are interested in the evolution of types.
We continued the exploration of the implicit corridor of the clinic. Where in "3x1" the waiting areas are integrated into the circulation, expanding it transversally and thus decreasing its longitudinal tension, this project explores how to integrate circulation "through" program as a plus to the spaces served.

Field Condition

When the programmatic bars are placed alongside one another to become an extended field and the façade is no longer an option for lighting the entire floor plan, new rules apply. “3x1” is a mathematical field condition with a characteristic rhythm that establishes the relationship between order, space and structure.

The mathematical field condition is linked to the notion of the continuity of a certain condition (function). It is called the “field of continuity” to the subset that satisfies the condition of continuity at all points. The points where the condition is not fulfilled are considered discontinuities.

“3x1”, as a continuous field, has some spatial and lighting conditions that are verified extensively on the xy plane in a sufficiently similar way, although not identically. The margin of difference between pure mathematical reasoning and constructed reality is, precisely, the margin of speculation that makes the translation from concept to space such an interesting conversation.

Given the accumulation of layers in the projective reasoning, it may be time here to also superimpose the idea of the underlying constructive thought that the artist Max Bill enounced in the text for his “Fifteen Variations on a Single Theme” (1938): “. . . although the exact placing of the spaces and surfaces of these figures was obviously done by geometrical methods, the controlling idea which produced the figures was neither mathematical nor geometrical.”

His work is about bringing to light what was hidden or, why not, hiding the obvious. Something we like to call “underlying structures” becomes the support for a certain continuity of exceptions: underneath a random image, there can be a system of order to be found and/or define.

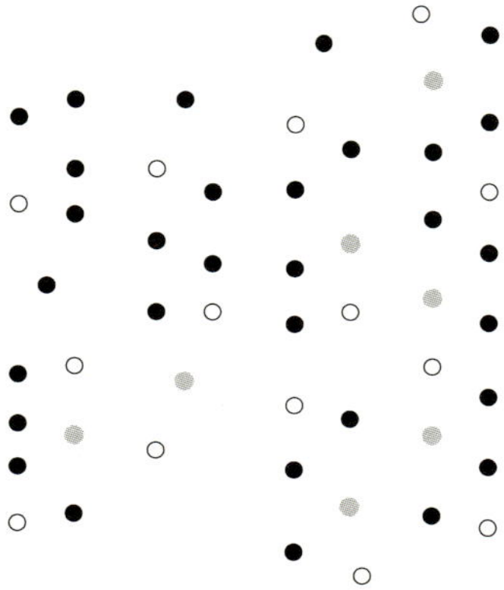

○ open out-door space: patio
● open in-door space: waiting area
● enclosed program unit: room

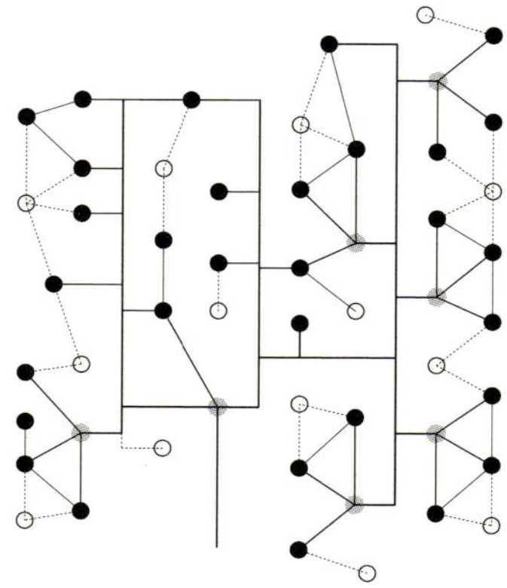

— main connection
— distribution to cells
— distribution between cells
···· cell-patio connections

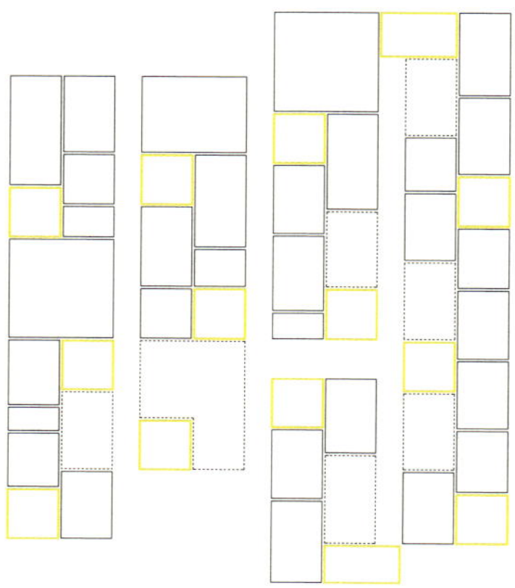

□ open out-door space: patio
□ open in-door space: waiting area
□ enclosed program unit: room

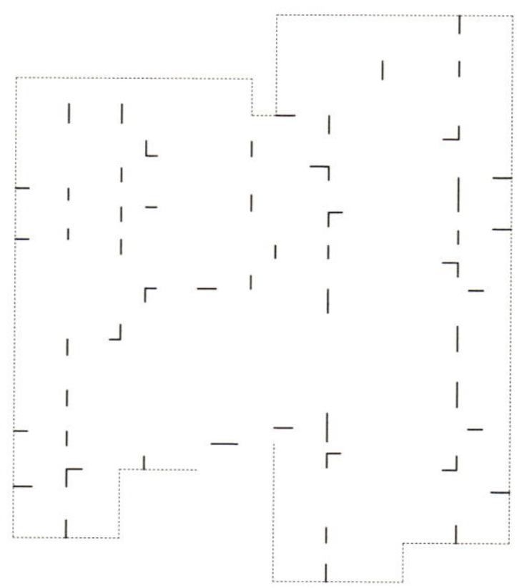

— connectors

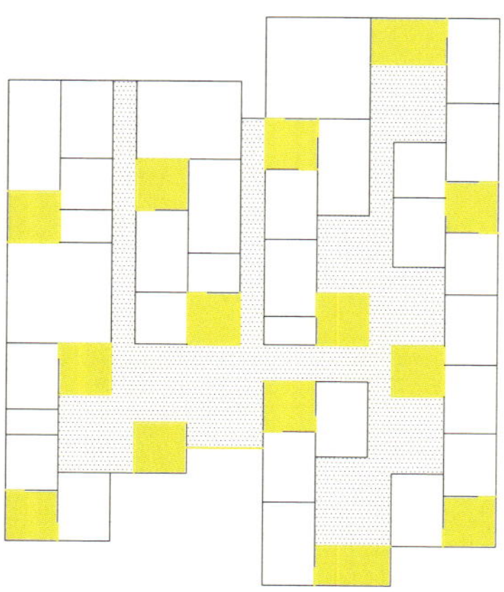

■ open out-door space: patio
■ open in-door space: waiting area
□ enclosed program unit: room

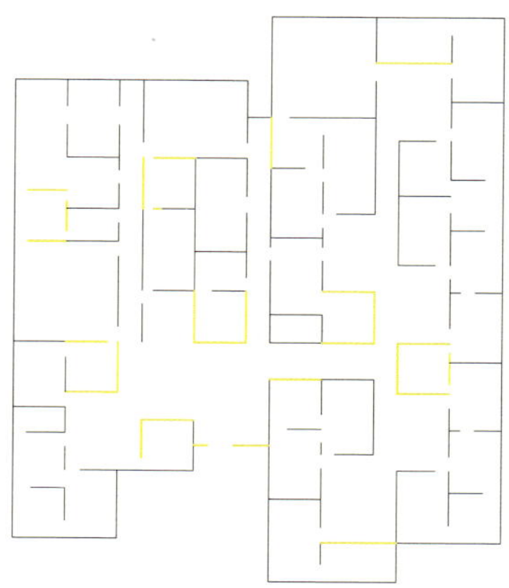

partitions

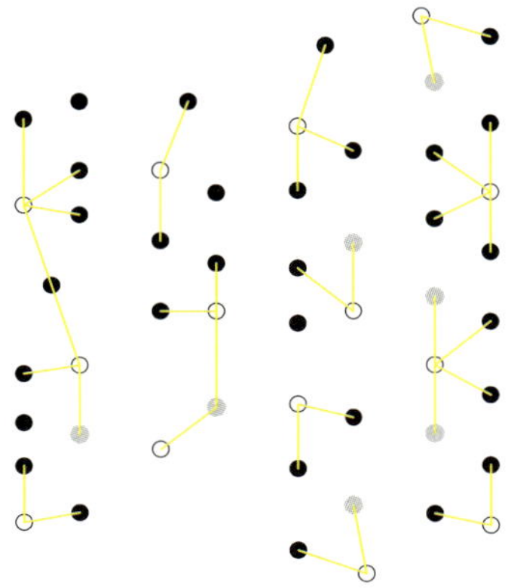

— direct lighting

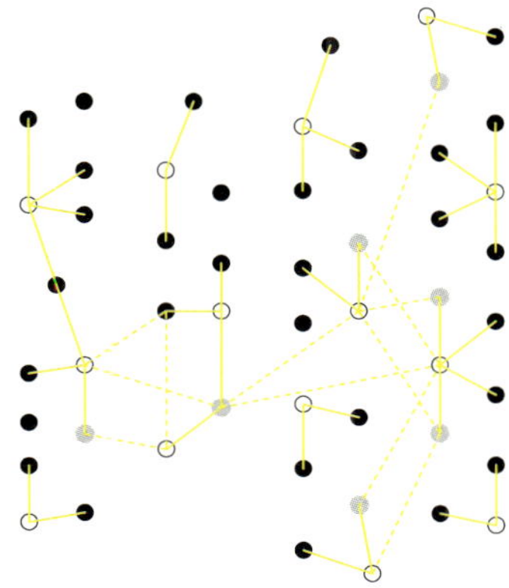

— direct lighting
-- indirect lighting

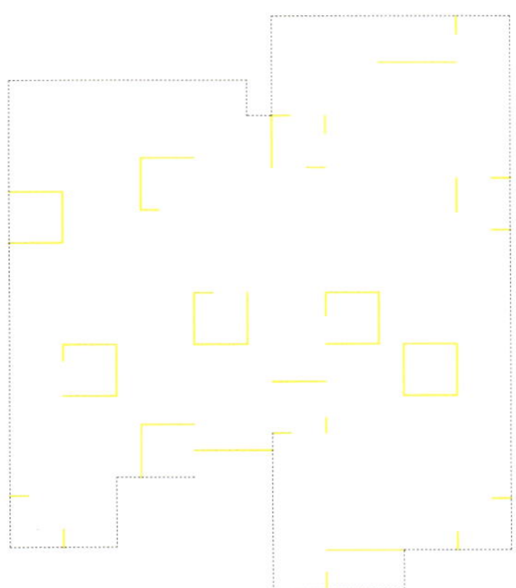

— glazing

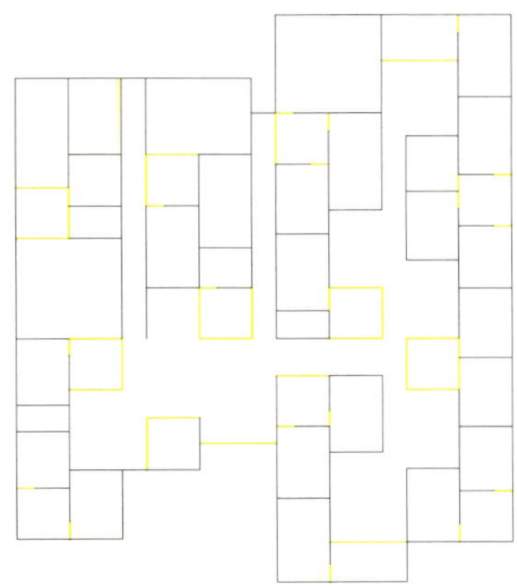

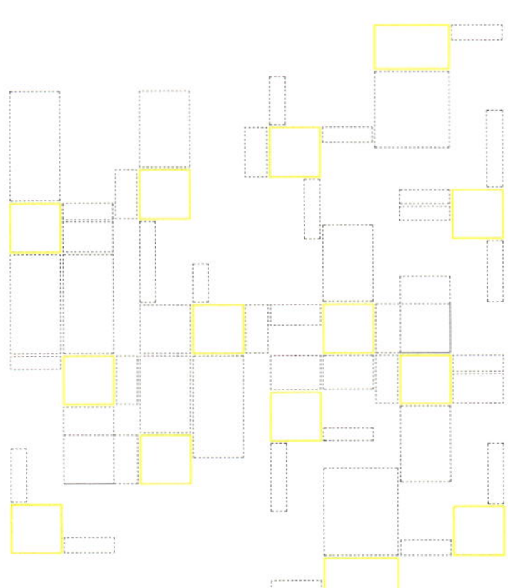

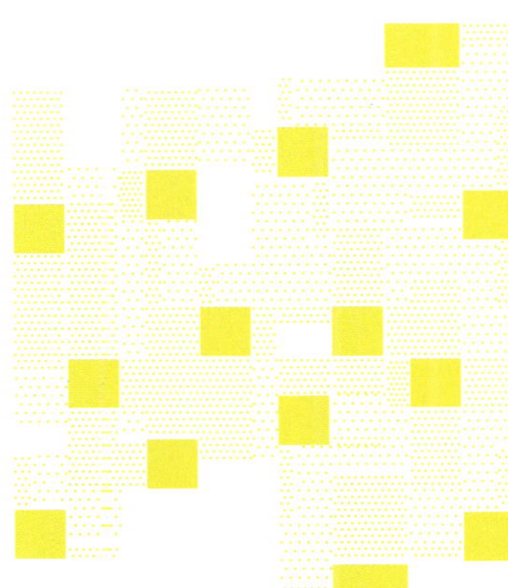

Order is not a synonym for control, but a capacity for relationship.
When considering relationships that are dimensionless, we are addressing questions of topology, also called the geometry of position, a branch of mathematics that deals with geometric properties in which measure is not involved. For two given components, the distance between them may not be relevant; what matters are the connections that exist.
The strategies for order that come with the study of continuity and the relative position in a dimensionless sense are to be understood through graphs and knots, maps and holes. Actually, graphs and maps are related, as dual representations of the same abstract mathematical object. That idea of duality is quite interesting as a vehicle to translate things into architecture. We sometimes have trouble visualizing the role of a "connection" in an architectural diagram, but its dual map (boundaries between the connected) somehow provides a visual answer.
Connections behave as the underlying structure for the plan solution.

Page 58:
3x1 dual configurations:

column 1:
components considered in a topological sense
function translated into spatial conditions
- white: open out-door space, patio
- grey: open in-door space, waiting area
- black: enclosed program unit, room

column 2:
programmatic connections graph
- physical connections (what links)
- partitions (what divides)

Page 59:
column 3 and 4:
Cells and space-light relationships
- direct and indirect lighting
- transparent versus opaque surfaces
- Spatial influence of the transparent in the spaces around (expressed by horizontal abatement) and its translation as a map of light gradation

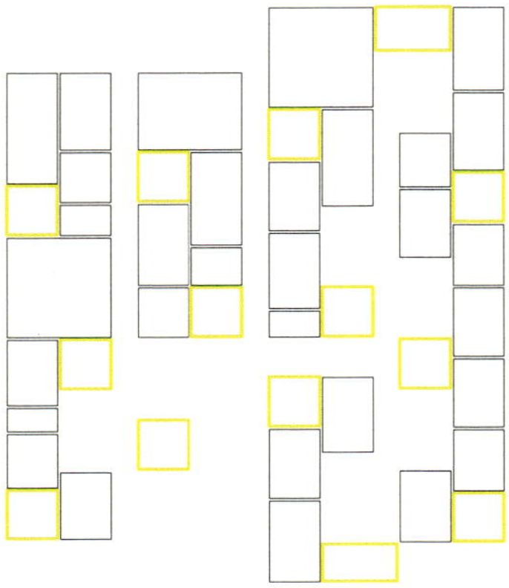
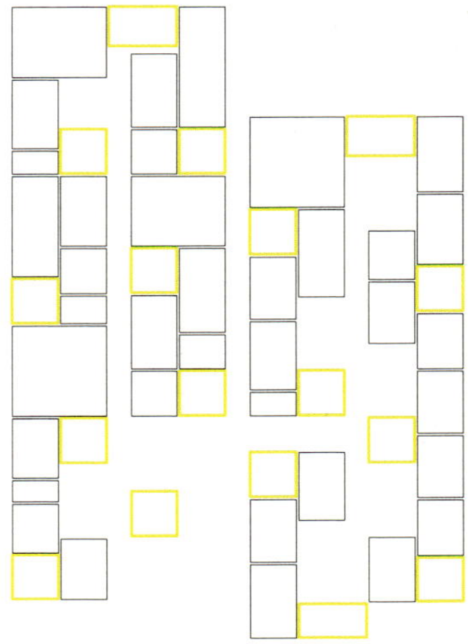
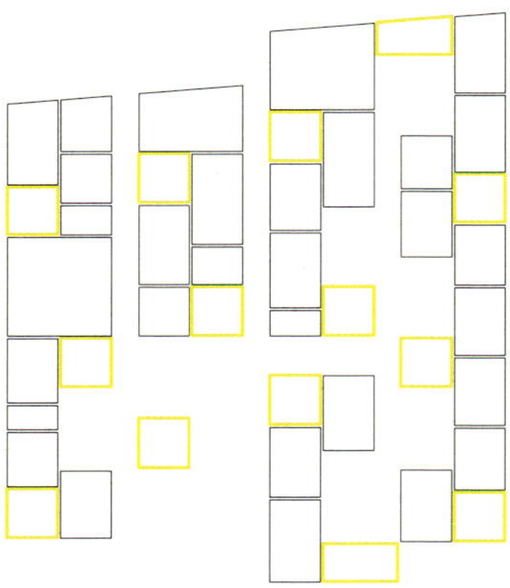
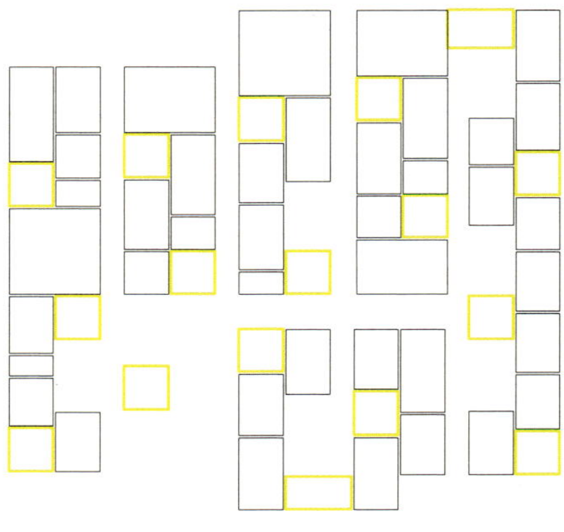

The cellular behavior of this collection of rooms (cells with assigned functions) is a bottom-up configuration.
Once the internal logic of how elements are juxtaposed is established, the same floor plan can be wider or narrower, shorter or longer, more or less regular or irregular, as in these derivatives of the “3x1” type.
The exact shape of the perimeter is not really important. The boundary conditions can coincide with the system logic (geometric) or they may be a clean cut that assumes a restriction imposed from outside. We have also seen cases in which an intermediate situation between the conditions of the system itself and those external to it is negotiated.
The nature of type becomes clearer here, understood from Quatremere de Quincy's perspective: type is an idea – the thought of an architecture that stands about the fullness of reality, a structure of form capable of multiple developments.

fragment (pag. 64_65)

Another way of understanding the field condition is as a potentially unlimited extension of certain conditions (in this case generated by repeating the same connections between cells). Paradoxically, this allows us to think of the building floor plan as a fragment of a higher rank structure, in which the ideas of order are much more evident than in the fragment.
Actually, "to fragment" is a very effective way of introducing or presenting randomness arising from an ordered system, like for example the first iterations of an algorithmic process or the first few digits of an irrational number like pi (3.14159).
The “3x1” pattern is generated by copy and translation, which is actually a type of symmetry.
It is more common to find symmetry in nature at micro scales than in the macro. Equivalently, in architecture, it is more common to find symmetry on the scale of geometric pattern generation (in floor plan underlying structures, in applied and decorative arabesques like in the Alhambra, or in modular components of a structure) than on a building or context level. Symmetry is therefore attributable as an aspect of the generative process, rather than to the whole.

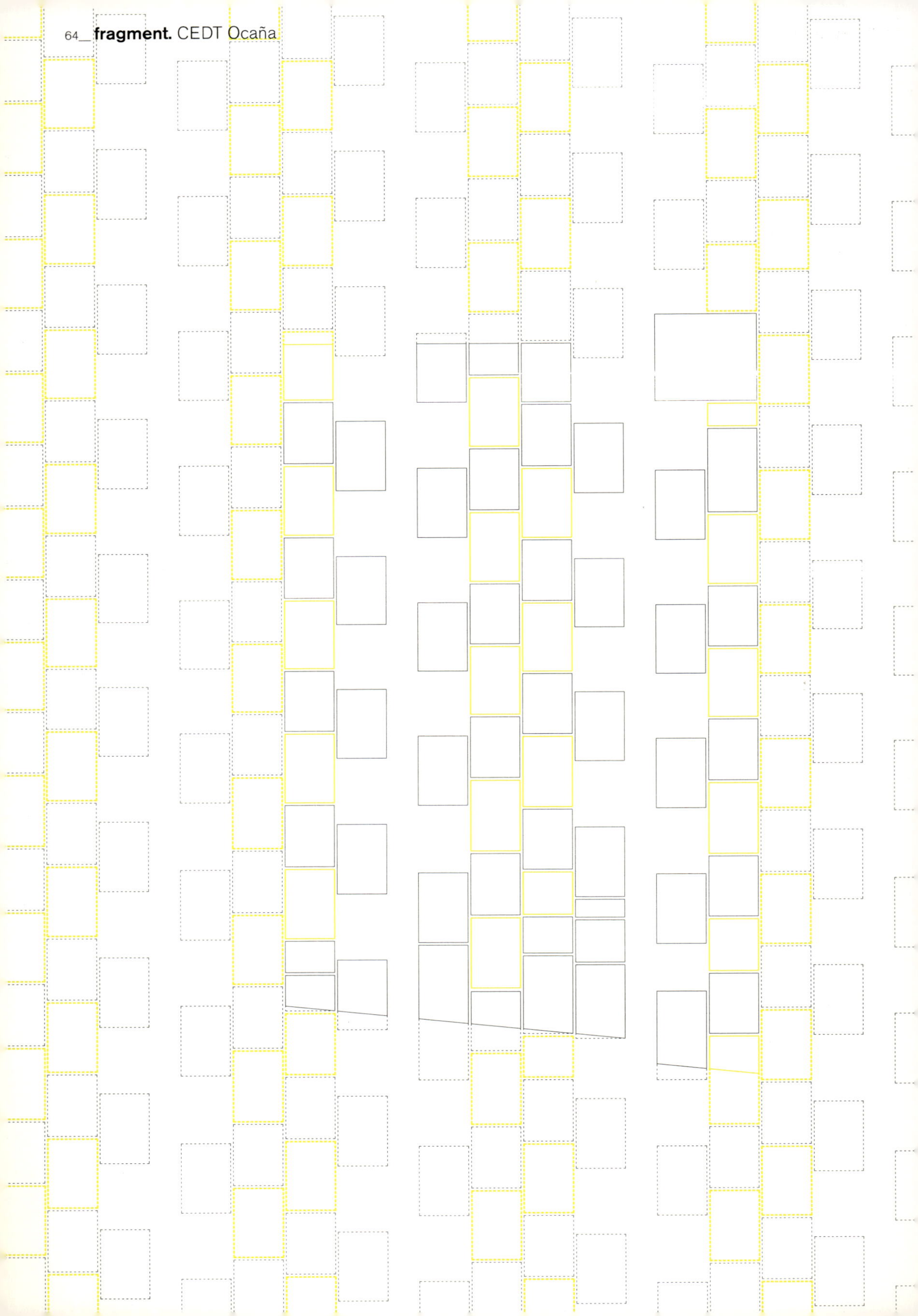

65_ **fragment.** 3x1

Patterns as tessellations help to better frame the idea of underlying structure: a configuration with abstract potential that may be the warp (though it is not necessarily evident) that supports the translation of a program into the spatial condition of architecture by being its "system inside solution". It enables a rich part-to-whole relationship that may vary with geometric or arithmetic criteria, but in all cases provides a direct and indissoluble link between the two.
An underlying structure is the weapon for establishing relationships between components of a larger system, and it spares us having to solve things individually. The underlying structure allows us to introduce a degree of regulated randomness, welcoming contingency and estrangement as a positive input into the process of providing thickness and depth to what is built.
For the House in Medellín there is an open logic diagram generation, according to which the various parts of the program are arranged on the pattern as support. The project solution begins by defining the pattern (rectangular semi-regular tessellation), scaling the cell size to suit the program (size matters), and defining the boundary condition (relationship between limit and extension).
The translation of the pattern into the 3D is something we will discuss further on.

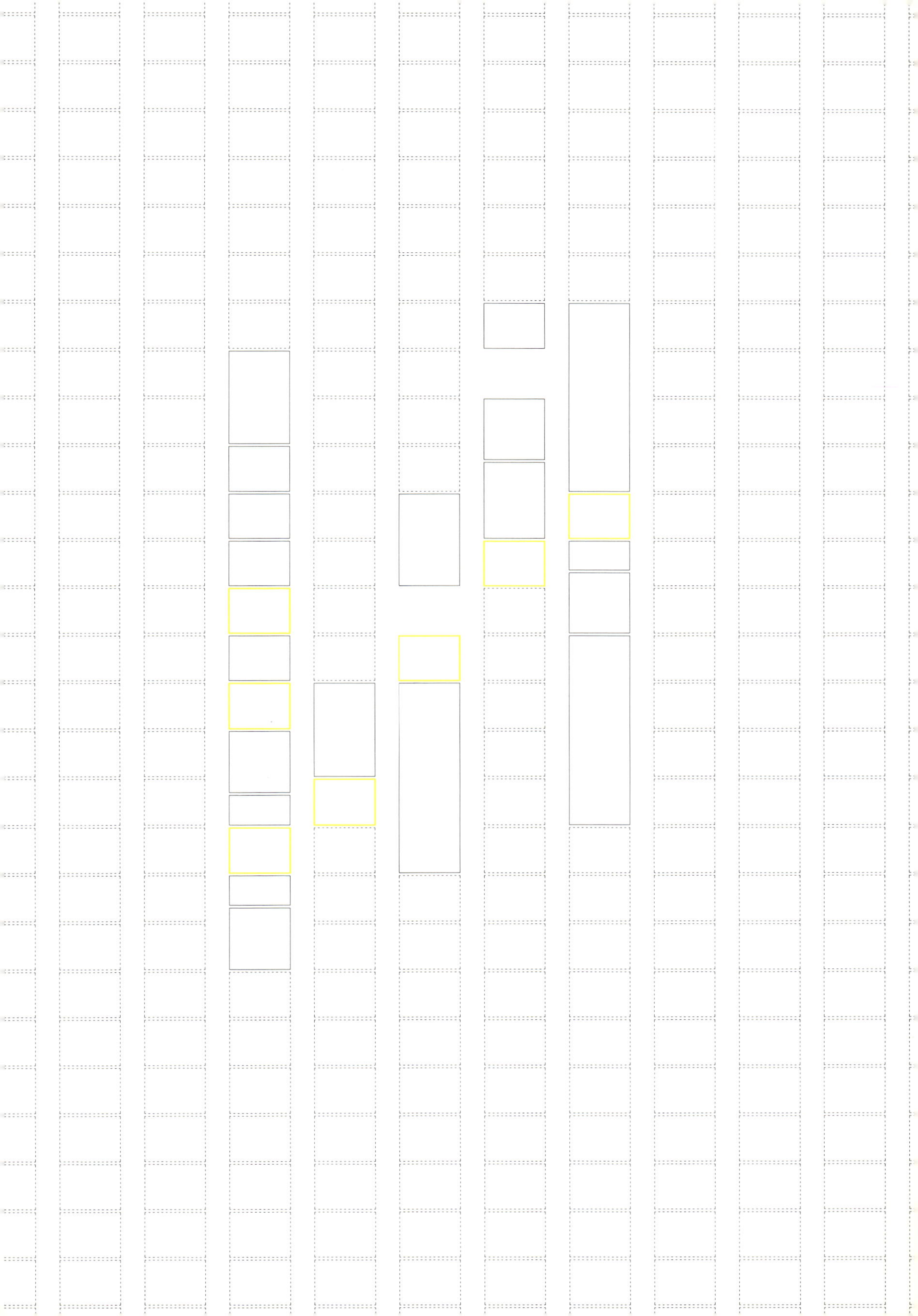

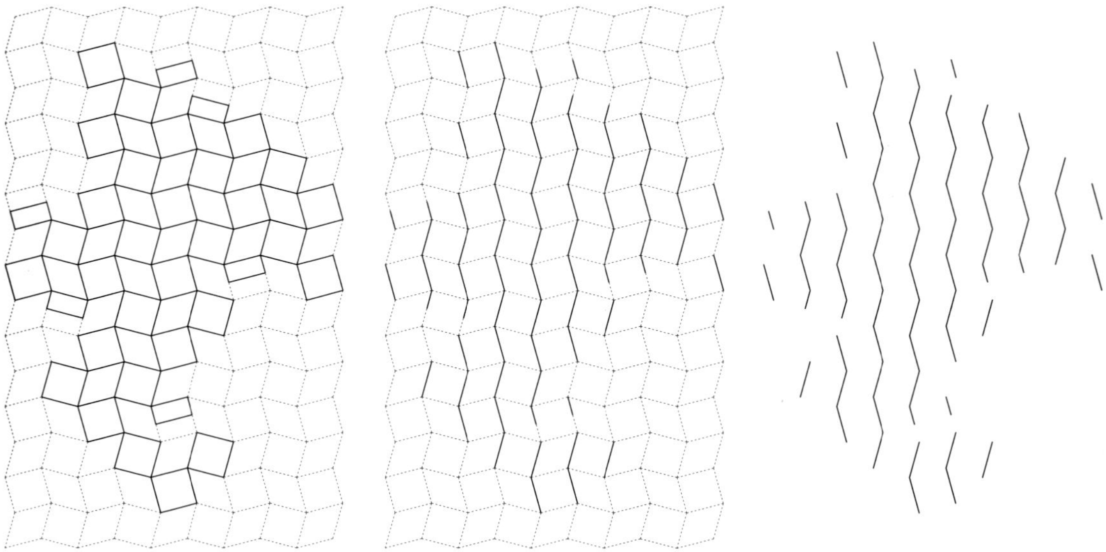

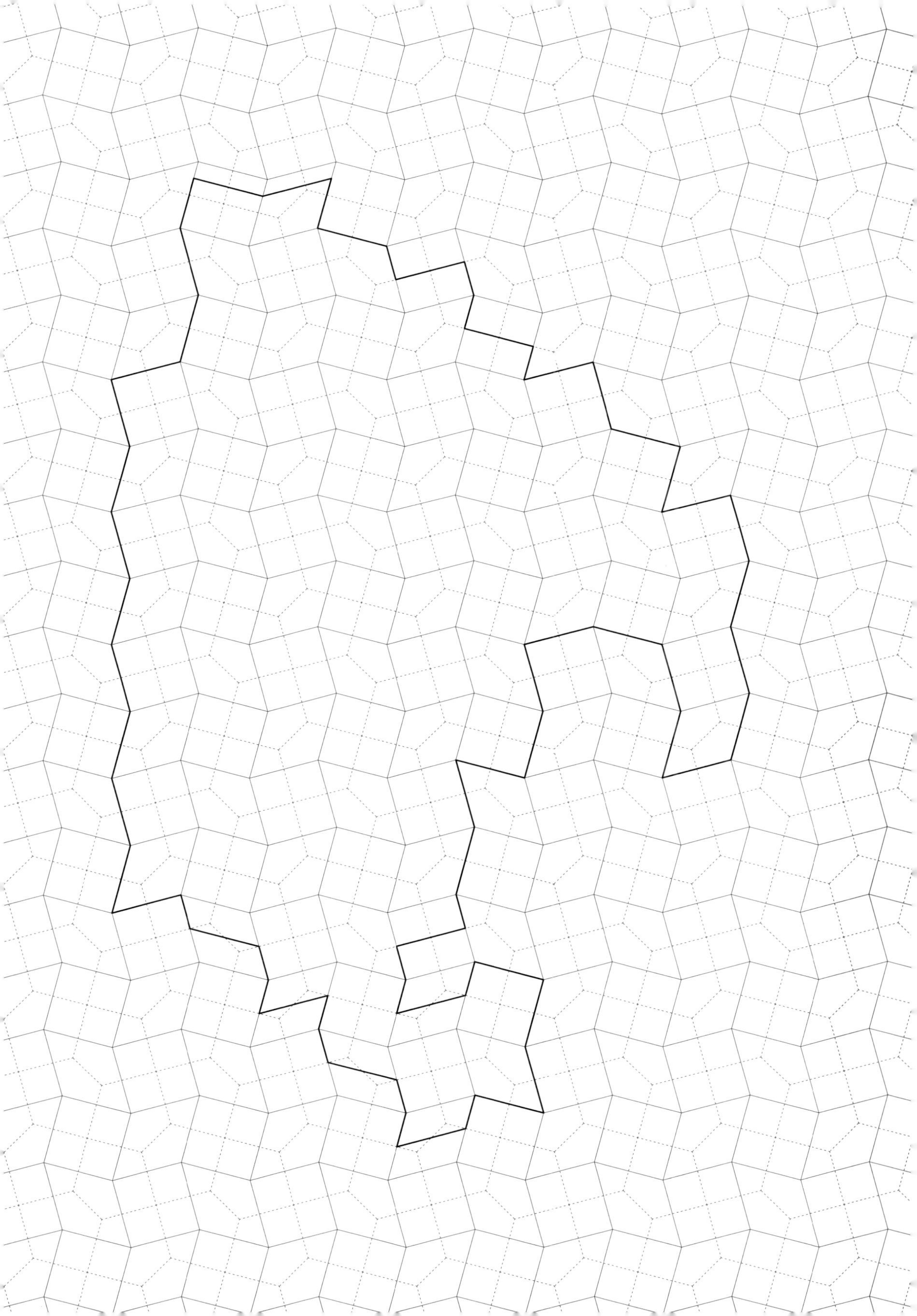

(pag. 68_69)

We are seduced by the role of order in architecture as a basic tool for building space. In the vast domain of the relationship between order and disorder, we try to find the hidden rules behind certain solutions, especially in built precedents like Musac (Mansilla-Tuñón), for example.
In a lecture at ETSAM, Luis Moreno Mansilla reflected (referring to Musac) on the geometric metaphor: "No metaphor is capable of producing architecture by itself; it ties you down or you just end up betraying it." He defended the subjective interpretation of the objective data of geometry: "Within a territory that is very limited, there is still great freedom to work, which is one of the most attractive paradoxes of architecture."
The geometrical strategy as a metaphor can be a powerful way of addressing order, however: metaphor meaning transport, like taking the bus for the trip we make from the world of ideas to defined architectural space. Thus, geometry is not the project itself but a useful way of getting there.
The mathematical field condition metaphor of Musac is a mosaic (the art of covering the plane with forms that do not overlap), actually two: the Archimedean tiling 3^2, 4, 3, 4 and its dual "Cairo tessellation" formed by pentagons of four equal sides and two right angles, which takes its name from its frequent use in the paving of the Egyptian city. (3^2, 4, 3, 4 means that at every vertex of the tessellation there are two consecutive triangles, one square, one triangle and one square). This set of guidelines supports the architectural solution and allows for introducing a certain degree of randomness in regulated patterns.
Regarding the necessary question about how these patterns can be transferred into architecture, Musac is an example of the pattern becoming the structural and spatial definition of the project. Bays are like streets, however subdivided in fragments or components, due to the lateral walls' sidesteps. The balance between the bay and the fragment is precise, beautiful and subtle and would entirely deserve the title of "geometry as the beginning of space".

(pag. 72_73)

Looking further into the relationship between order and the structure of a building (spatial structure and load-bearing structure), all examples shown here have a clear structural directionality that "combs" the plan in one direction.
"3x1" (6) is a mathematical field condition with a syncopated rhythm due to the circulation "aabaa", where Musac (3) has an "aa" rhythm, and the house in Medellín (7) has an "aba" one. These calculated intervals or frequencies have a direct consequence in the relationship between circulation and program, which in all these cases is defined by structure; Musac and the "aa" rhythm presents a disposition in which program and circulation are the same thing (it is a museum) and the load-bearing structure is almost 100% coincident with the spatial one (there are no partitions).
The spatial conditions happen over the basted line of the structural order as alterations of the basic rhythm. Over the basic "aa" of Almere (4) we also find 2a, 3a, 4a, etc. In Musac, due to the pattern geometry, relations are diagonal like in √2aa. Over the rhythm "aba" of the house in Medellín, these possible relations happen: a, ab, aba, bab, etc.
The regular grid is "played" allowing for spatial interaction between adjacent structural bays, and spaces can therefore be part of different bays at the same time. This provides a freer sense of directionality and questions the direction is which the space is tensioned. That is how the field condition is highlighted, not only because of the extensiveness of the plan but also of the spatial quality.

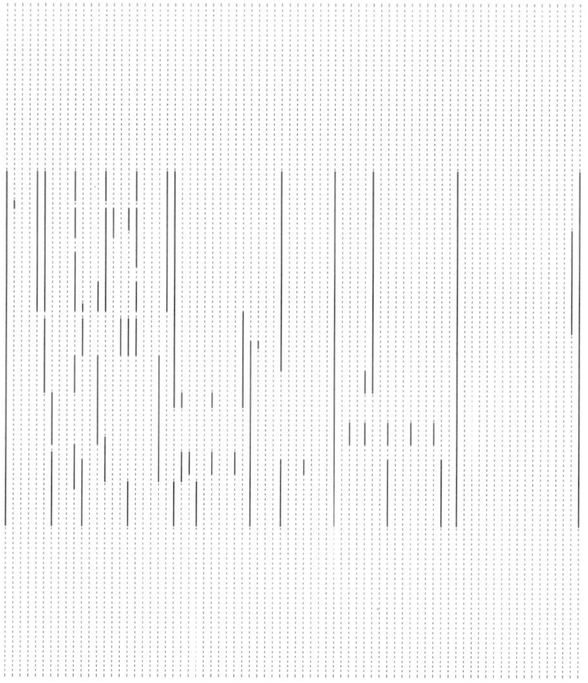

1a

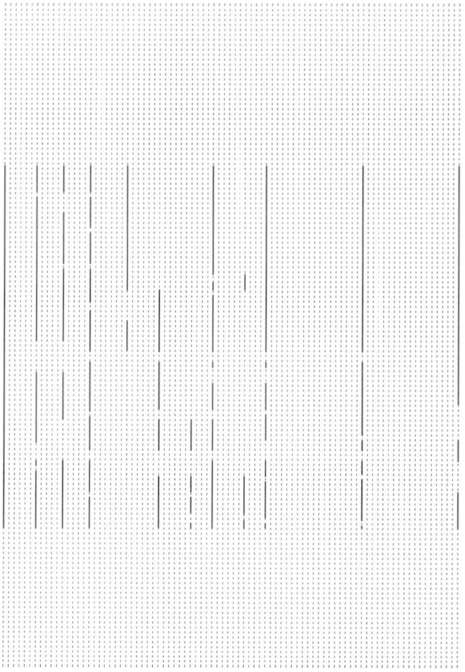

2a

1b

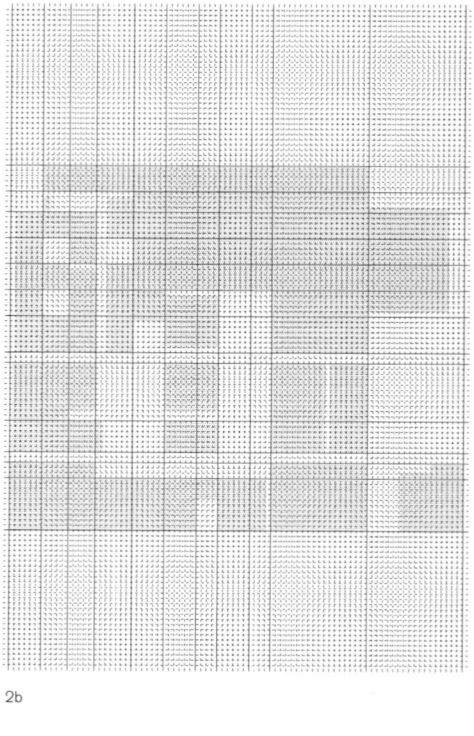

2b

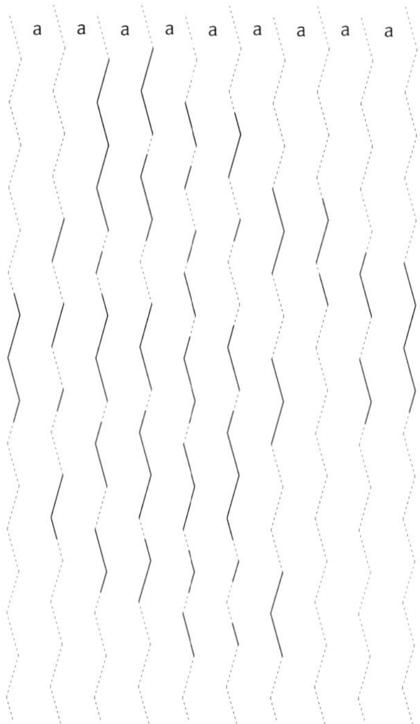
a a a a a a a a a

3

6a 5a 5a 7a 6a 6a 4a 6a 4a 18a 18a

4

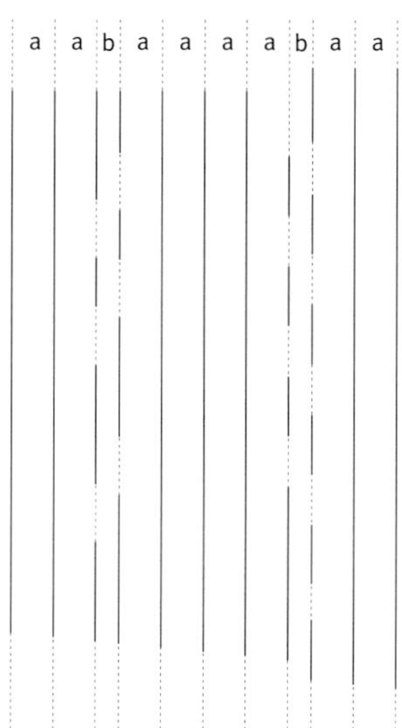
a a b a a a a b a a

5

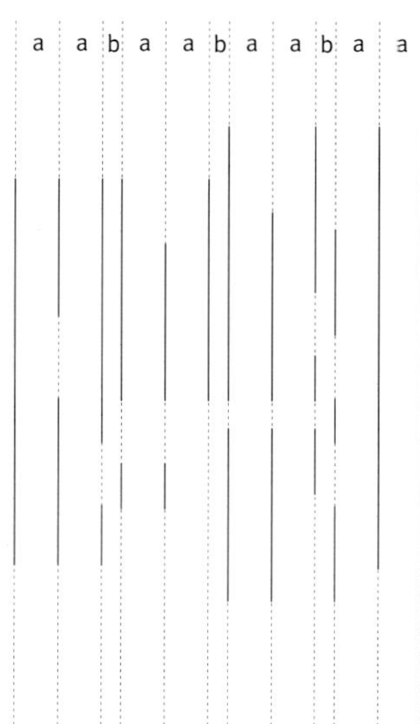
a a b a a b a a b a a

6

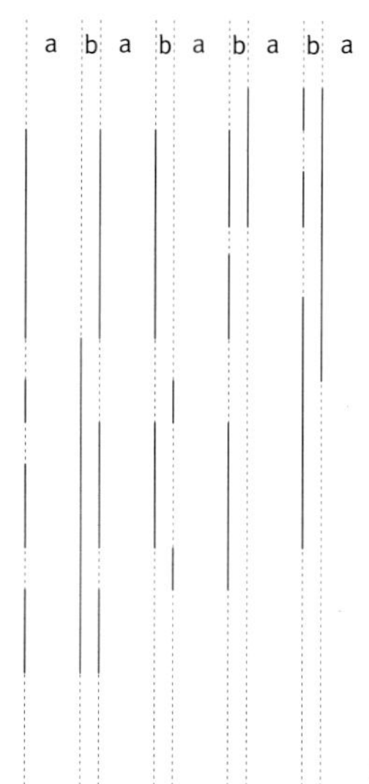
a b a b a b a b a

7

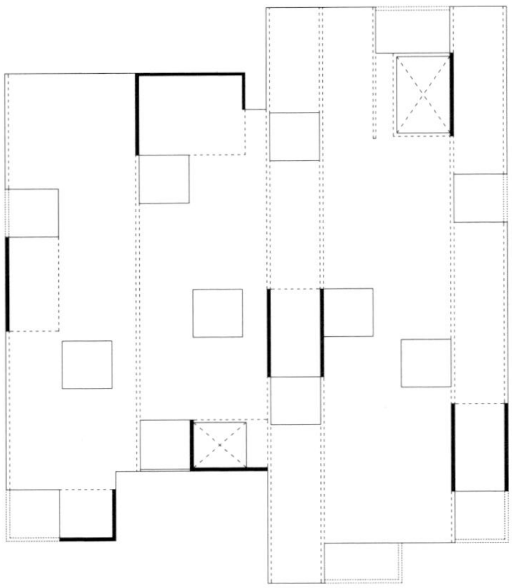
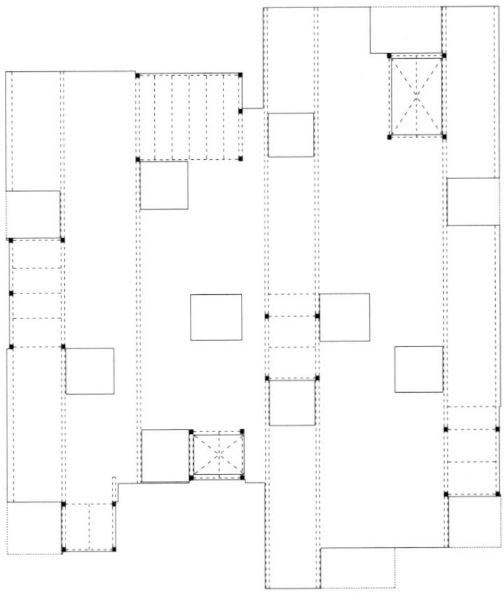
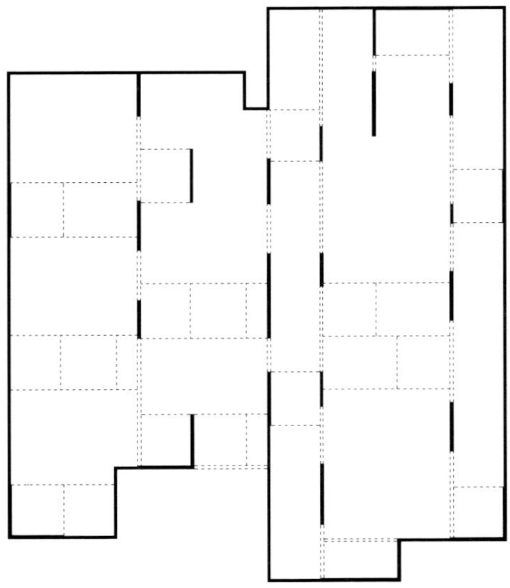
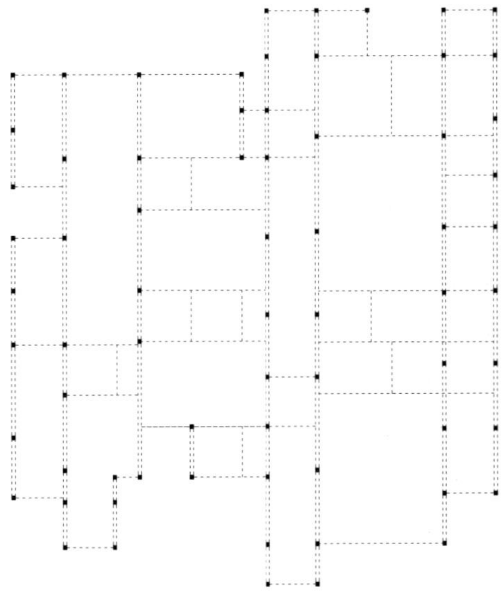
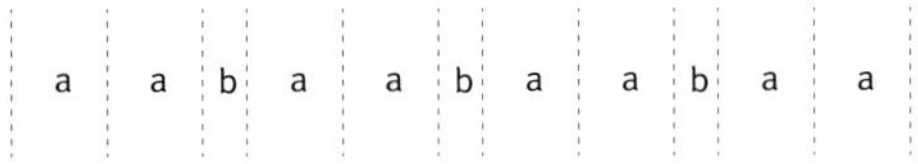
a a b a a b a a b a a
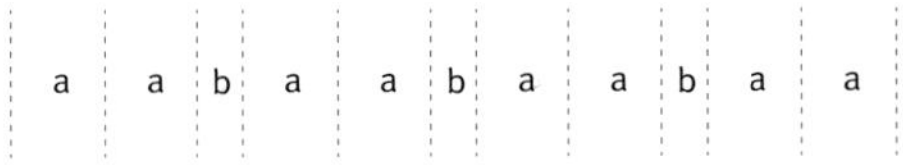
a a b a a b a a b a a

There is no harm in admitting that this clinic project was not thought out from the beginning in terms of gravity (structural gravity), but in terms of spatiality. Good proof of this is the fact that two different structural solutions are used for the three individuals. On the left, S and U with concrete load-bearing walls; on the right, V with steel frame.
Both solutions follow the same logic, though; over the "aabaa" rhythm of the double-double loaded corridor, the structural bays' dimensions are aab, a, aa, ab and aba. The aab and aba large spans allow for the absence of supports in the patios' exposed corners. End of corridor patios are "ab" wide (large=typical+circulation).
Starting with the load-bearing iterations, the structural disposition is key for making decisions on the specific type of enclosure that each side of a patio may have. Walls are concrete only if they are load bearing or if they are part of the outer skin. Thus, there are no concrete walls perpendicular to the linear structural portals other than the façade. These non-bearing walls are simple cladding covered in ceramic tiles. Together with the transparency of the glass surfaces, this "structural secret" makes the specific finishes of each patio quite unexpected. That same reasoning is extended to the added volumes on the roof, which are made out of concrete only when there is concrete (load-bearing or façade) underneath. The uneven placement of the load-bearing walls in relation to patios and volumes (and vice-versa) makes the structural trace hard to follow as well as any possible anticipation of the reason for each wall's material quality.
Robert Somol's words come to mind when, in the introduction to Peter Eisenman's Diagram Diaries, he assesses the different positions in the conception of form as the relationship between space and structure that are presented in the investigations by Colin Rowe and John Hejduk or Eisenman himself, in which the binomial form-structure prevails over spatial intentions in what Somol calls "objectification of the structure". Comparatively, one might say that for the V clinic (right column), though a lintel structure, it is a space without supports (hidden out of sight) and it could be described as a structureless space. This condition of lightness is reinforced by the quality of translucent material and reflection of the envelope to the outside.

form (pag. 76_77)

Although built on the same underlying system, the structural, spatial and programmatic strategies of "3x1" do not coincide. They are not exactly the same thing: structural bays are different than program bays or bars. The important issue is what is translated into physical space and what is not.

1. - outer volume, outer shell
   - circulation and waiting areas, possessed public space
   - skin, exterior wrapping

2. - voids, horizontal windows
   - Circulation, waiting areas and patios; appropriated public space
   - program, programmatic bars

3. - light-cells; light and its area of influence; patios and waiting areas
   - three dimensional matrix of independent components (parts, cells, units, elements)
   - program-cells

4. - structure as parallel load-bearing walls
   - structure as metal frames

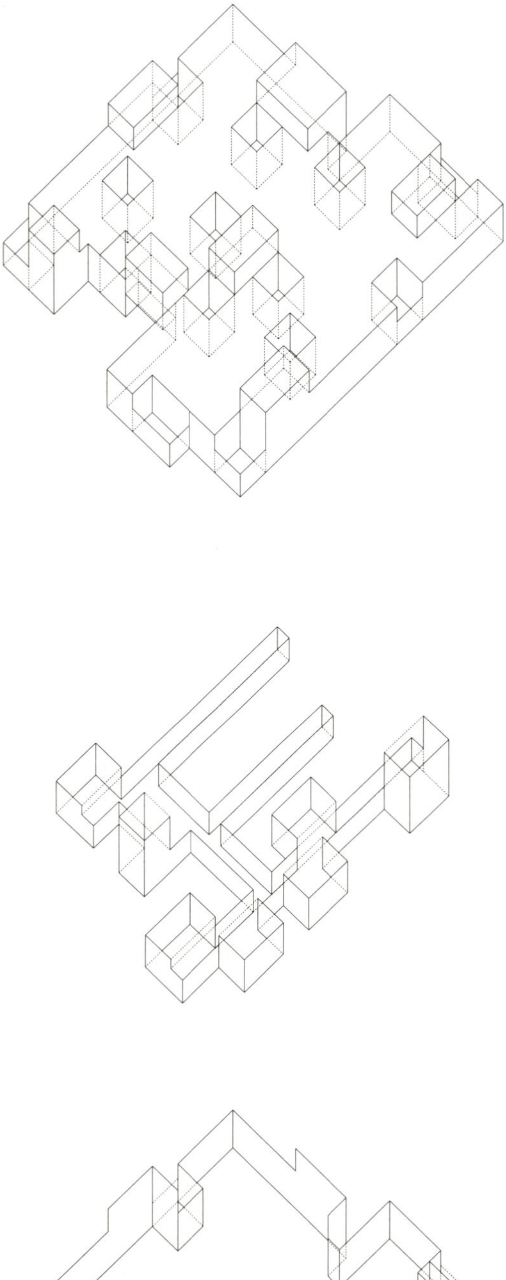

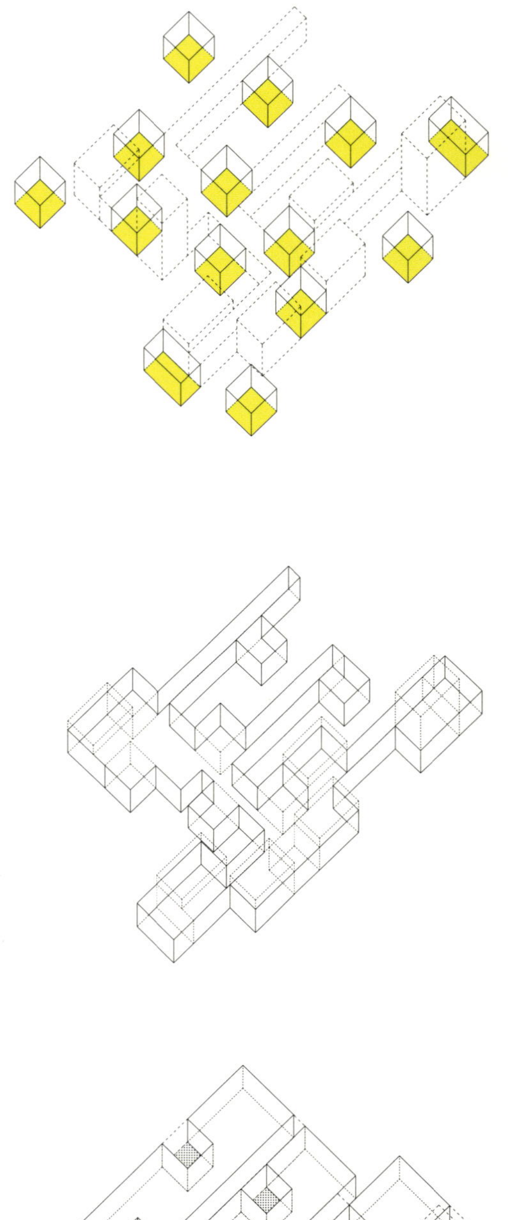

1

2

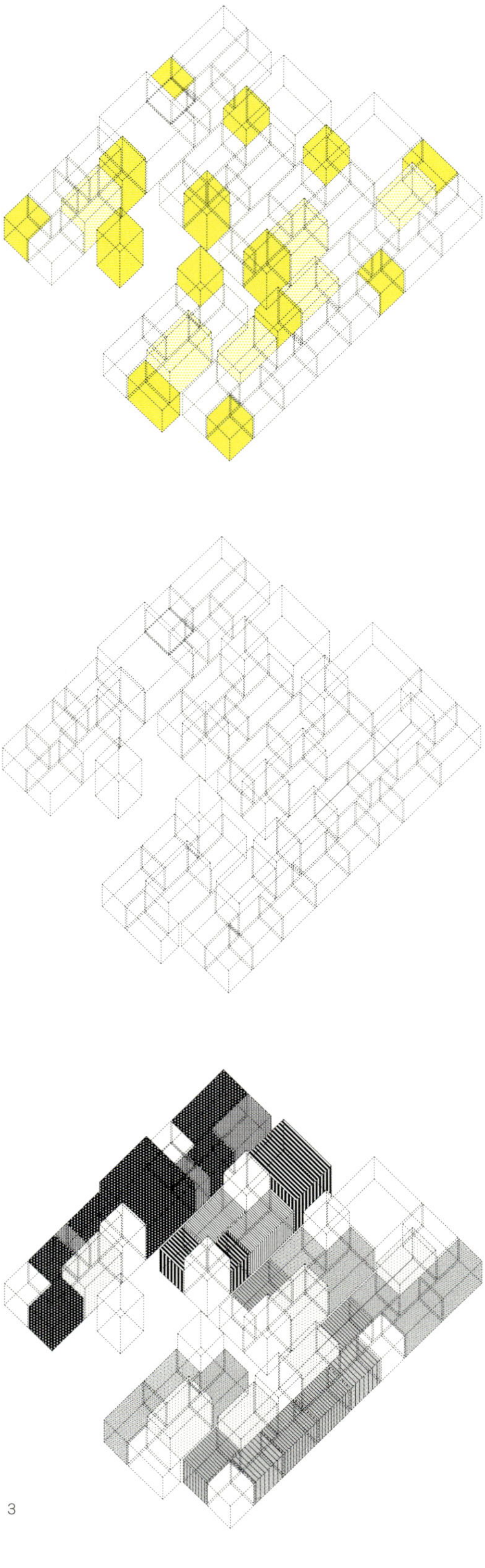

3

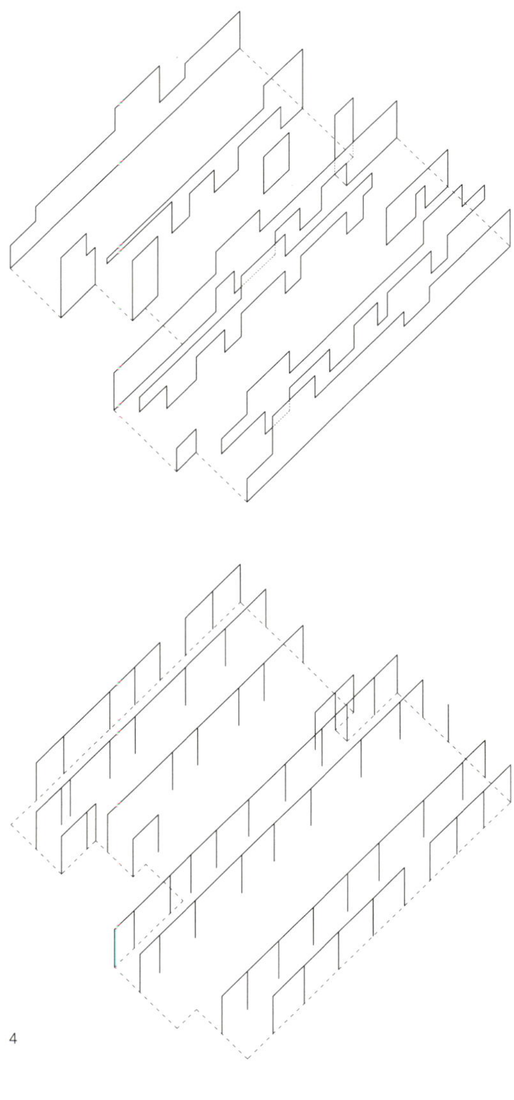

4

Difference and Repetition

Building the same building three times becomes a learning process in itself: what is the same but different, how different can the spatial translations of one plan be, what is the consequence of the material physicality of what is built, are some of the questions that arise. The question of the one and the many, across scales and components.

We may understand it as the opposite of dealing with the idea of absolute and uniqueness; rather, the relationship between generic and specific. The question of the one and the many describes the relationship of each one of the individuals ("the many"), where "3x1" is the one concept or oneness that describes them all. Therefore, at different scales, there is a certain "many" also understood as diversity and a "one" as unity.

Repetition is quite an effective way of creating content: from photocopying or replication to complete distinction, there is the fertile world of tension and dialogue between what is, in a certain sense, equal but also different. This dialogue is presented here in the form of sequences: sequences of drawings as ideas, as possibilities, as decisions, as instructions, as the place for thought. They are drawings made, as Enric Miralles might have said, "not to accumulate data but to multiply it, to allow for the appearance of what we had not thought about".

Here, the difference of repetition happens to be illustrated with three buildings but – as we said before – that is not important, there could have been two, or four…

Only the trained eye can read subtle differences in the envelope in the floor plans: structure that is the same as enclosure, versus wrapping, versus hiding structure in the layering. We can also see in more detail how the main spatial differences are due to the presence or absence of color (the effect of patios in space) and material qualities of the envelope (skin/enclosure).

The three clinics have the exact same floor plan. It serves as a demonstration that the spatial understanding of the third dimension is not something implicit in its orthographic representation, or that what we draw in plan is not the same as what we perceive. The secret of the floor plan as seed for space is actually my own "lesson of Rome". It is also a reversible thought: How is it possible that the same floor plan can have three very different spatial realities and vice-versa? (I like reversible ideas.)

Back to Max Bill: "... Once the basic theme has been chosen – whether it is simple or complex – an infinite number of very different developments can be evolved according to individual inclination or temperament."

The trilogy of clinics has something of a recursive function as well: the individuals can be understood as iterative loops in which the result of an iteration becomes part of the statement of the following. Based on a hypothesis A, the idea is to reach a result that contains A but becomes Z.

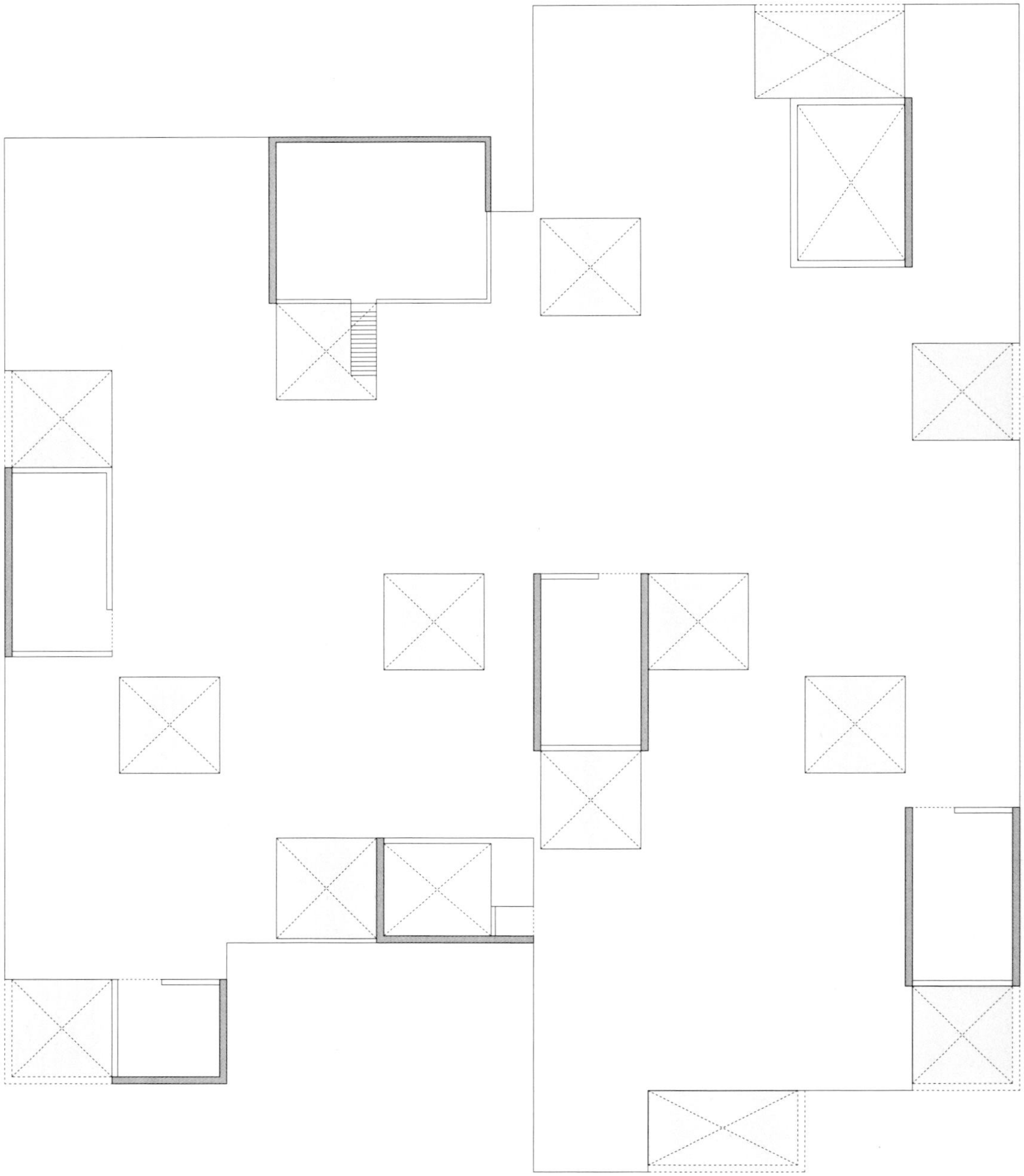

S; exposed, uncovered, laid bare, left unprotected.

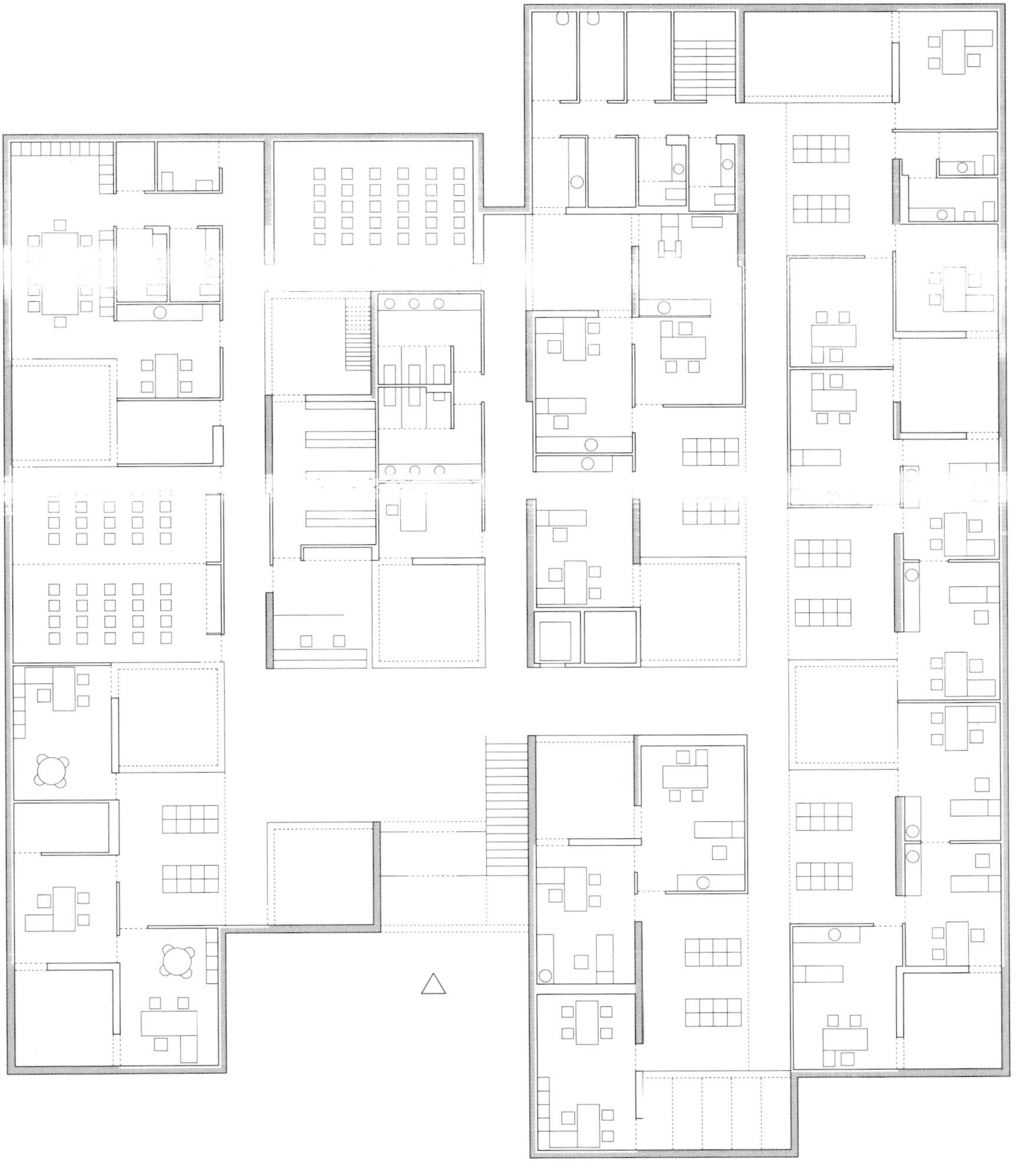

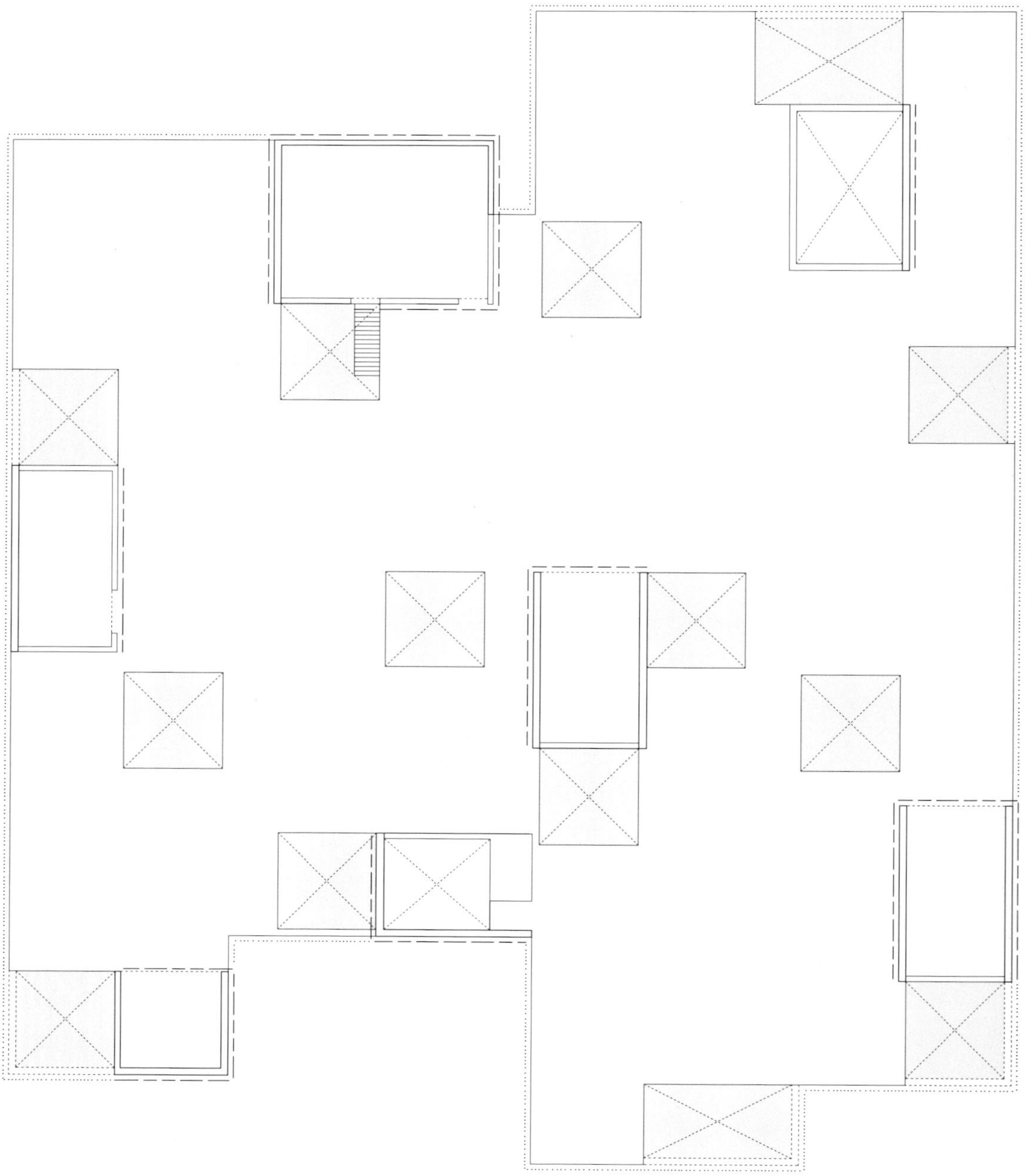

U; concealed, veiled (which qualifies or corrects).
Idea of arrangement or improvement of the same

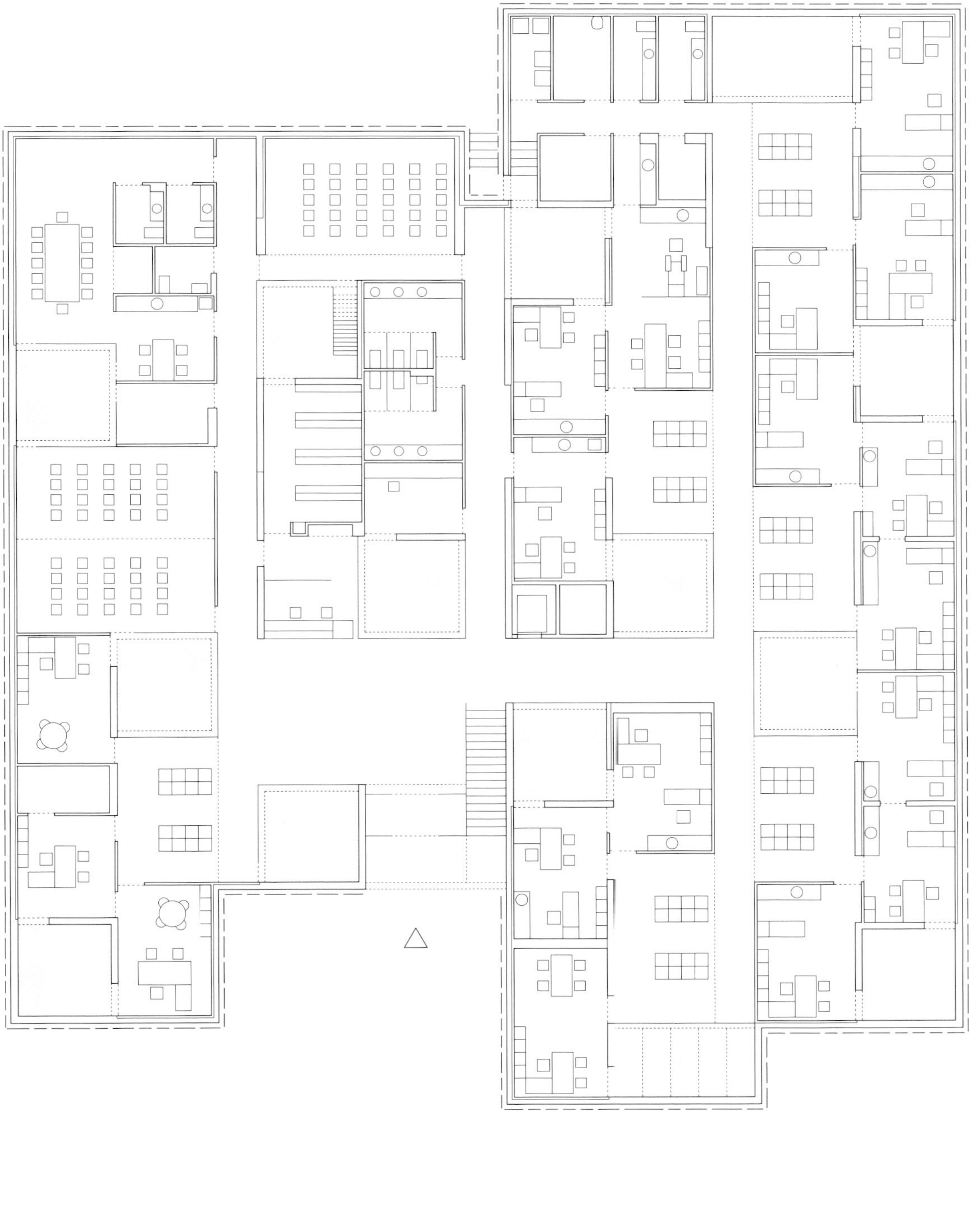

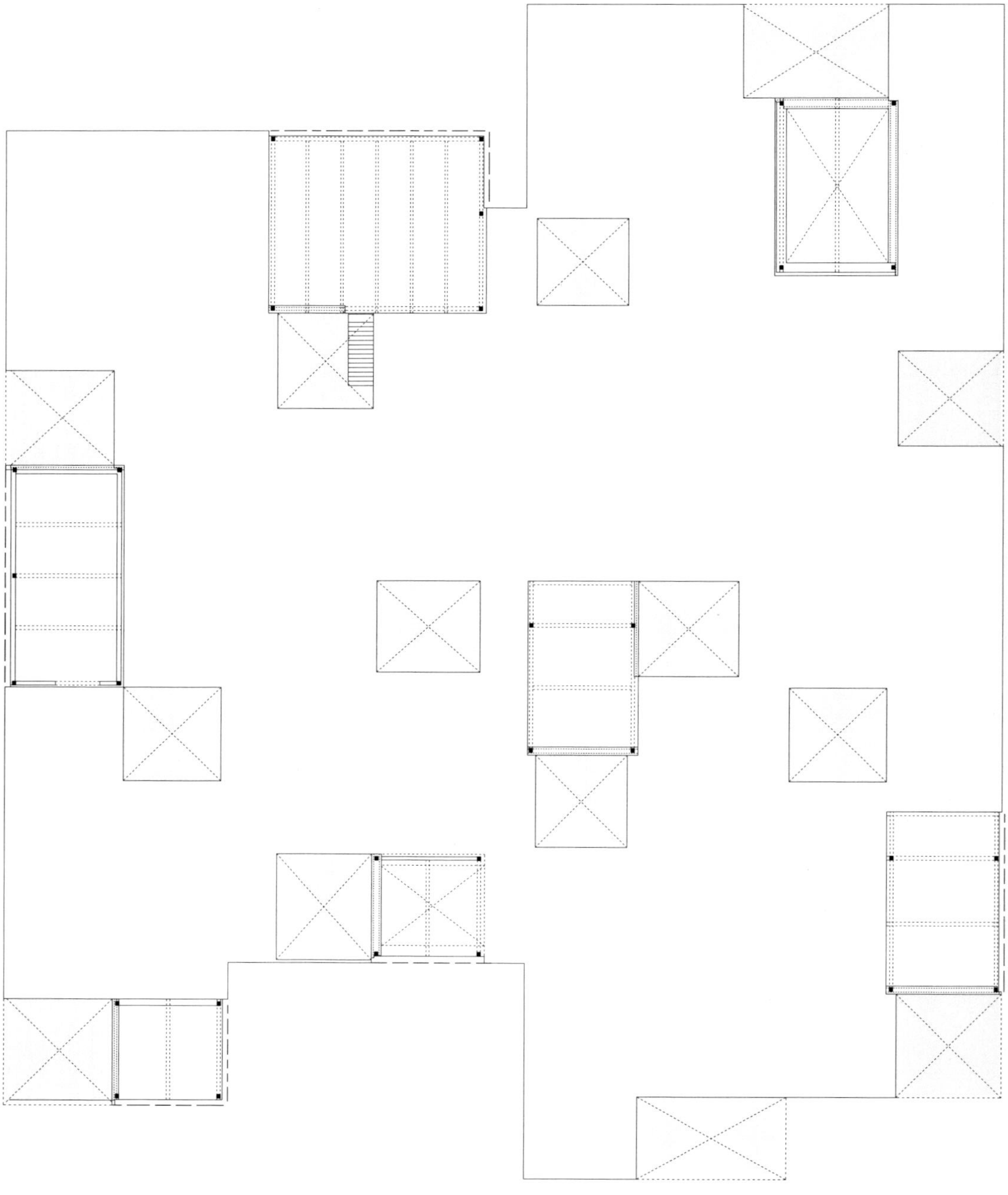

V; hidden, occult, not visible.

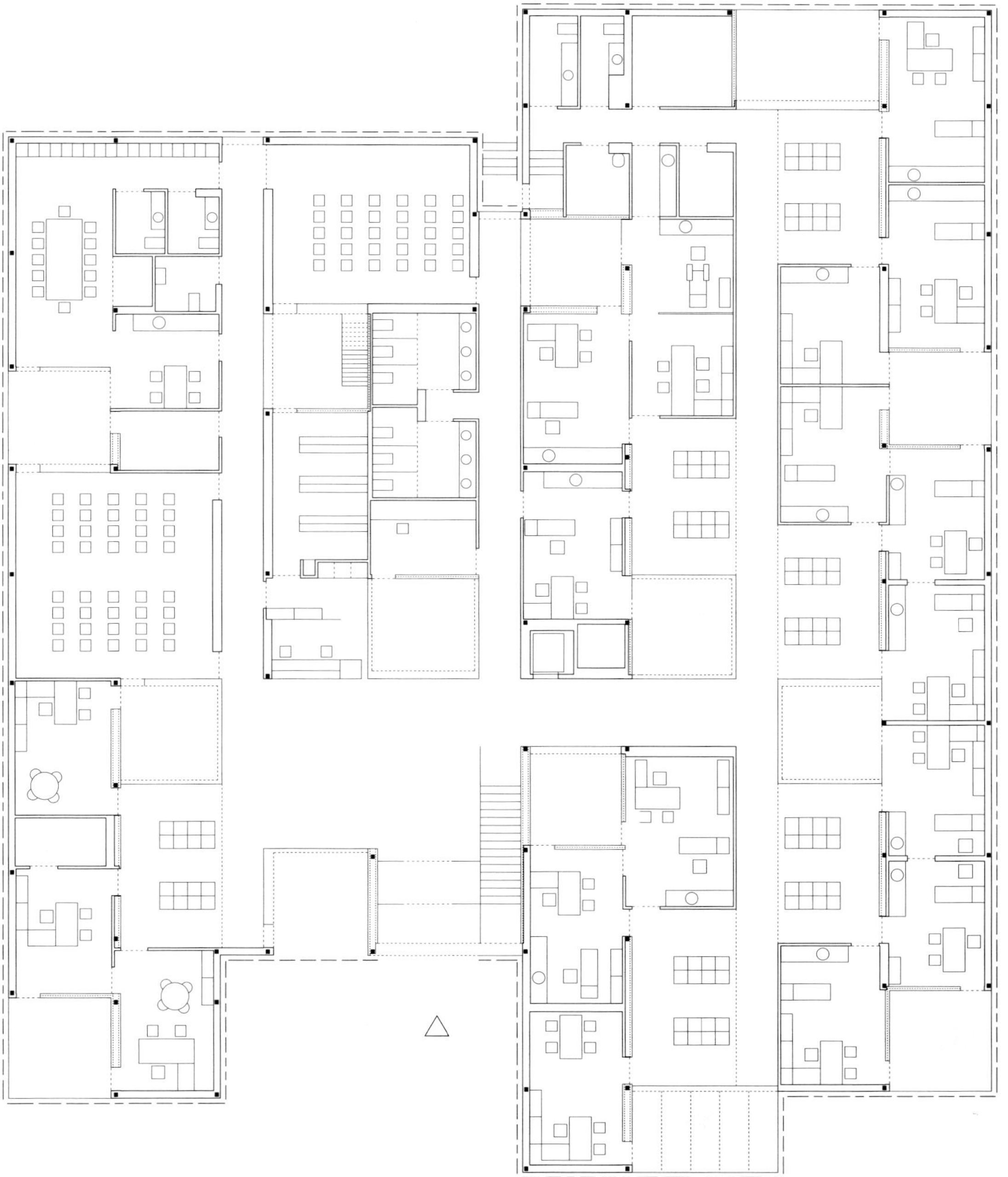

The dark blue in the S patios creates a vertical relationship and fixes their placement in space, as entities within a larger scenario. (X and y are fixed, z is the vector of spatial tension.) The here and there of these blue pockets tenses the public space as a collection of events or moments, in between which we move, from one to another and another. There are no identical patios among the fourteen of the clinic, a multiplicity as diversity rather than repetition.
Back to the idea of secret: all building logics may have one, one way or another. For S, the secret laws of disorder are due to material, dimensional and structural reasons and don't belong entirely to subjectivity. It is a kind of "controlled subjectivity" embedded in the process of making (the active procedures within formation, as Somol says). This decision making based on process is open to the surprise of the unforeseen.

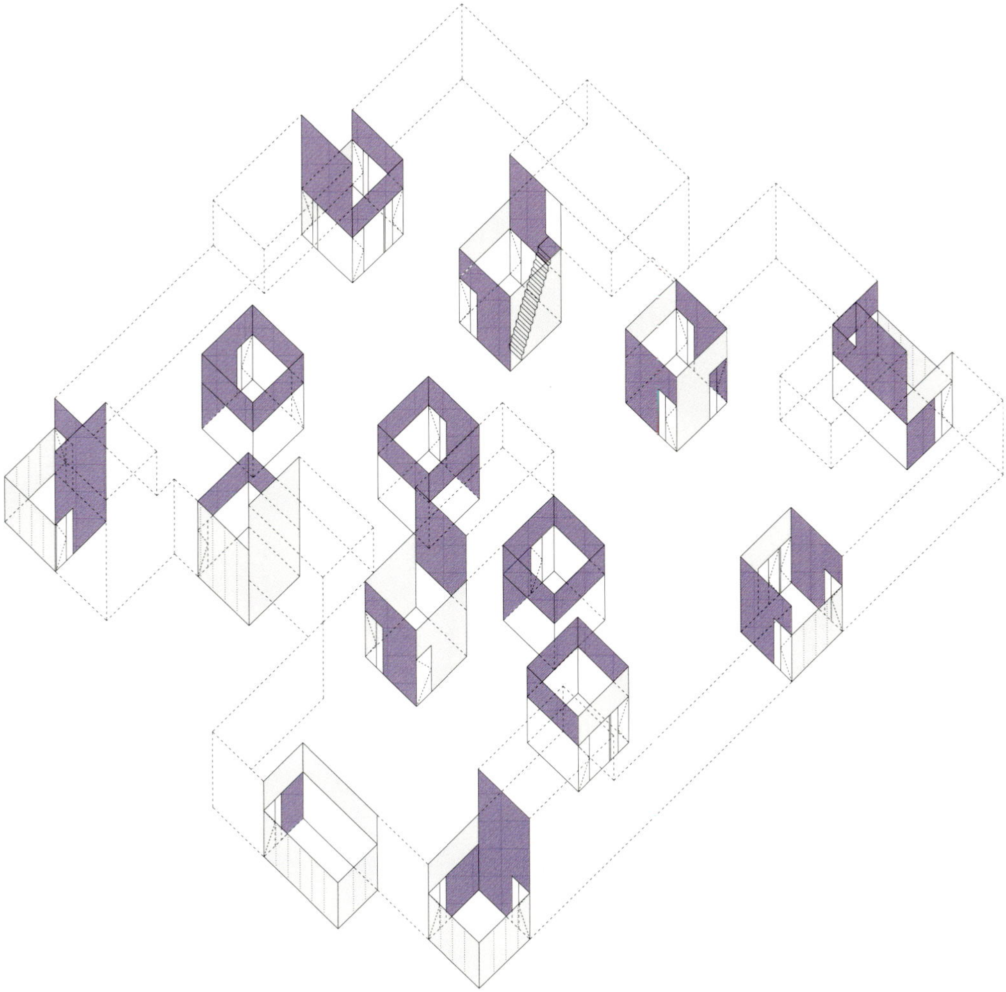

For the U case, it is possible to read the interior space as a more horizontal and abstract one in comparison to the previous case. The only material difference from the previous one is the white ceramic tiles instead of dark blue. The white tiled surfaces in the patios merge visually with the white inner walls of the waiting rooms and corridors, and the difference between inside and outside is not that clear anymore, blurring the boundaries and making the vertical condition less evident. There is a certain estrangement that comes along with this fuzziness: what you can't see clearly, or what is not understood or revealed.
The question of nesting (how things fit into each other) is important here, since the perception of patios as entities or components is enhanced or diminished according to the public space around them.

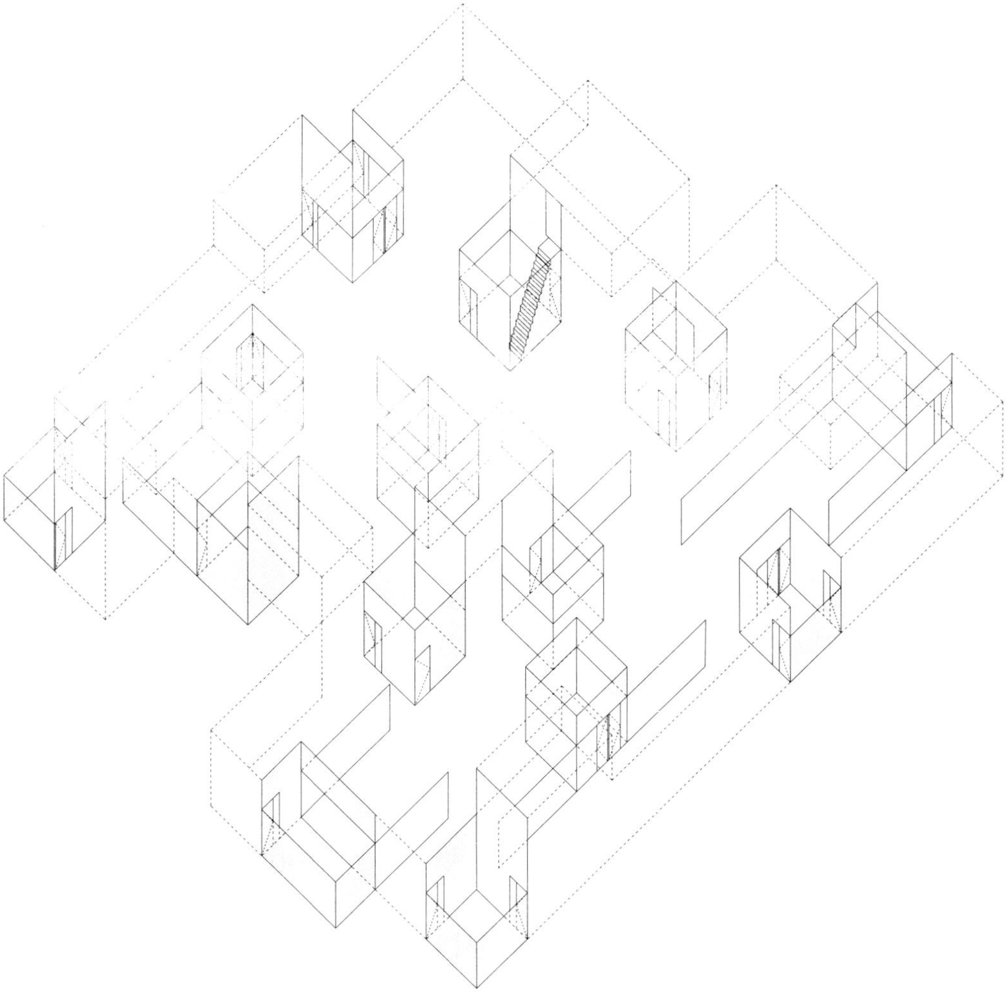

The third derivative of the same disposition, also a very different spatial condition. Replacing the opacity with translucent materials, the result is more atmospheric, and x, y and z are more balanced. Although imported from fractal mathematics, the idea that a space can be more or less three-dimensional is a concept close to architecture. If we consider that a point has no dimension ($D = 0$), a line or curve in the plane is $D = 1$ and a plane as surface is $D = 2$, we understand how the fractal dimension of some complex curves approaches 2, as they are more "superficial" than a simple curve but do not cover the plane completely; we can build an element of dimension 2 (plane) with one element of dimension 1 (line). Following on that, we could say that, despite its undeniable volumetric condition, space can be more or less three-dimensional according to its characteristics.

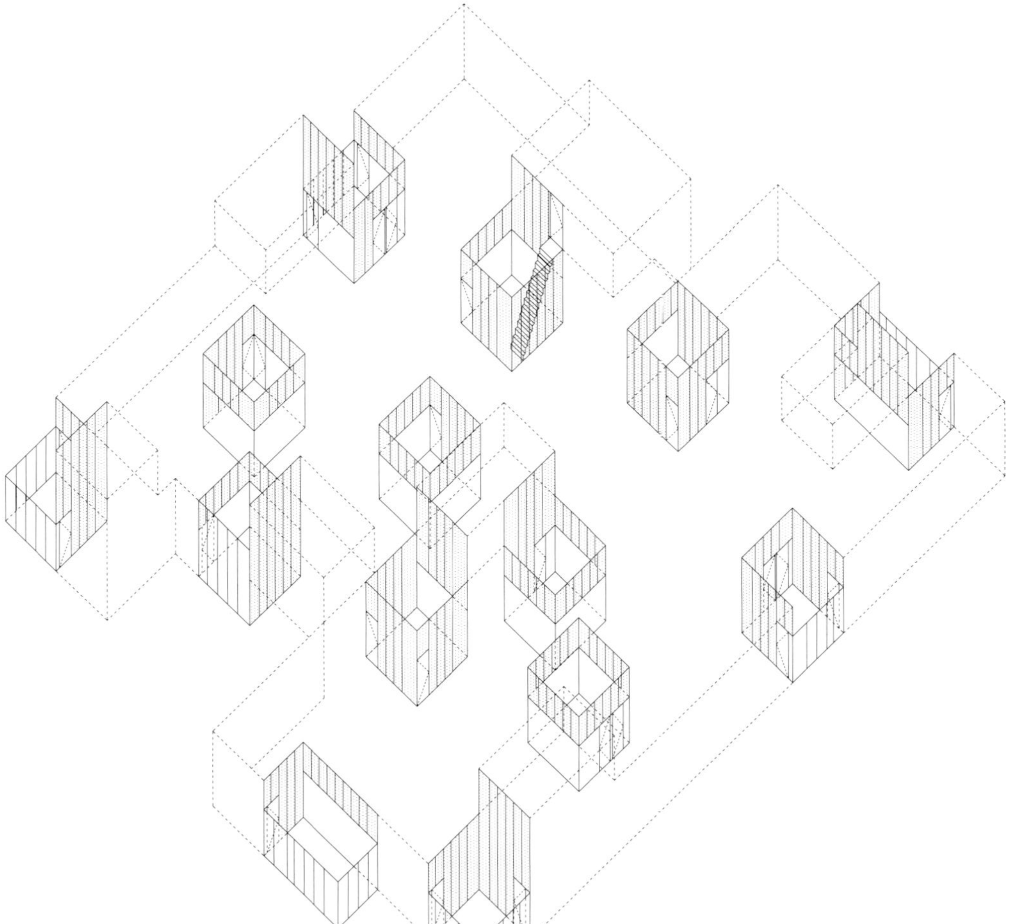

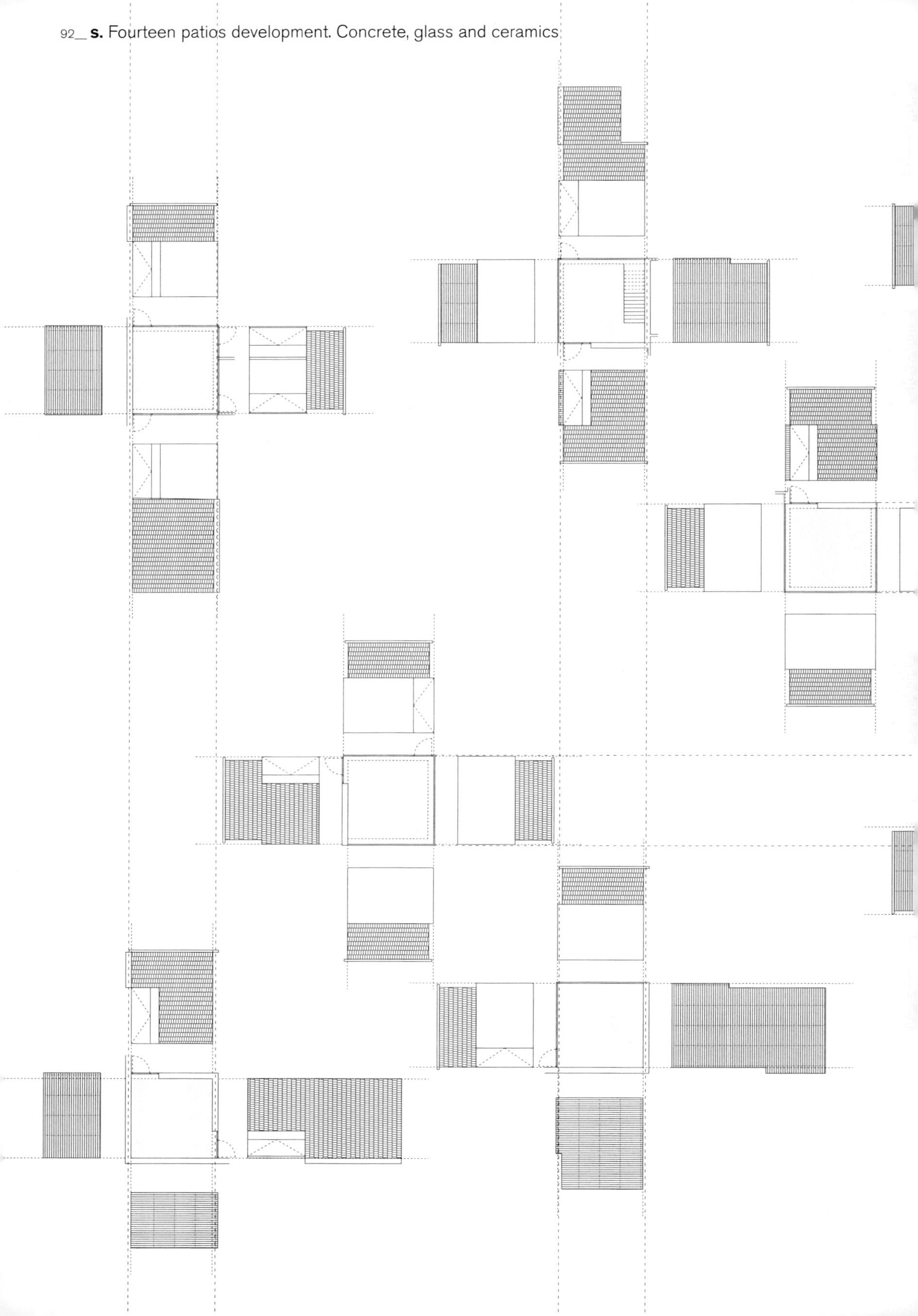

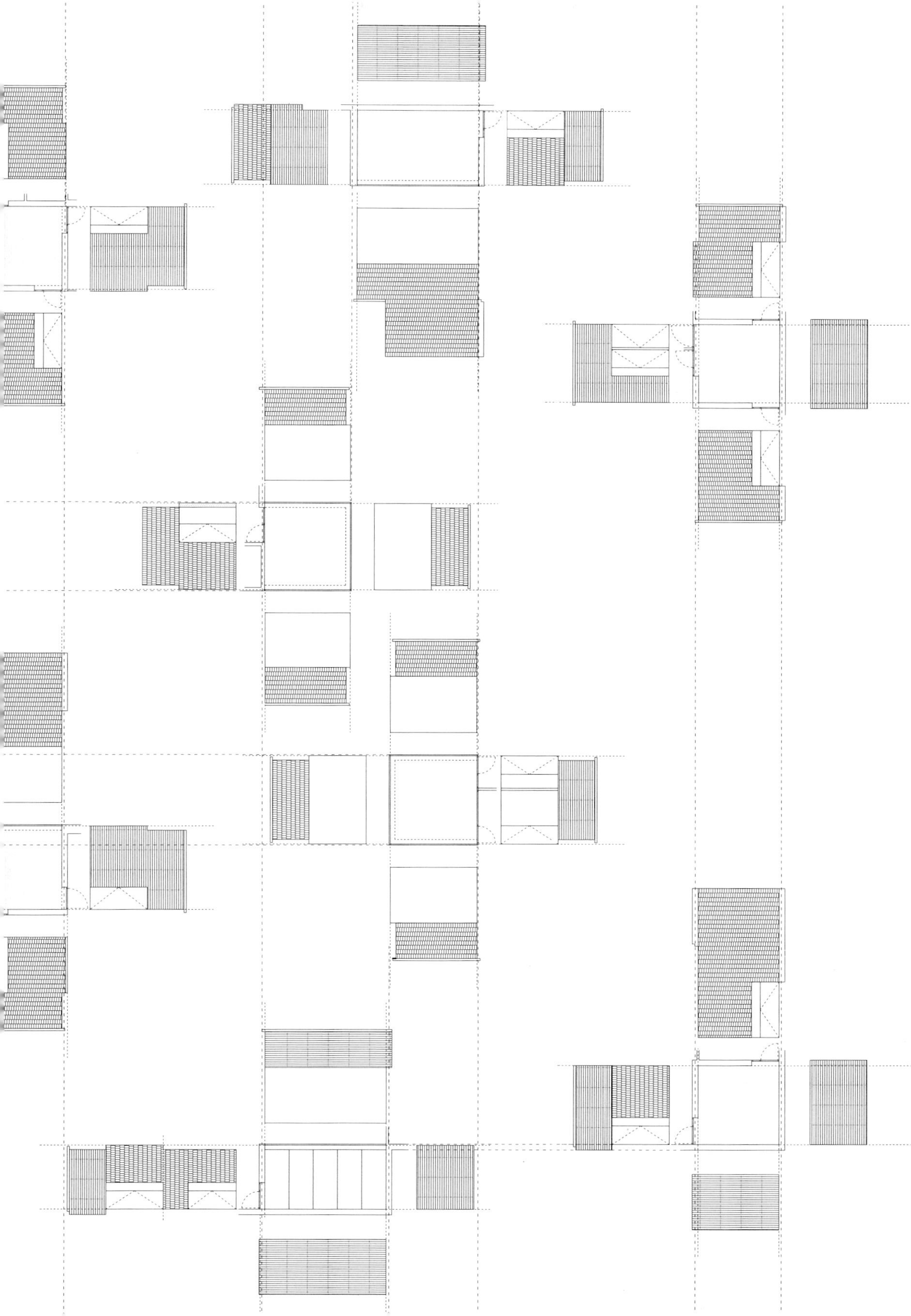

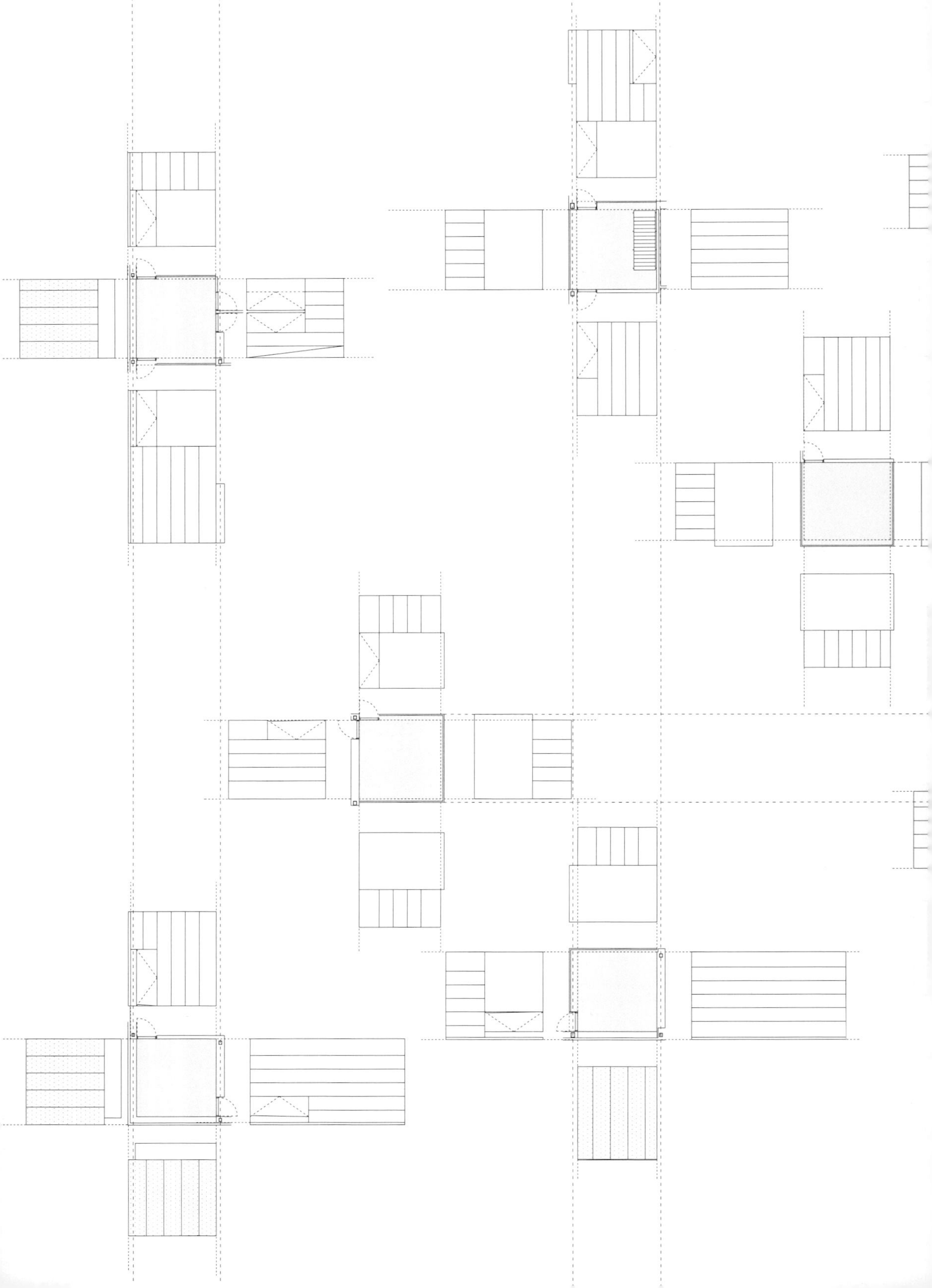

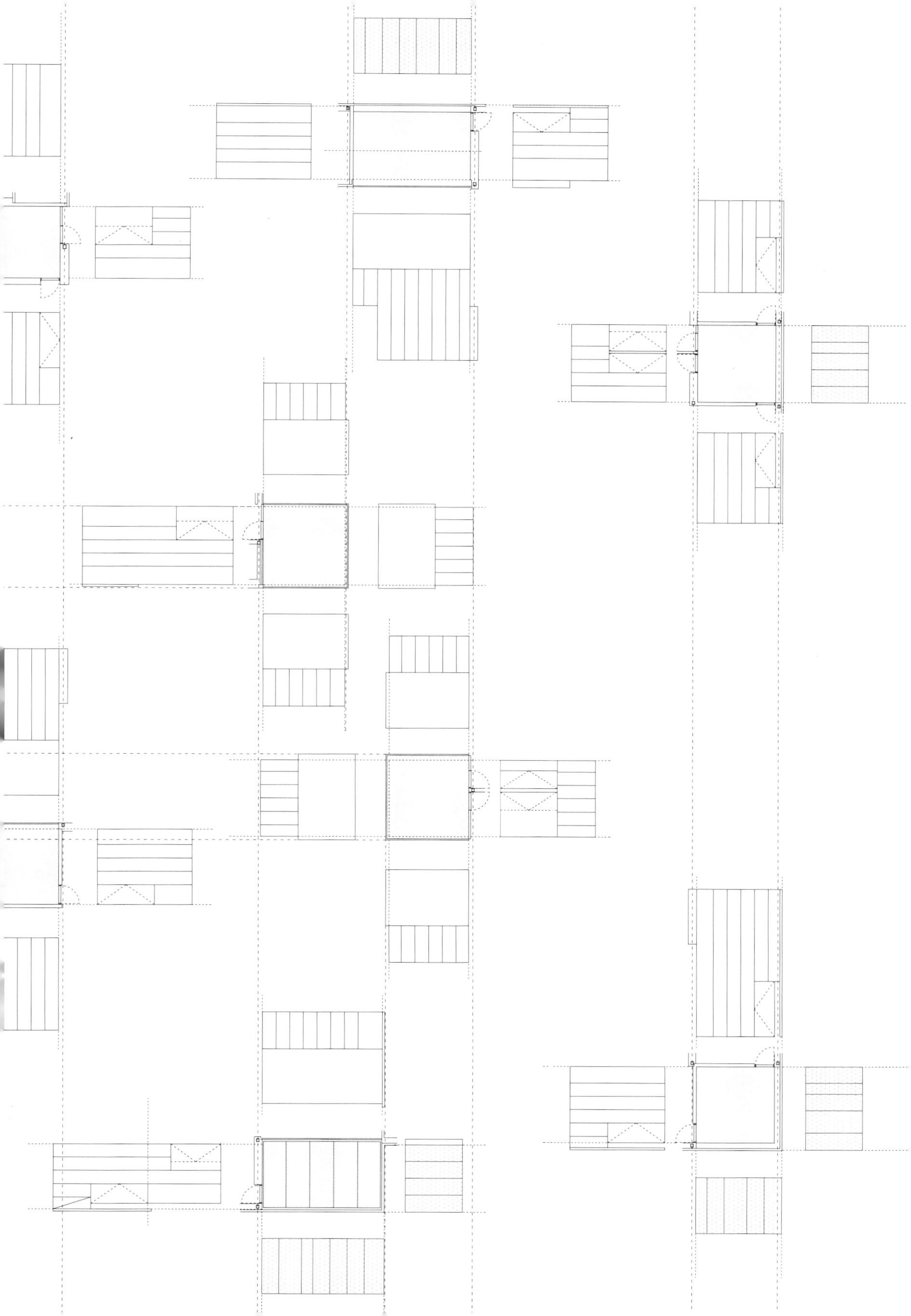

The Scarless Merger

However many different components or parts a project may have, we tend to erase their independency in favor of the whole. It is like the hand to arm continuity, where there is no clear division between one and the other. Like a typical condition in human skin, when we build the idea is to cut and join things in parts so they look complete once the parts are put together.

Turning back to the question of "the one and the many", we see that while considering the individuals versus the collective, it also speaks of the fact that an individual (such as man) is made of many organs but is still one man. To use more specifically architectural terminology, we work with ideas on the part-to-whole relationship, trying to investigate what the glue is that keeps different components together in a coherent whole.

unfolding (pag. 98_99)

That is probably why we often work with unfolding drawings or developments, which bring in the idea of a continuous wrapping or skin.
This is the script, or maybe we should say the story board, for *clinical*; there are five variations but only three buildings, although they are all possible ends:

1. Generic abstract continuous windowless mass
2. S. Concrete formwork using wood planks
3. Spiral pattern
4. U. Golden metal skin
5. V. White glass

It expresses the paradox of an architecture with no clear front or back. All four sides of the box are similar and the skin pattern goes all the way through in continuity. There are three different scale readings superimposed one onto another; the outer shape (figure), the part scale (panel), and the piece scale or texture (wood plank, mesh opening). There is also a pervasive sense of surface: neat and tense planes that read as something overlaid (layering as the opposite of weaving).
As a result of the whole skin process, we like to talk about identity: that of the individuals, but also how that multiplicity can be understood as a cohesive identity too.

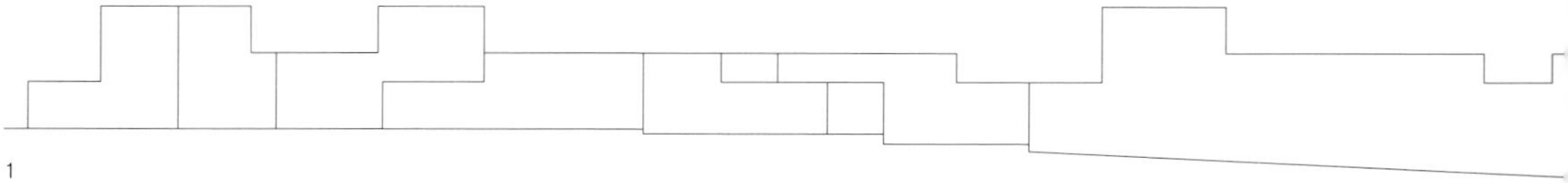

1

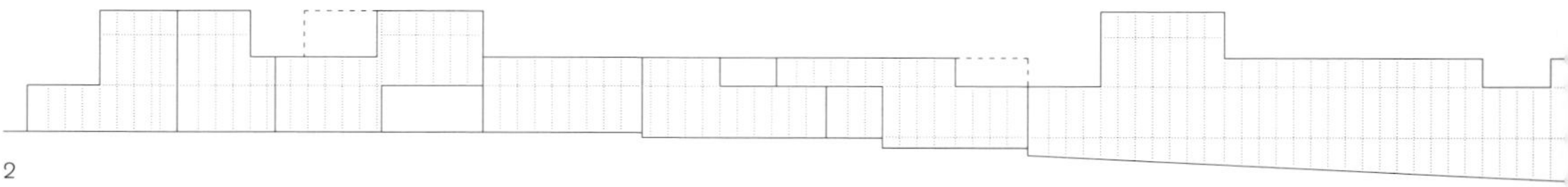

2

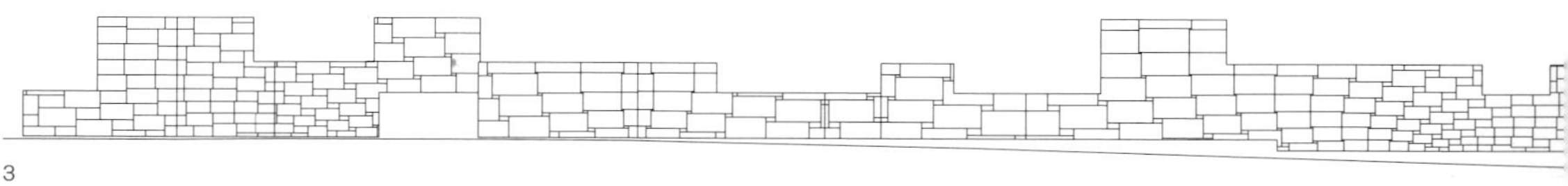

3

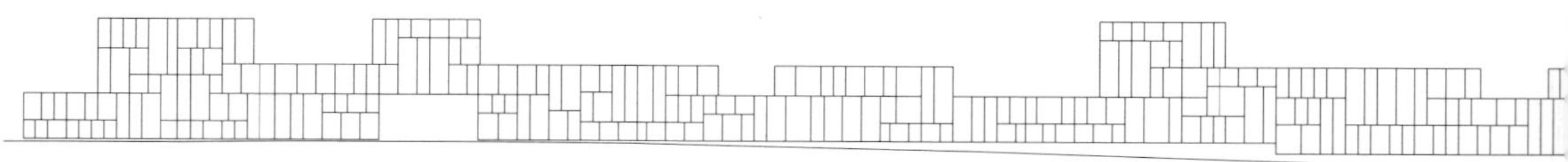

4

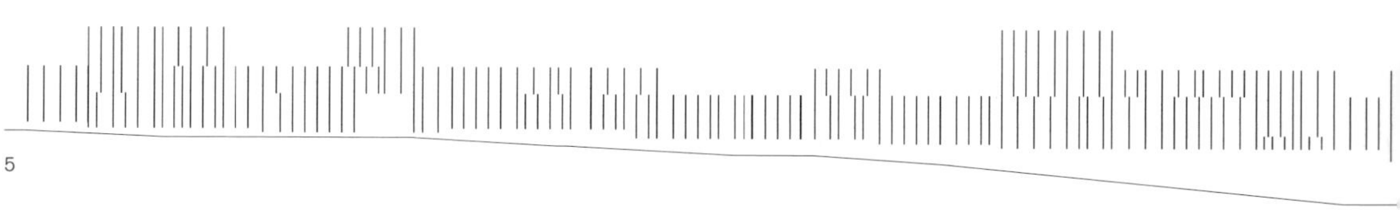

5

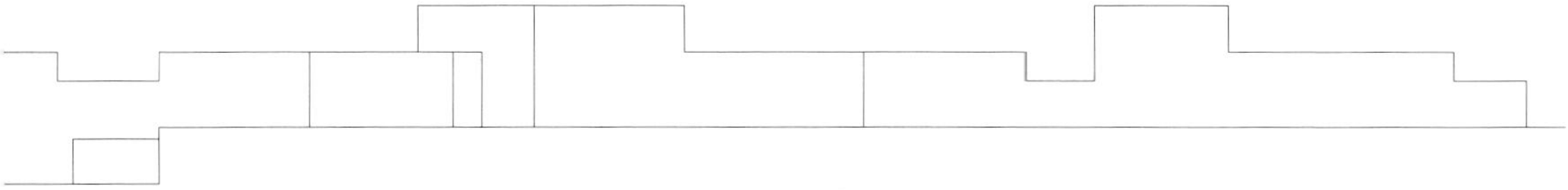

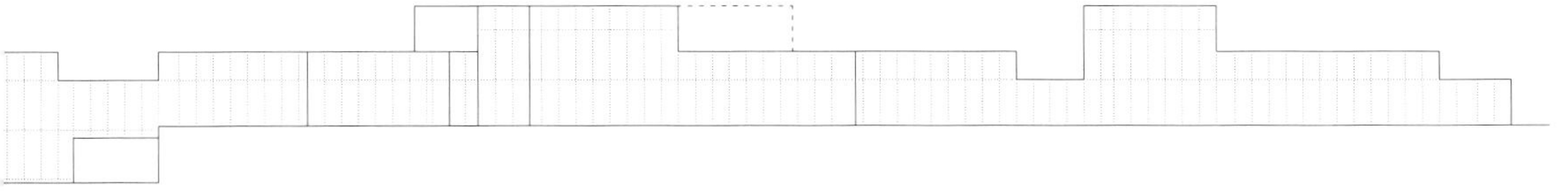

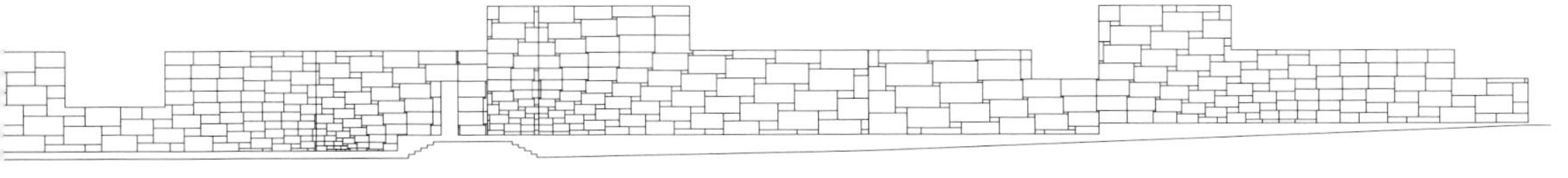

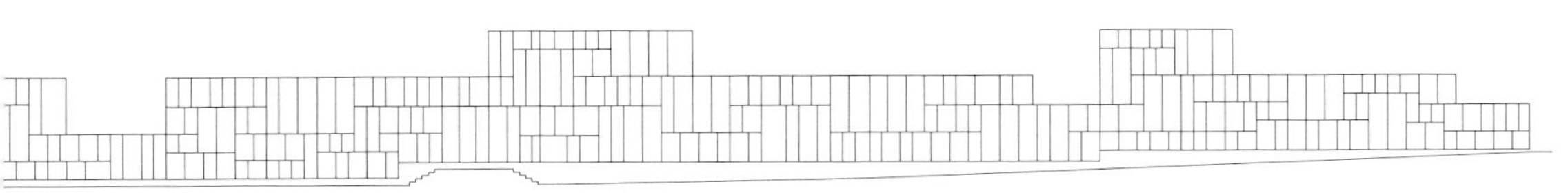

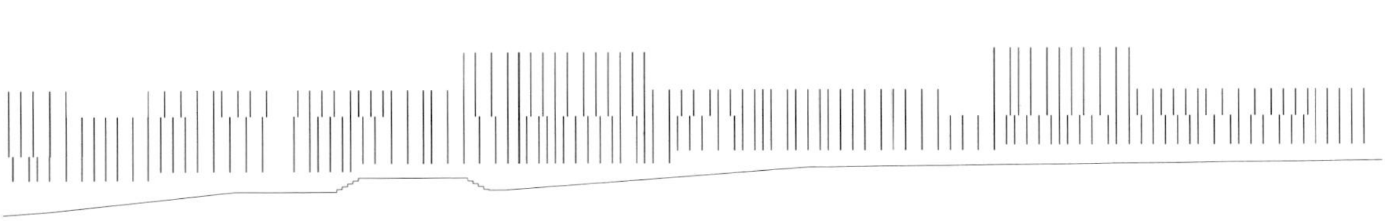

In terms of the volumetric condition, what matters is not so much the architecture of the fragment as the relationship between fragments. And this is the graphic quote referencing the lesson learned from Alvaro Siza: blurring the formal independence of the parts. In the Carlos Ramos Pavilion (Porto Architecture School), we see how the strategy works: depicting a more or less abstract object, assembled out of geometrical forms, with few recognizable building elements such as doors and windows and roofs and treating all surfaces with the same finishing. The perception at human height, unaware of the overall operation, dissolves the articulations and the unity of the image prevails over the diversity of ingredients.
We have already talked about Le Corbusier's Sun and Medusa drawing. Following on that, another more extreme and recent example of that scarless merger is UNStudio's "Manimal" icon (a hybrid of human, lion and snake). It is a fusion of the parts, where it is no longer possible to distinguish what belongs to whom; on the one hand it is a new creature; on the other hand maintains familiar features from its predecessors.
Translated to architecture, this seamless collection of elements brings some vagueness to the real, which questions tradition in a non-confrontational way. There is always something familiar to the built volume, and yet it is novel.

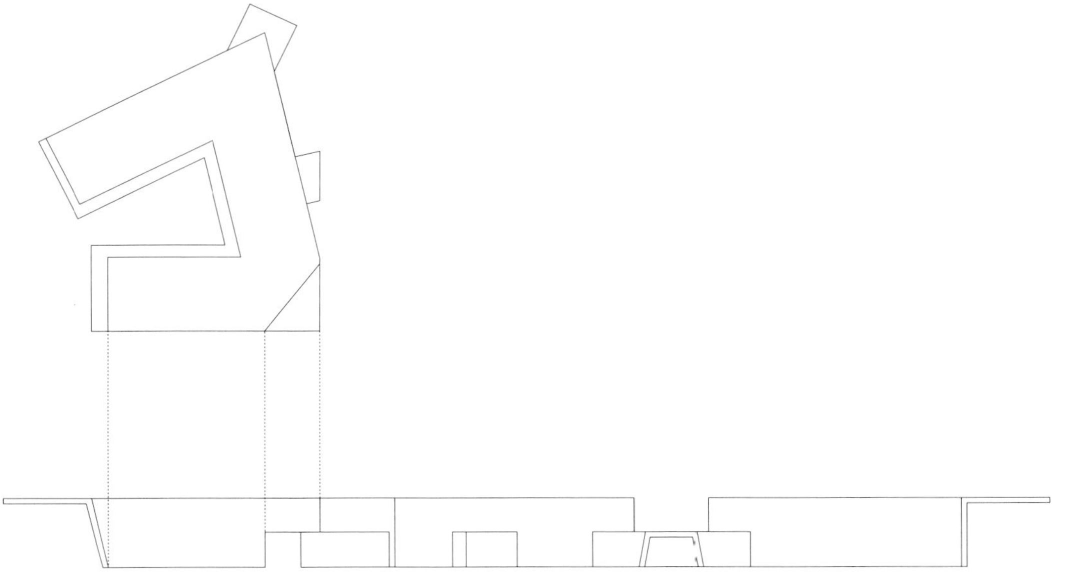

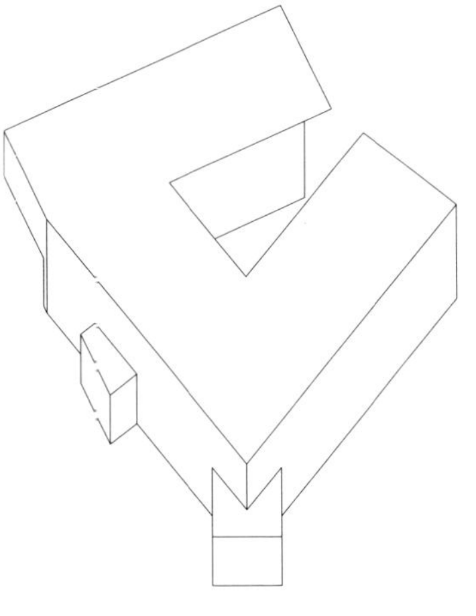

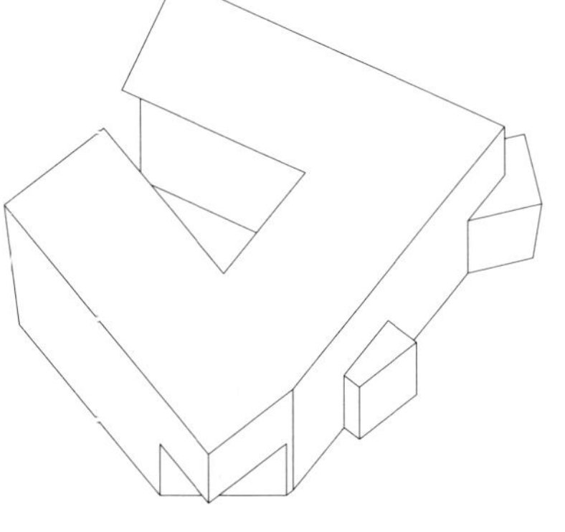

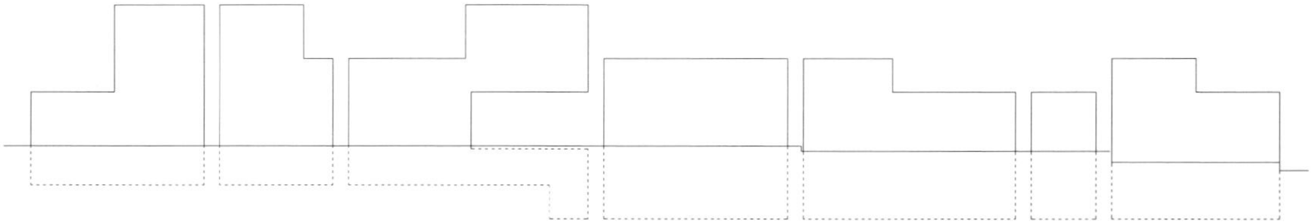

S

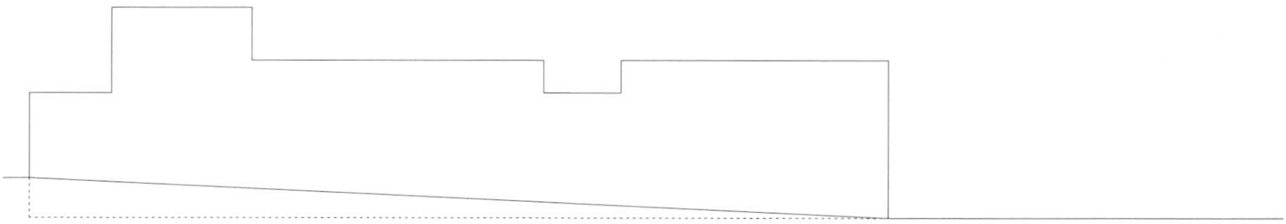

E

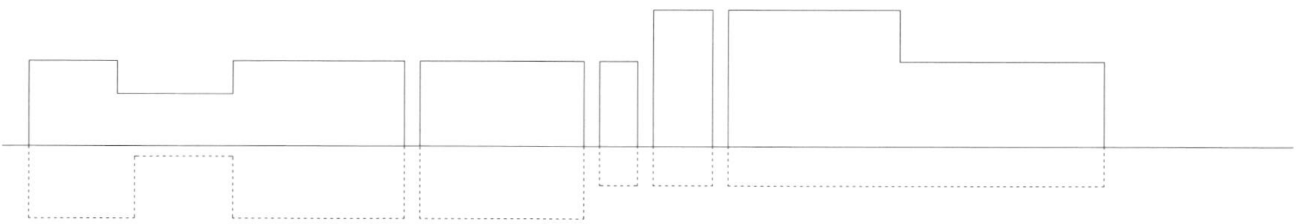

N

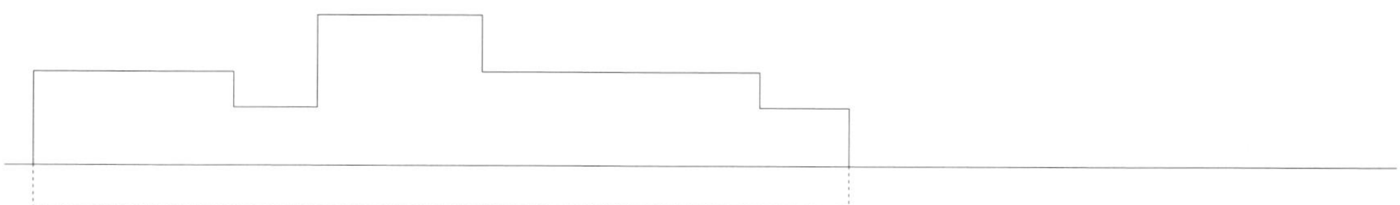

W

In the journey between the generic abstract continuous windowless mass to the specificness of the trilogy S, U, V (concrete physical presence), we find many questions; some are related to the idea of abstraction and how it is manifested (preserved) at different levels (intermediate scales) once we start incorporating contingency into the building process.

Aristotelian thinking tells us why science, by definition, is abstract, because it aspires to the generality of a law, a relationship or a concept, and not the uniqueness of an existence. But architecture, in its particular way of thinking, is constantly moving between the general and the singular. Enric Miralles expressed that distance between the project and concrete architecture concisely: “what should not disappear and what appears”.

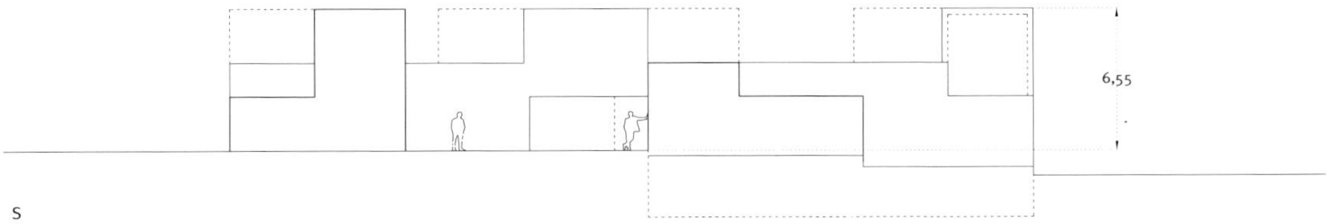

S

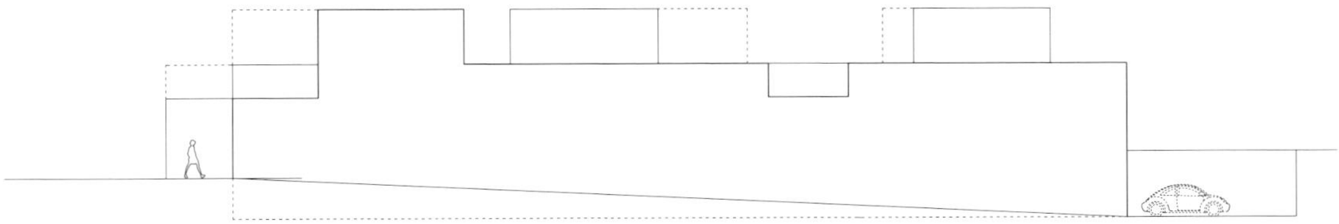

E

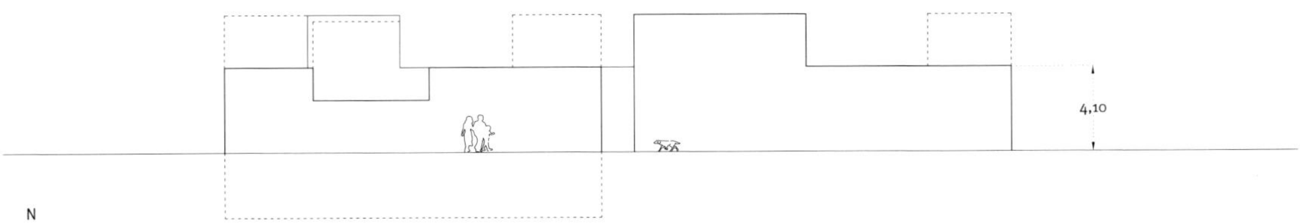

N

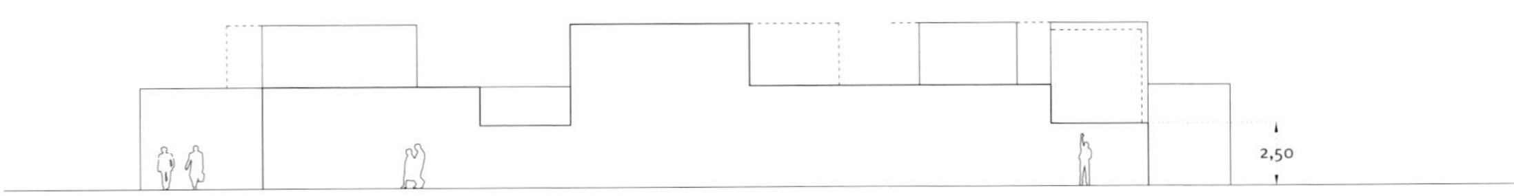

W

As simple as they look, these are the elevation drawings of the walls to be built. At its maximum degree of abstraction here, the question at stake is the relationship between shapes and volumes: the "L" shape, the trimming in and out on the base line of the roof plane, the sliding volumes with no intersection, etc.

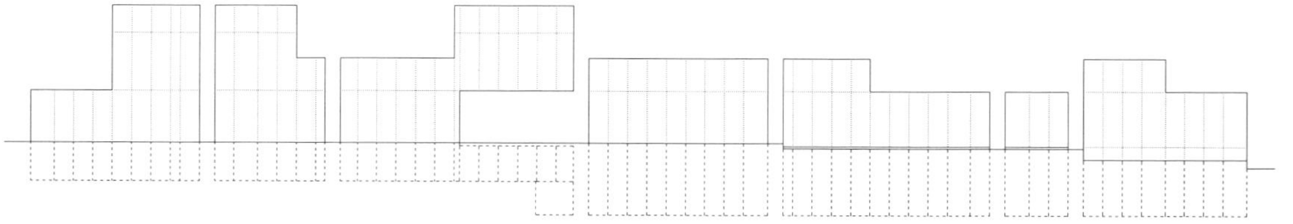

S

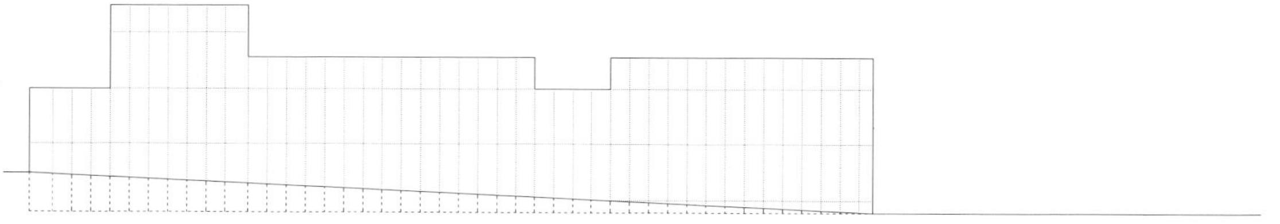

E

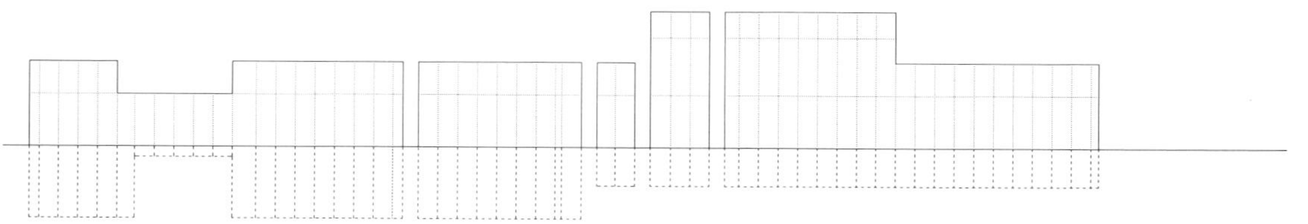

N

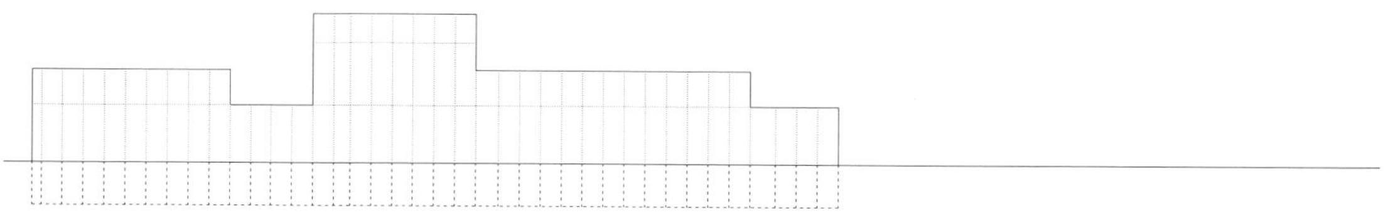

W

The abstract continuous windowless mass is conceived for S as a solid and heavy façade. The skin is enclosure and structure at the same time.
Walls are made of reinforced cast-in-place concrete. The construction system is based on the use of standard forms as coffer and uses only one panel size to module the whole building. Some adjustments and negotiation were necessary in order to merge two foreign logics: that of the project's initial silhouettes and that of the modulation which, applied as an afterthought, did not match the overall dimensions.

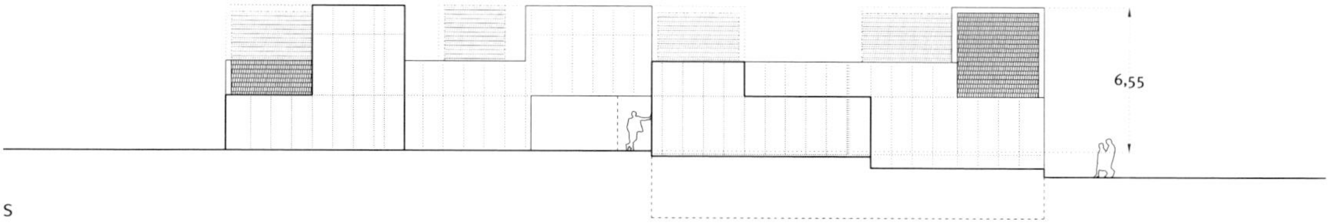

S

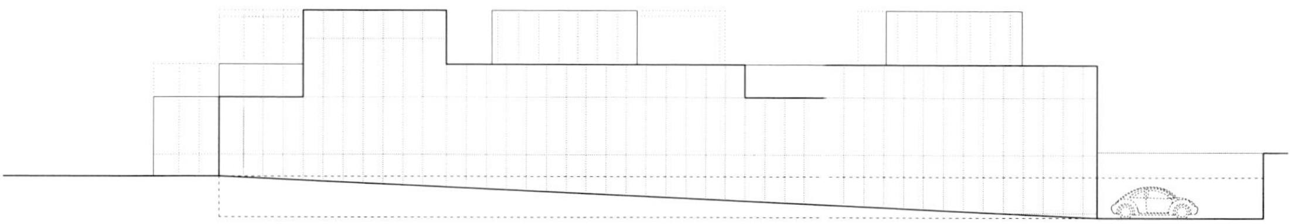

E

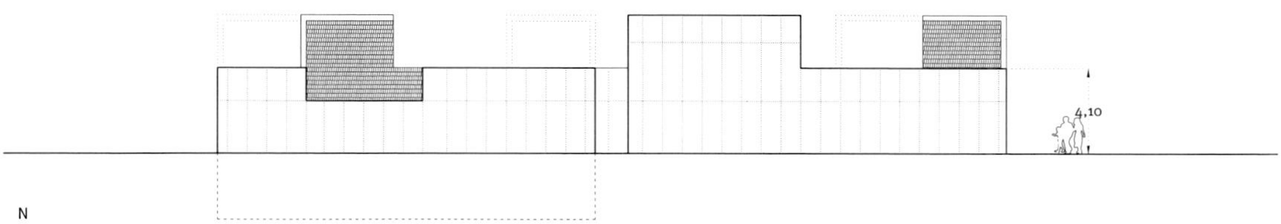

N

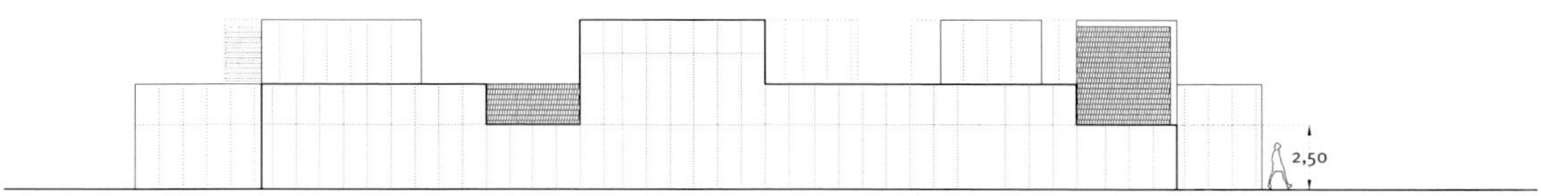

W

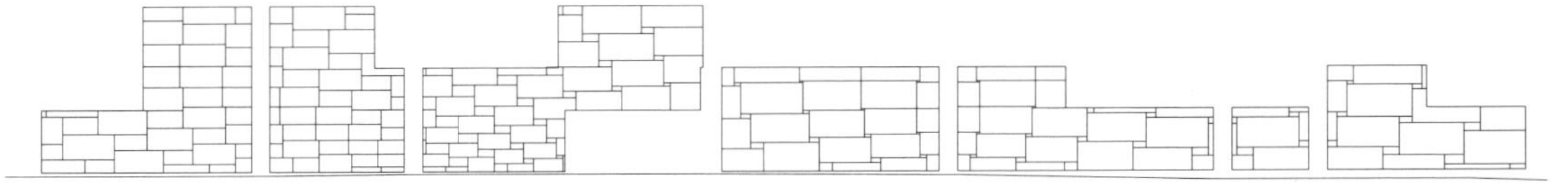

W

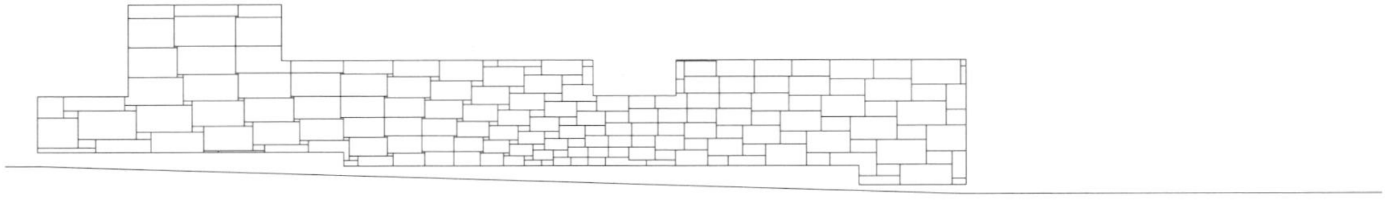

S

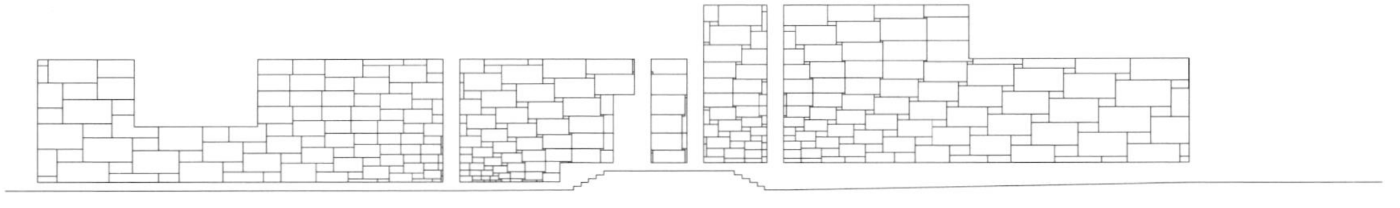

E

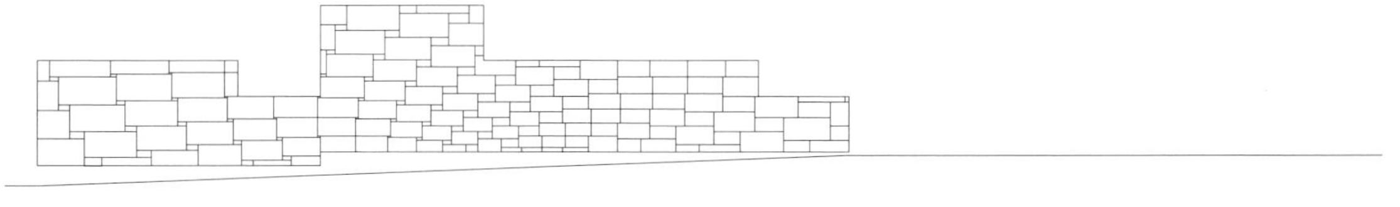

The windowless mass intended for U is a thin and golden layer to hide what could not be shown, but with a little extravagance. We thought about cutting out the figures from a given pattern as if we were using stencils, fostering the idea of virtual expansion without framing.

The mathematician Marcus du Sautoy explains in his book on symmetry how rotational symmetries with motifs on spiral shapes (such as the Alhambra mosaics), which generate a direction, create the impression that the scheme continues to repeat itself beyond the wall, producing the effect of a moving image, suggesting the infinite expansion of space.

This first pattern iteration for the golden mesh was not built: even though the pieces are all rectangular, the physical execution and placement seemed too complex and we couldn't afford delays in construction at that point. We did however save the pattern in our minds for the future as we begin to better understand its behavior and richness.

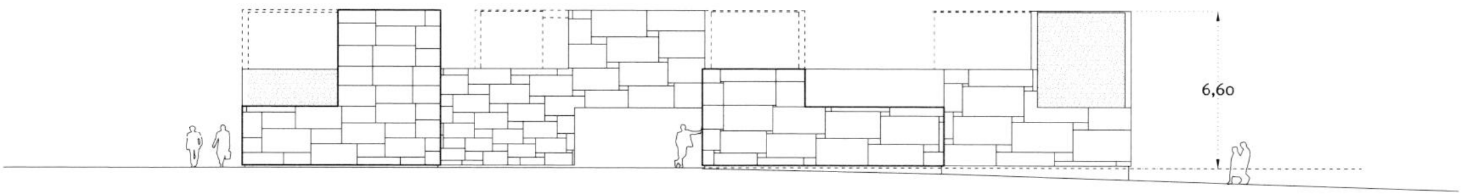

W

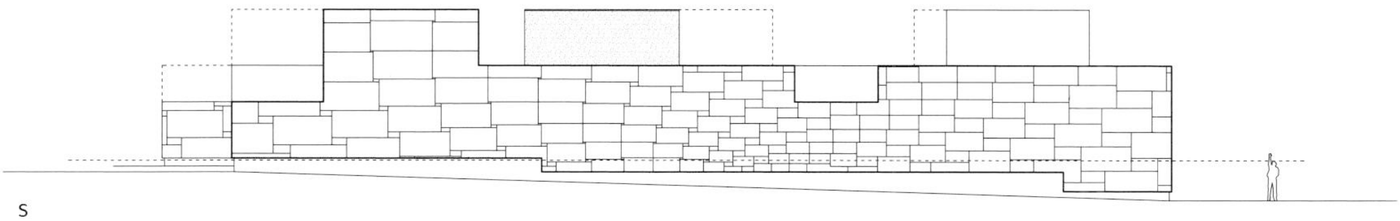

S

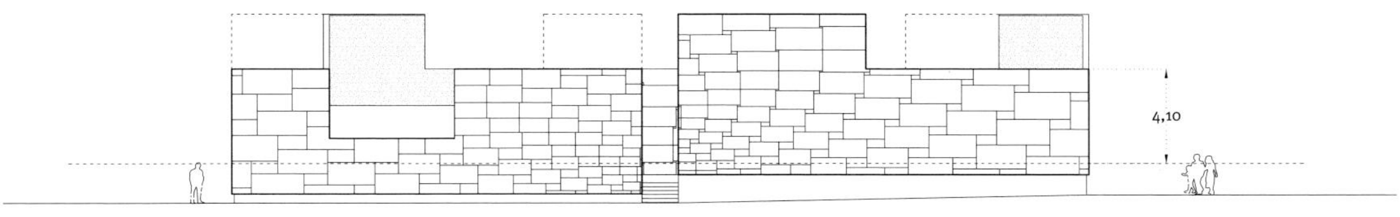

E

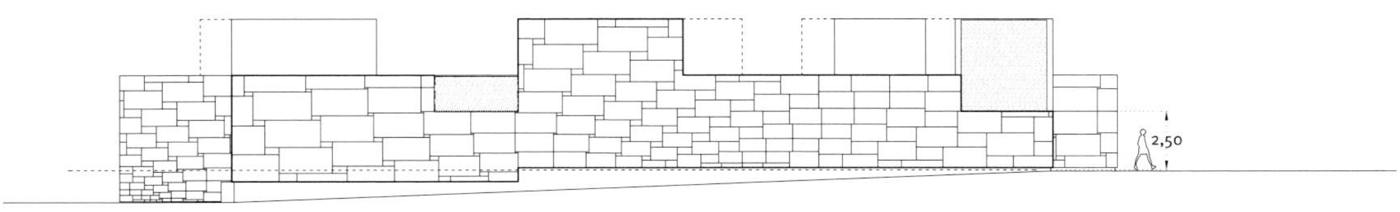

N

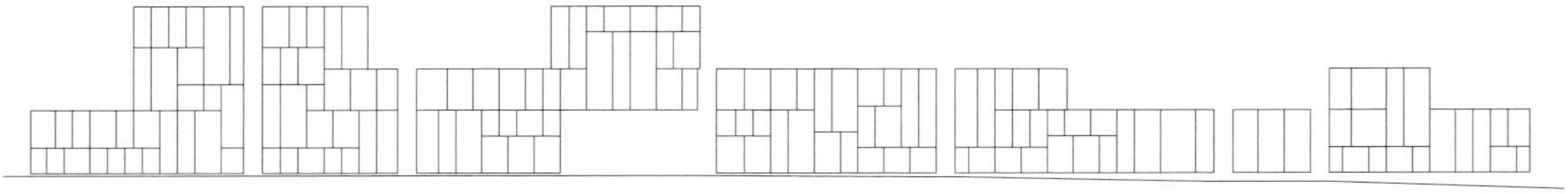

W

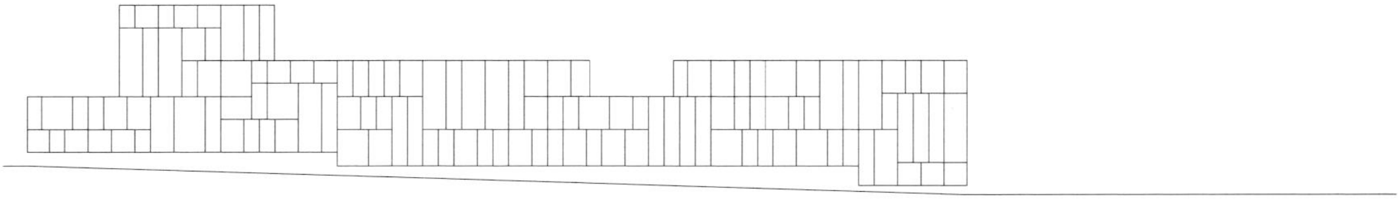

S

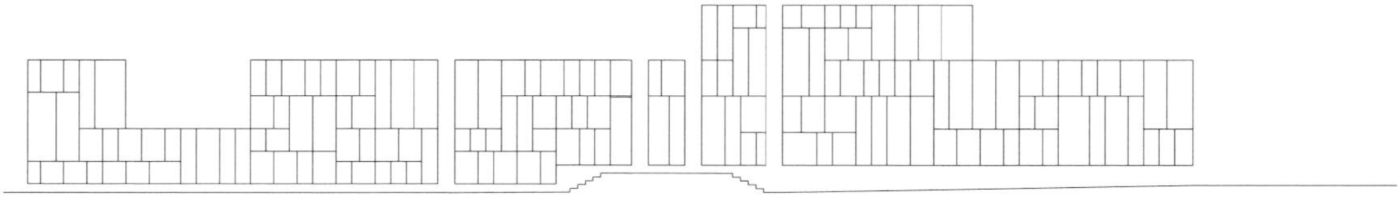

E

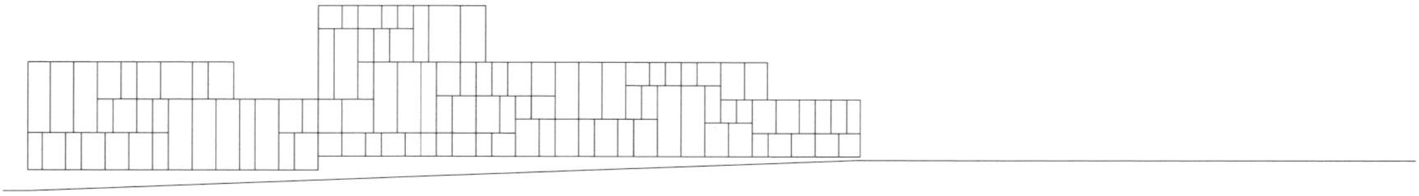

N

The final gold box of U uses the mathematical rule of the greatest common divisor. There are three sets of related dimensions of panels that allow for laying different free sequences one on top of another which only align vertically at certain moments, whenever they sum the same.
To maintain the idea of the impenetrability of the façade, we arranged different panel sizes while avoiding building a grid. The layout combines different heights and widths in a way that makes it hard to see how many floors or levels there are in the built mass, pursuing a balance between horizontal and vertical.

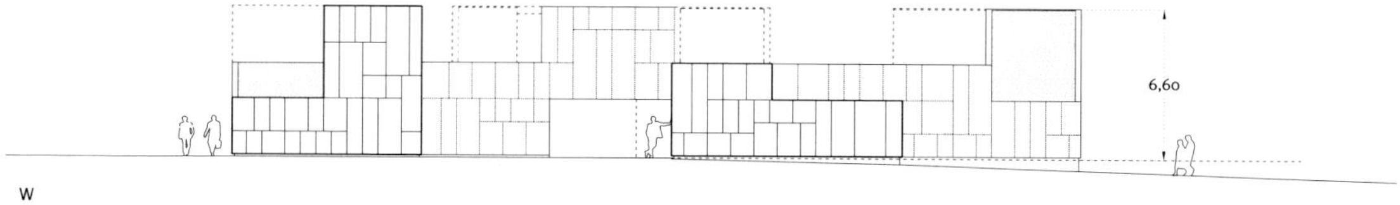

W

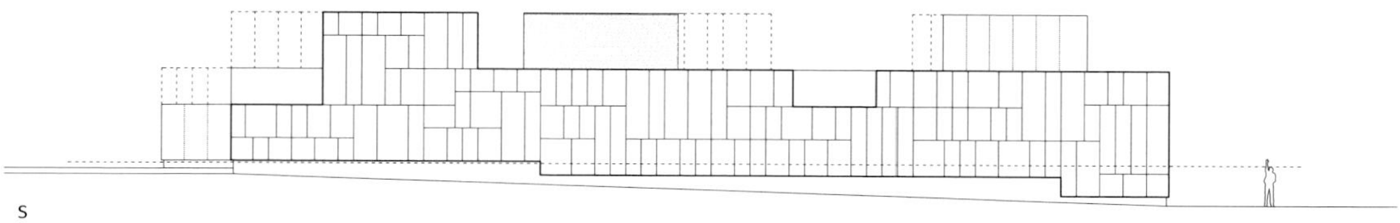

S

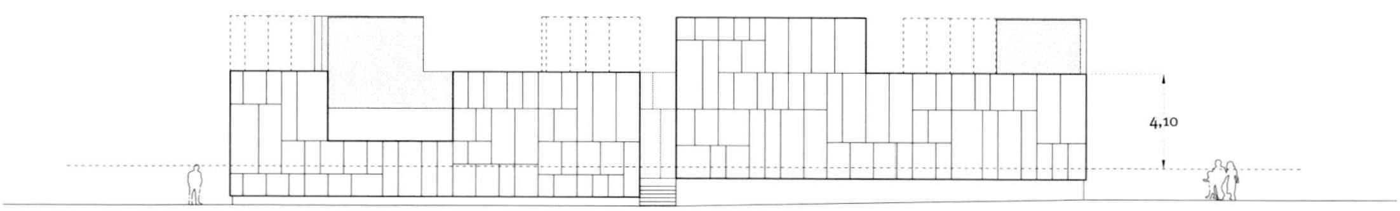

E

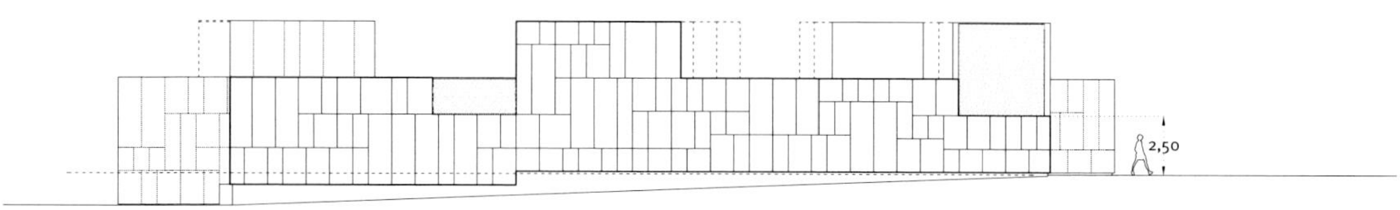

N

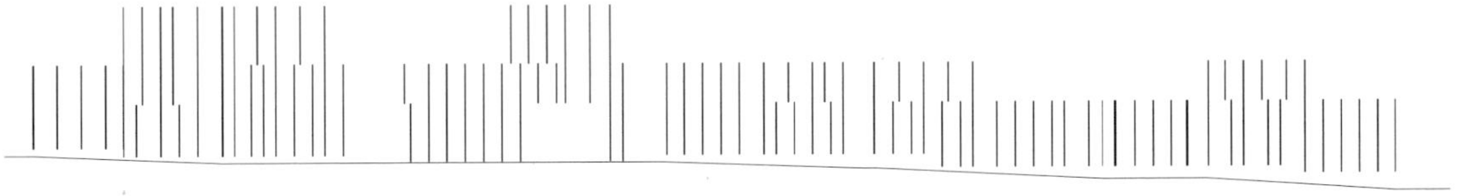

S

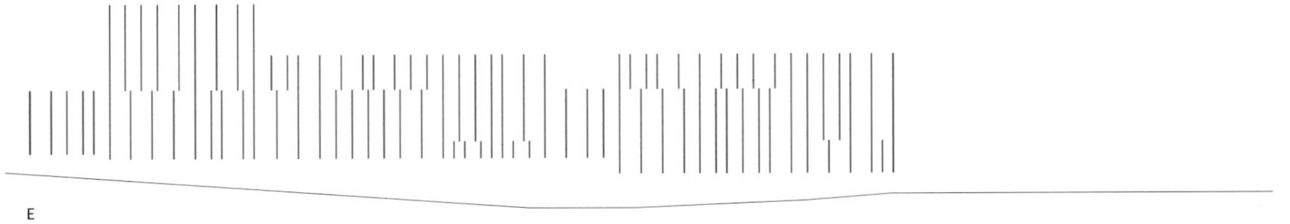

E

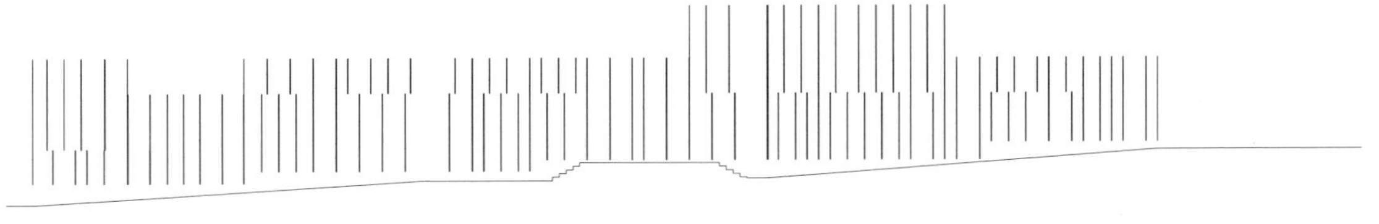

N

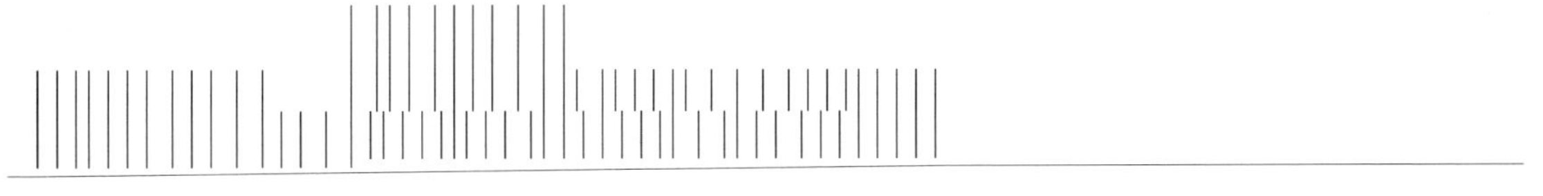

W

The V windowless mass is made out of glass, so the original hermetic image is not a heavy presence, but a disappearing lightness by reflection.
The glazing works with the same rules as U paneling but in a different proportion: three fixed widths of panels with a greater common divisor and the alignments every time they sum the same. Two finishes of white glass with different degrees of opacity add a secondary reading to the shapes and volumes (without competing). Denser on the top, lighter on the bottom, the distinction of the two relates the “patios” to the outer skin more closely than in any other variation. Volumes fade by deleting the perimeter frame.

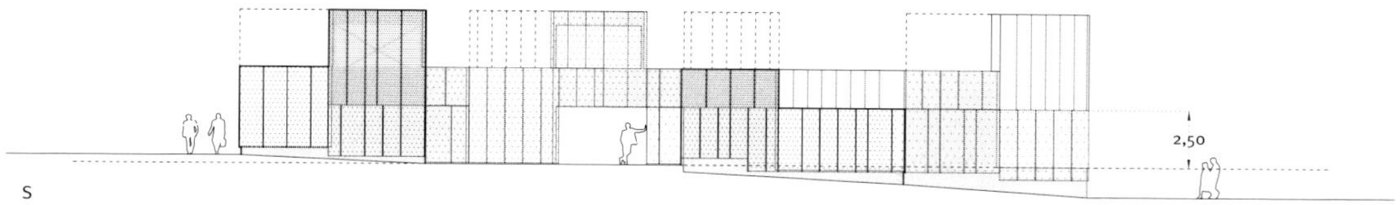

S

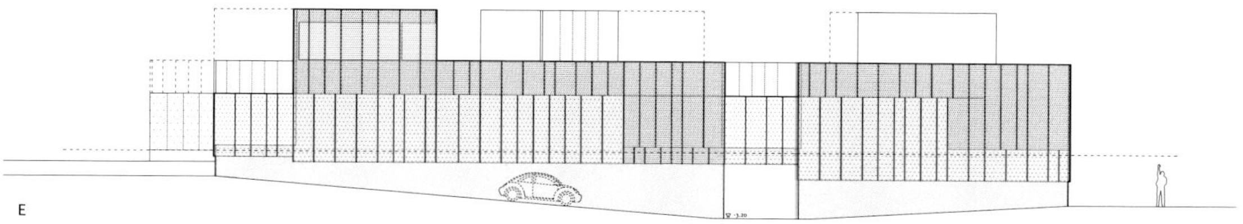

E

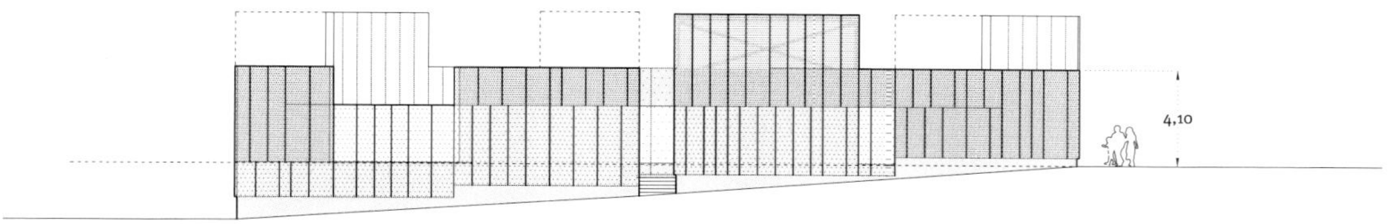

N

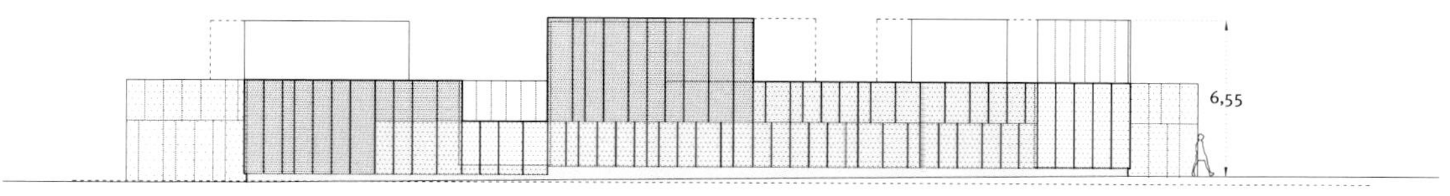

W

There is an intended ambiguity in the definition of front and back of the building as an urban object, while also avoiding big differences between left and right. It is only fair to explain that this intention does not come from the will to diminish the frontal arrival (and the understanding of the "box" object as building) but from the will to prevent the unfortunate "rear" connotation of the building as something less important or less desirable to look at.

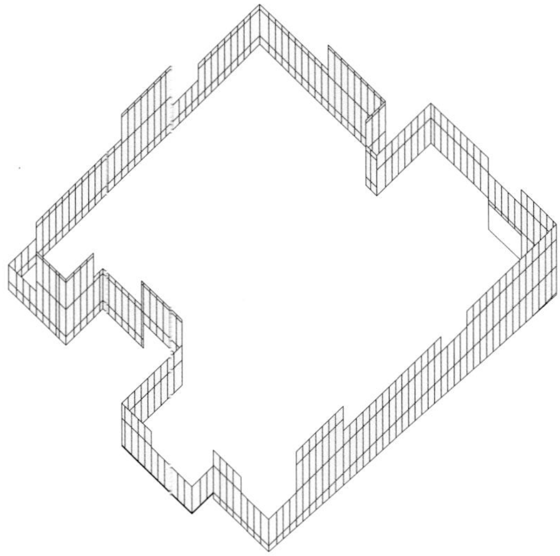

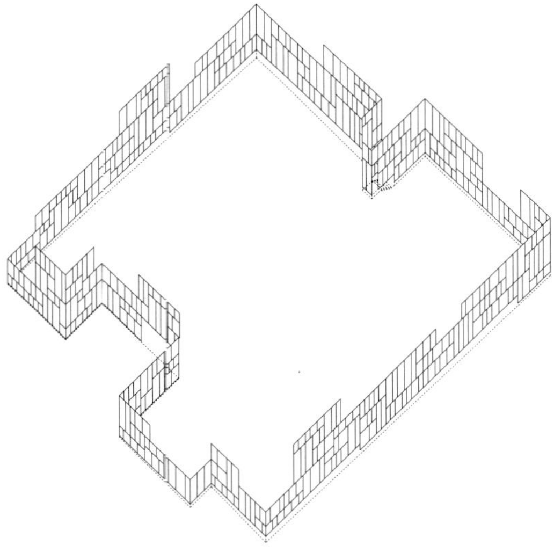

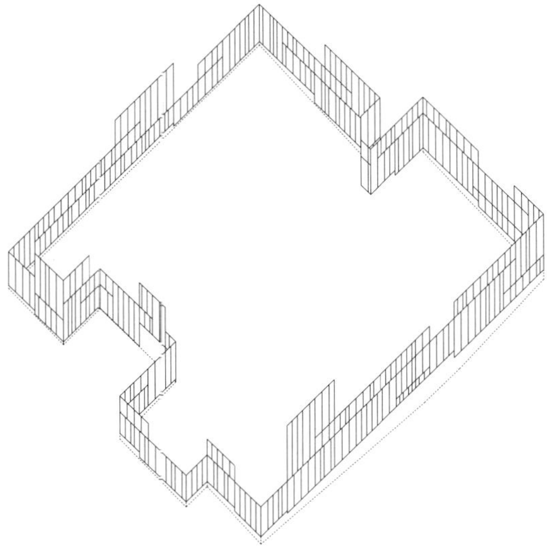

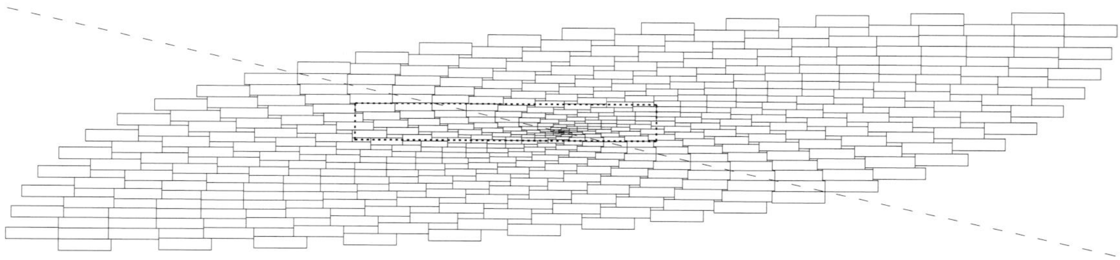

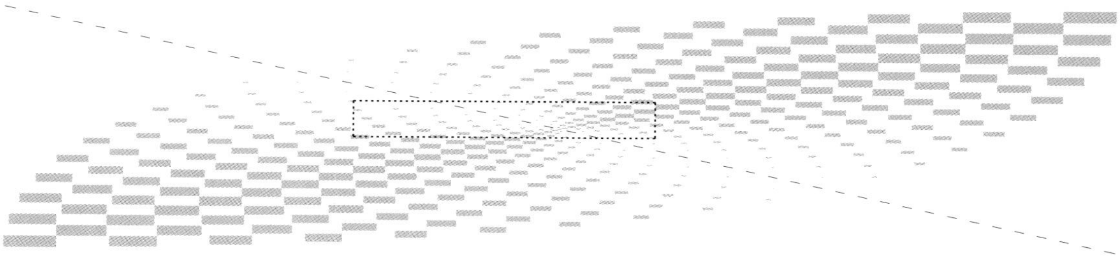

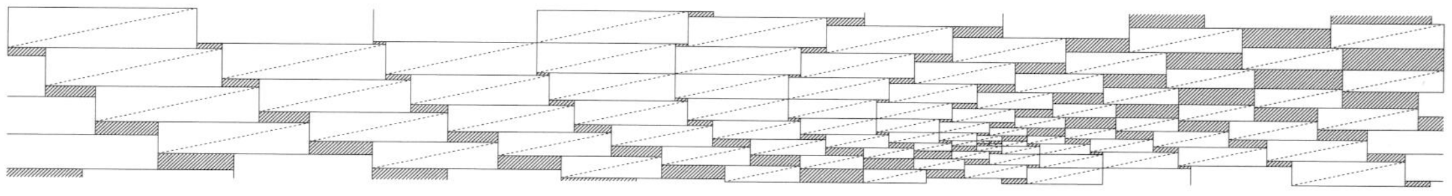

We enjoy investigating how to cut something into pieces in a discrete manner, so it will look complete when joining the pieces back together in the construction. To solve the cutting/joining issue of the golden skin of U, we worked initially with a spiral net formed by proportional rectangles.

Bottom left. We found the drawing of this fragment of a spiral in the Actar book called *Verb: Matters*. Marta Malé-Alemany and José Pedro Sousa held an installation at SCI-Arc in 2013 entitled (e) 3_emergencia.efecto.entorno. They described the initial parametric drawing as a mosaic of a rectangular pattern that repeats at a progressive rate: "This field reveals its potential extending endless with proportional contours and hidden symmetries arranged in rotations. It offers a system of variable parts arranged in identical modes."
We were seduced by this beautiful pattern and entertained ourselves finding those underlying symmetries. In the process, we learned that it was indeed a fragment of a spiral that could vary in shape and width according to the type of rectangle used as initiator. Unfortunately, we have not been able to find the mathematical name of this spiral yet; it has to have one for sure.

Right: These are the two complementary sets of rectangles that could vary in proportion for similar but not identical nets, like the whole spiral can be fatter or slimmer and still have the same pattern conditions. Different local symmetries are involved in the pattern.

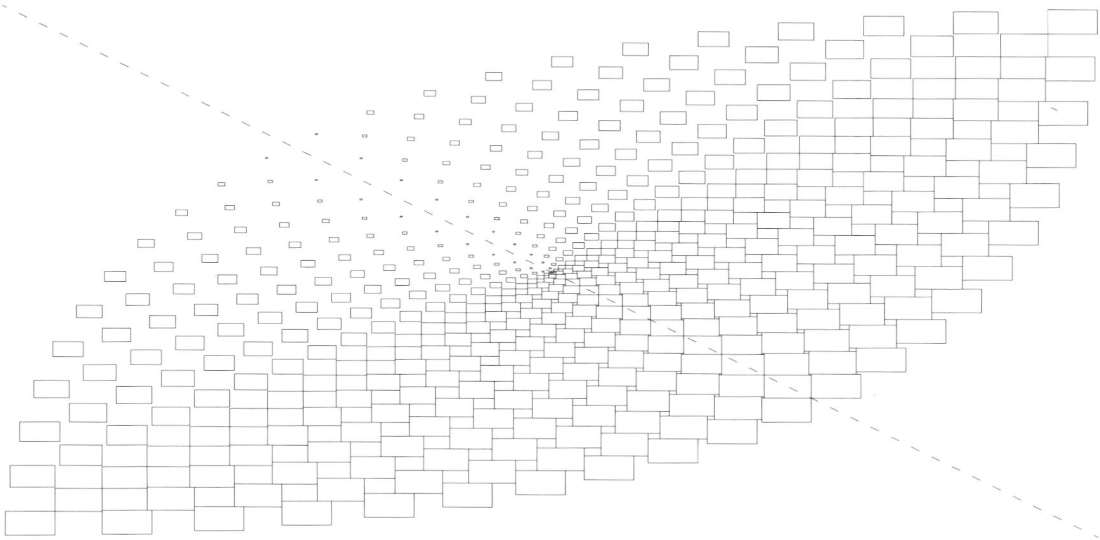

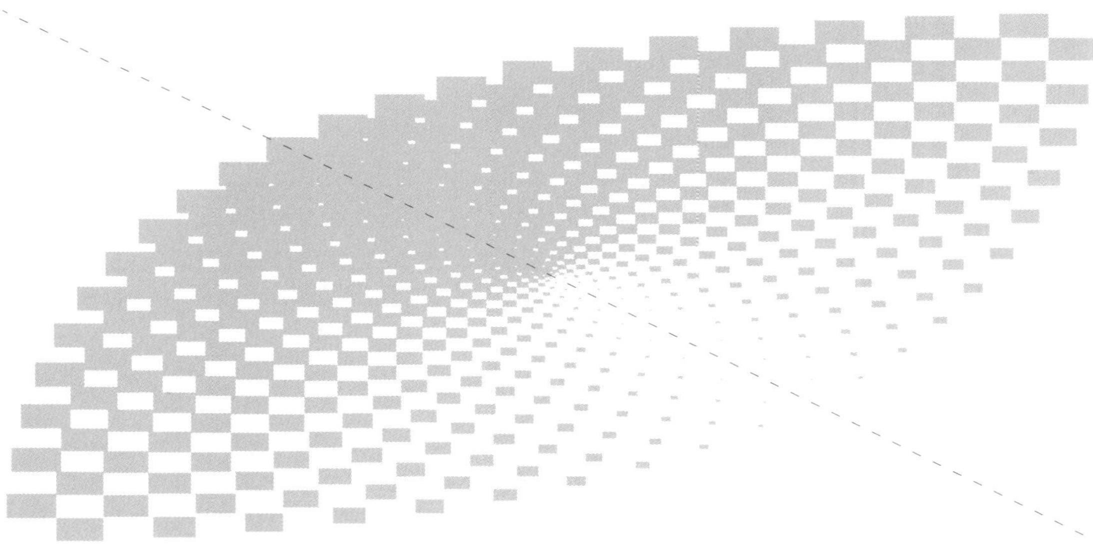

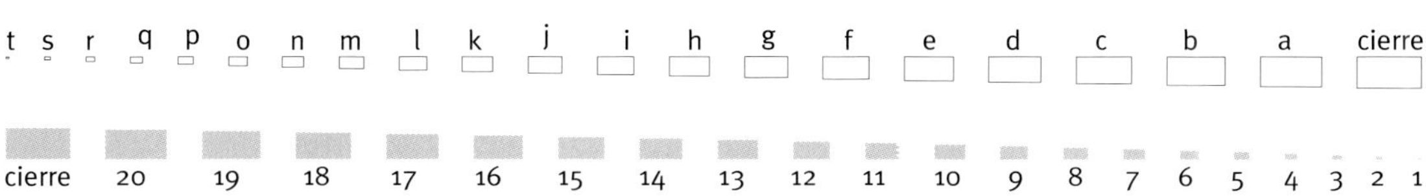

20=a, 19=b, 18=c, 17=d, 16=e, 15=f, 14=g, 13=h, 12=i, 11=j, 10=k, 9=l, 8=m, 7=n, 6=o, 5=p, 4=q, 3=r, 2=s, 1=t

1

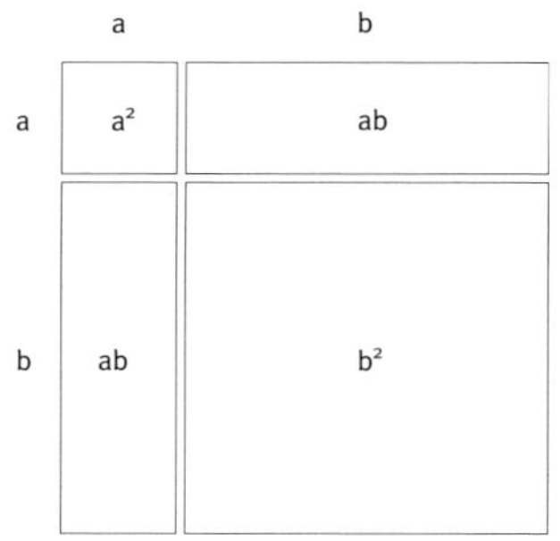

2

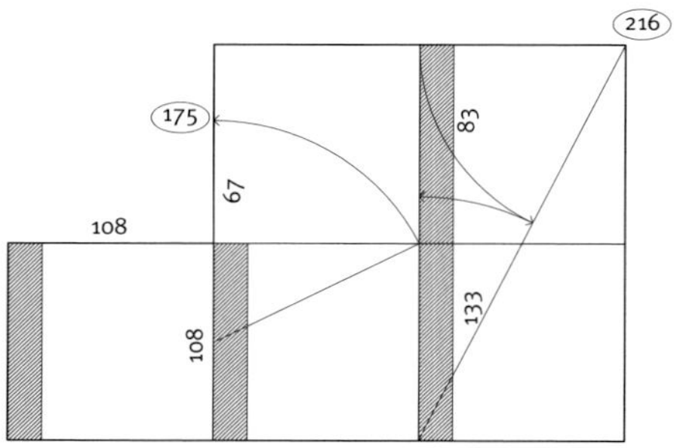

Le Corbusier again helps as a reference, with the "Modulor" system of proportions that he defined by using a Fibonacci sequence (2).
Modulor is the result of merging two views of the same reality that is man – from geometry and from algebra. Like two sides of the same coin, from one side, geometry is related to plastic intuition and to aesthetics, from the other side, the numbers game, rigor. Different measures of the Modulor's sequence are related in golden section: "the short is to the large as the large is to the whole".
Gregory Bateson, in his book *Mind and Nature* (1979), also gives a good example for understanding the role of mathematics in design logic and its translation into architectural space. He says that "every schoolboy knows" this equation (the square of a binomial): (a+b)2=a2+b2+2ab, but many "schoolboys" do not know the geometry behind it: that is, a collection of four independent but somehow related parts that are contained in a greater whole and also the idea of length and width that implies (1).
This brings us back to the concept of harmony as a combination of elements, the recognition of what is hidden.

3. Proportional initial set of rectangles for the golden spiral net; 1, 2, 3 and 6.
4. First iterations of the net construction.
5. Spiral net fragment at a point where it is still soon to understand the spiral behavior.

3

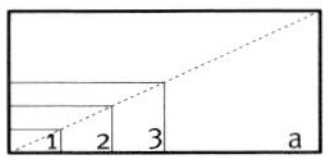
1
2
3
a

4

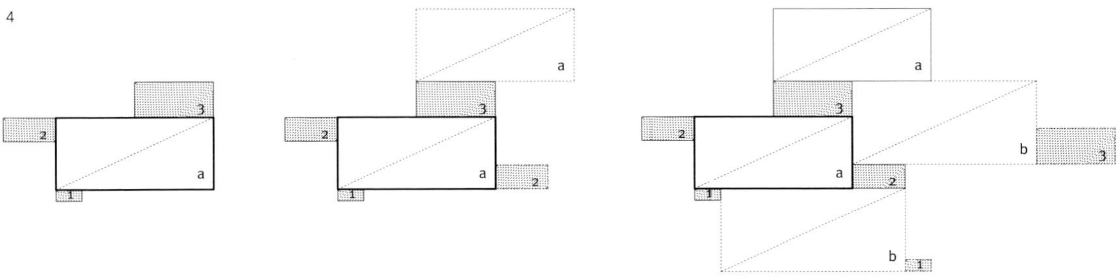
3
2
a
1
3
a
2
a
2
1
a
3
2
b
3
a
2
1
b
1

5

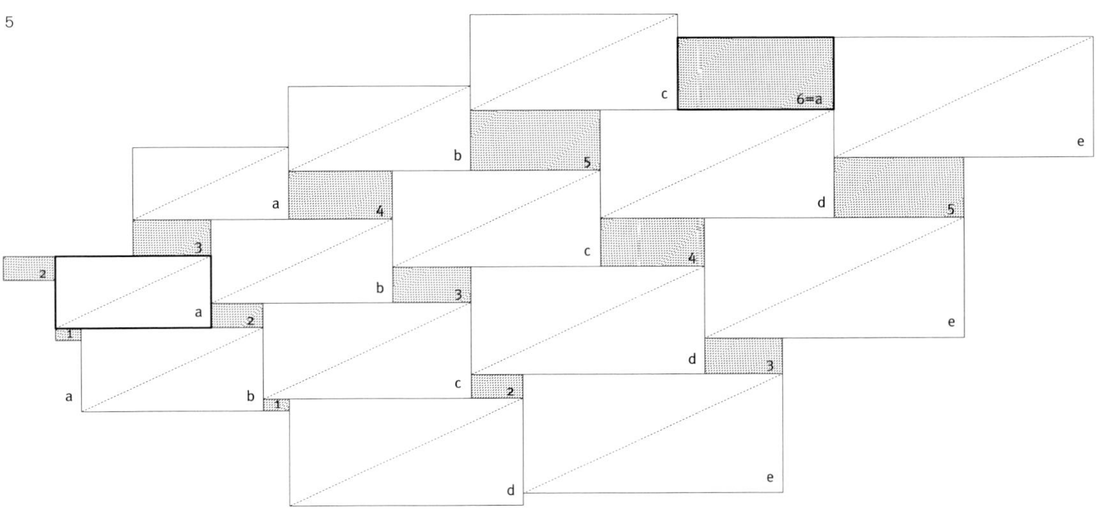
c
6=a
e
b
5
a
4
d
5
3
c
4
2
b
3
a
2
e
1
d
3
a
b
c
2
1
d
e

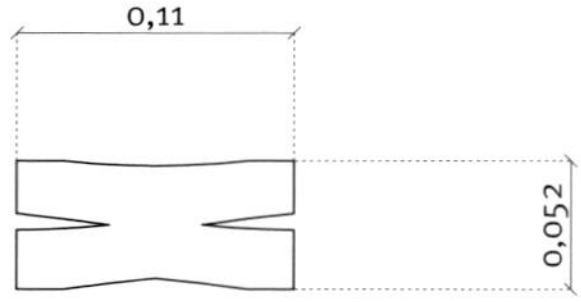

m

1

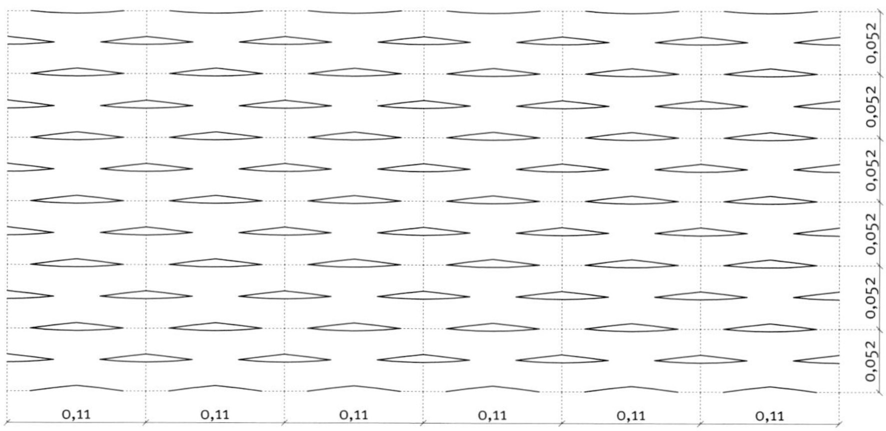

2

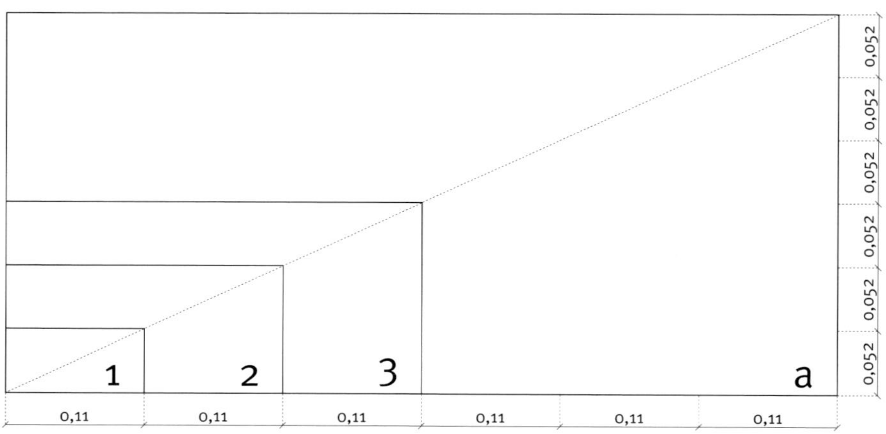

The golden expanded aluminum mesh (1) has a powerful texture with a clear pattern, 11 cm wide by 5.2 cm high; in both golden iterations explored for the U case, the panel dimension is always a multiple of the pattern module. Therefore, the mesh texture goes over the paneling without interruptions in pattern.

2. Spiral net panels logic. Proportional rectangles (11/5.2).
3. Greatest common divisor logic family of panels. Panel width is multiple of 11 and its height is multiple of 5.2 and they are divided in three groups of 66, 99 and 132 cm. They create relationships like the large one is twice the small one, large+small is twice the medium size, etc. (n3= 2n1, n1+n3=2n2, 3n1=2n2).

3

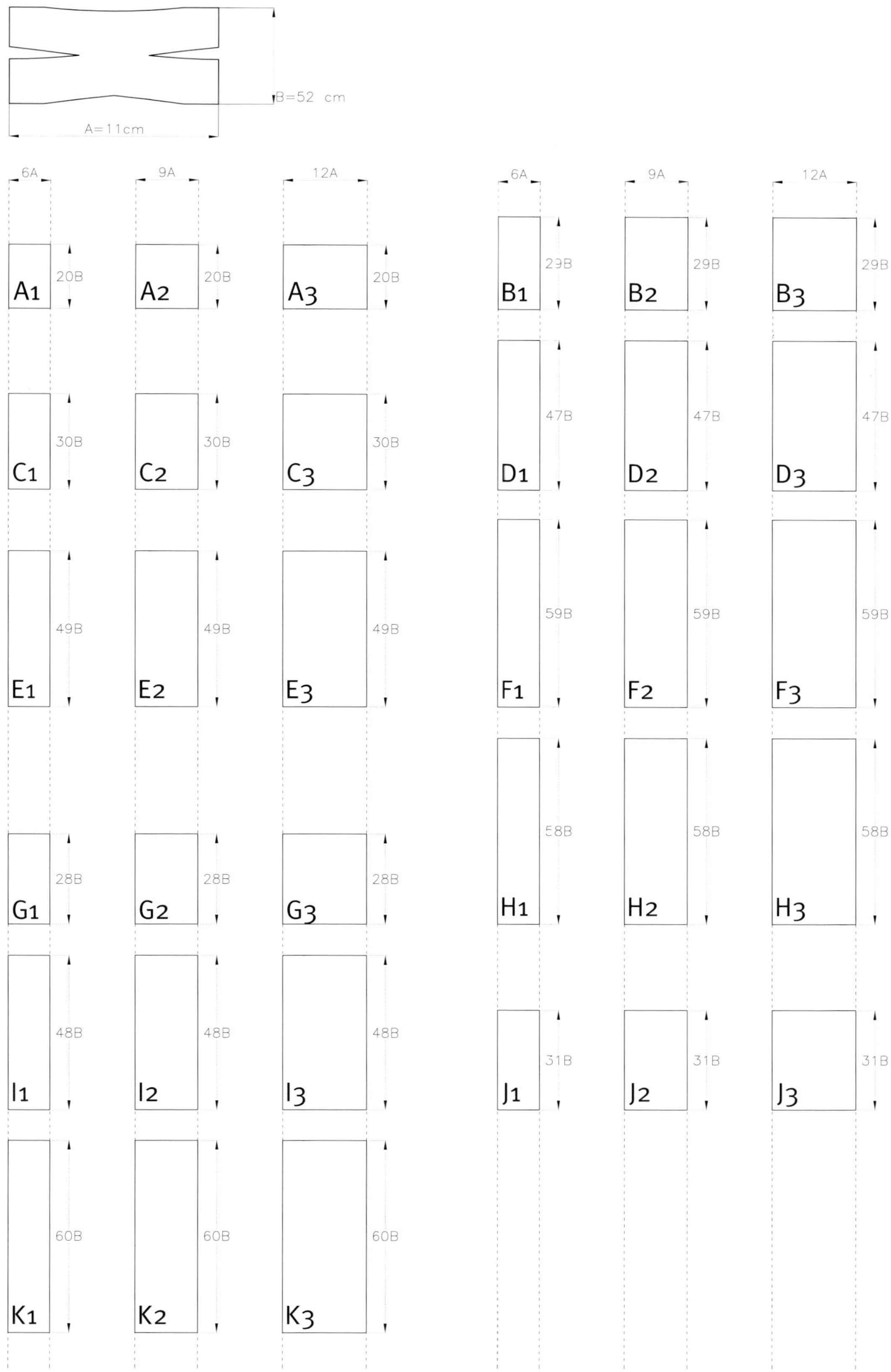

B=52 cm
A=11cm
6A
9A
12A
6A
9A
12A
A1 20B
A2 20B
A3 20B
B1 29B
B2 29B
B3 29B
C1 30B
C2 30B
C3 30B
D1 47B
D2 47B
D3 47B
E1 49B
E2 49B
E3 49B
F1 59B
F2 59B
F3 59B
G1 28B
G2 28B
G3 28B
H1 58B
H2 58B
H3 58B
I1 48B
I2 48B
I3 48B
J1 31B
J2 31B
J3 31B
K1 60B
K2 60B
K3 60B

There is a certain type of architectural drawing that behaves as instructions for the building process, a coded graphic representation of the secret laws of disorder, which certainly talks about the distance that exists from intuition to the laws of disorder hidden behind an apparent randomness.

1. U concrete wall silhouette to be dressed. Traces of intersection with perpendicular element and changes in depth.
2. Golden aluminum studs grid fixed onto the concrete
3. Expanded mesh panel disposition

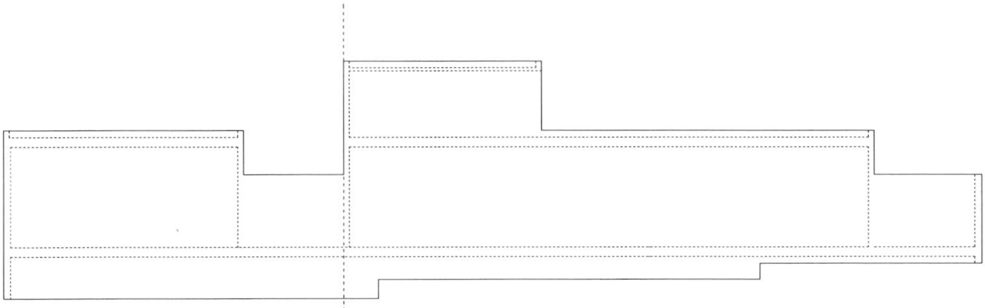

1

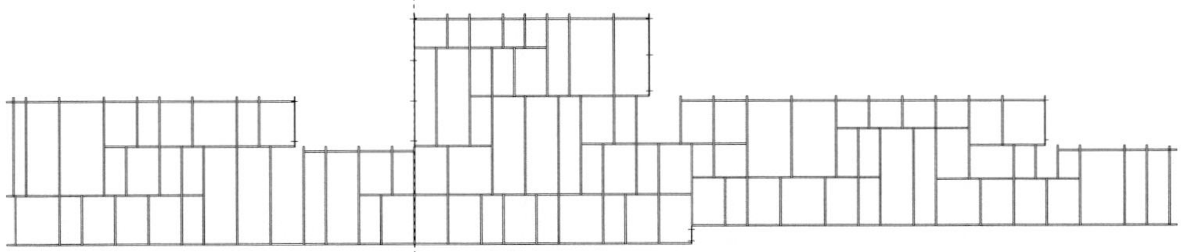

2

◄ ► SETTING-OUT ORIGIN

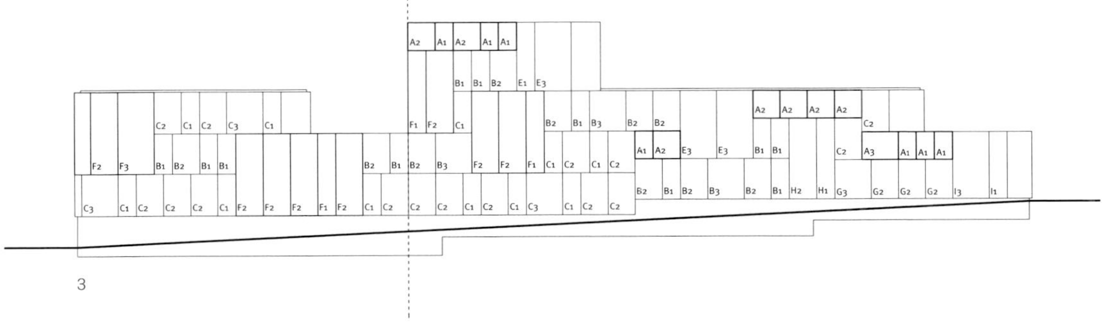

3

1. U brick wall silhouette to be dressed. Traces of columns and intersection with perpendicular element.
2. Anodized aluminum studs fixed onto the plastered brick wall. No horizontal frames.
3. Glass panel disposition with two different degrees of translucency.

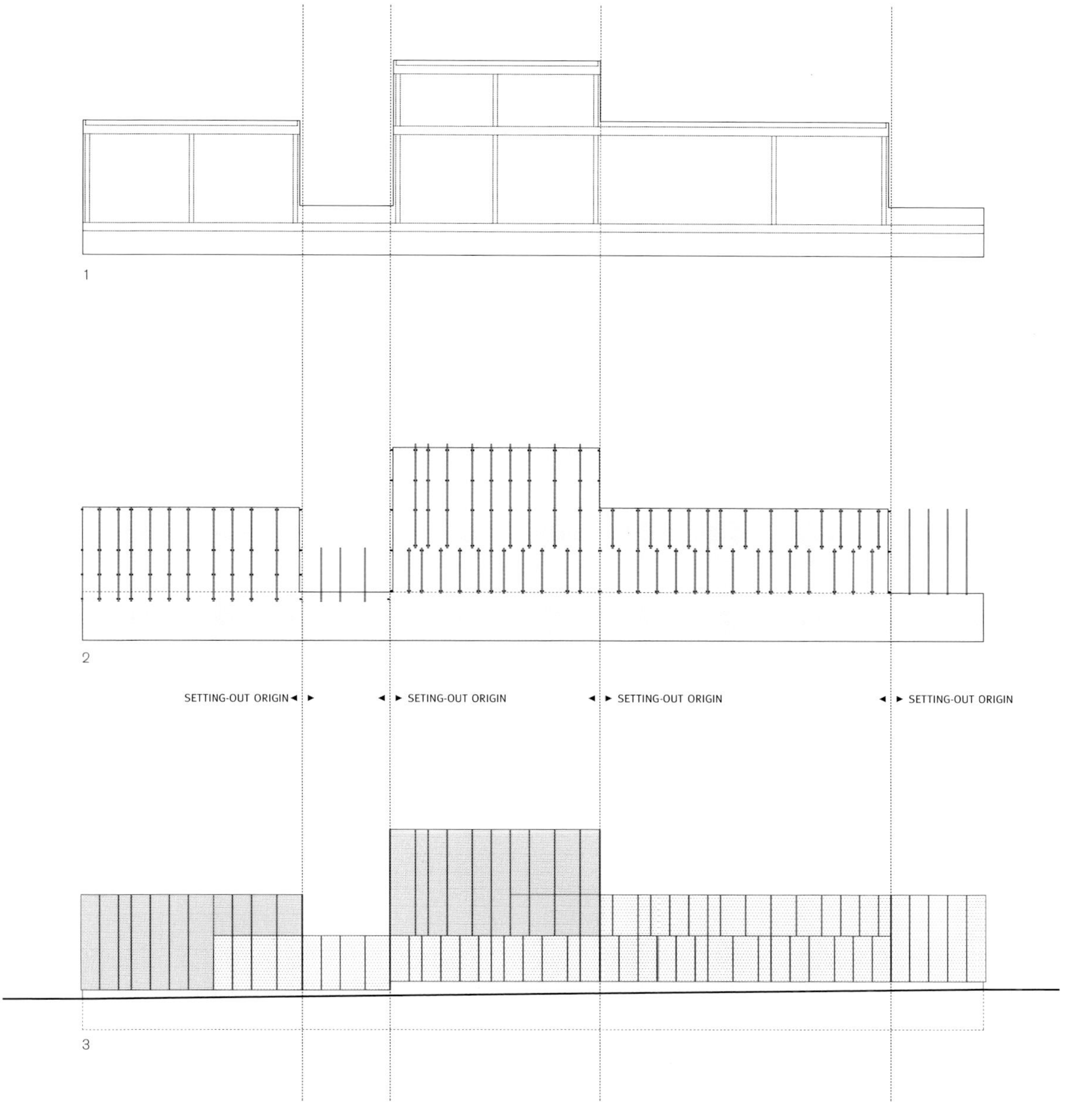
1
2
SETTING-OUT ORIGIN
SETING-OUT ORIGIN
SETTING-OUT ORIGIN
SETTING-OUT ORIGIN
3

The idea of heaviness in S is reinforced in the construction by the rough texture formed by the horizontal wood planks of the concrete formwork. Using a standard form size of 90cm in width and 2.70m in height, the vertical modulation is set to align panel joints with the elevation cut-outs avoiding incomplete pieces or pieces with a bite.
For the non-matching parts there are adjustments of 30 cm, meaning that there are never parts smaller than 30 cm and, on the other hand, panels are enlarged up to 1.20 at the most. These deviations are obviated by not being placed in the cut-out points. A layer of wood planks of 90 cm wide by 10 cm high over the standard panel is the last instruction in the construction process which, all together, results in a non-standard rough skin made out of standard components.

1. S concrete wall silhouette. Traces of intersection with perpendicular element and changes in depth.
2. Formwork paneling and adjustments
3. Wood texture pattern

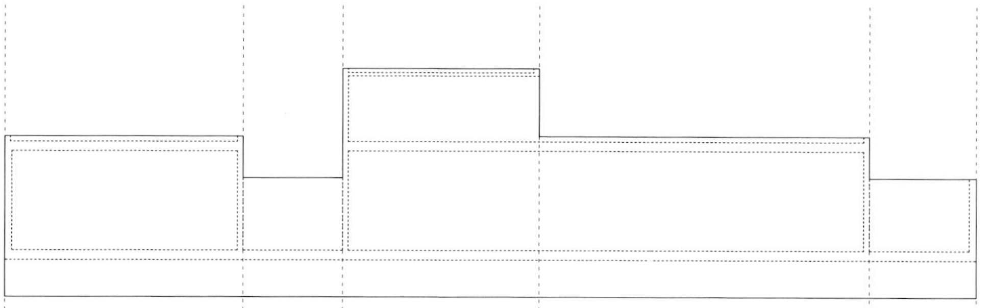

1

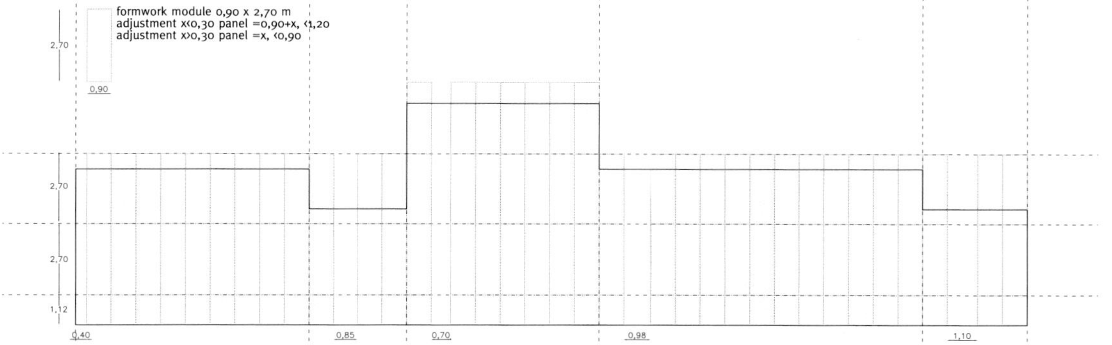

2

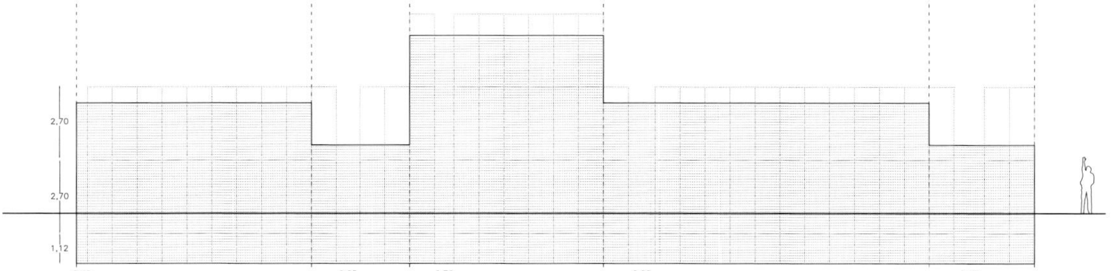

West elevation (modulation)

3

Towards the Nonstandard

The nonstandard appears when varying from the usual. It is about questioning the given status quo and, from there, the role of the discipline-based creativity of architectural design. It involves the consideration of certain ordering systems and their specific way of addressing gravity, scale, and the width and depth of what is being built.

Rethinking the standards means looking at things from different angles, without bias. It is not a start from scratch though, but a way of establishing new or renewed links with architecture, history, the past, technological backgrounds, etc. It entails a negotiation with "the real", with the physicality of architecture, and with architectural space that is synthetic and strategic and bounces constantly between speculation and pragmatism, intuition and calculation – an experimental branch of architecture supported by construction.

The work method here is based on abstraction as the consideration of things that do not appear in isolation in the real (sensitive) world. A non-ordinary or extra-ordinary consideration of the material aspect of the construction and its spatial consequences approached from within the discipline.

As for the nonstandard rough skin made out of standard components of S, the wood planks are nailed onto a standard form. The very standard quality of the plank itself (basic construction) makes the finishing surface uneven, as planks have small deviations in depth. The small changes in depth translate into lines of shadow that add a certain vibration to the concrete. The identity of the built mass comes from the balance between the strict order of the vertical alignments and the subtle unevenness of the wood traces.

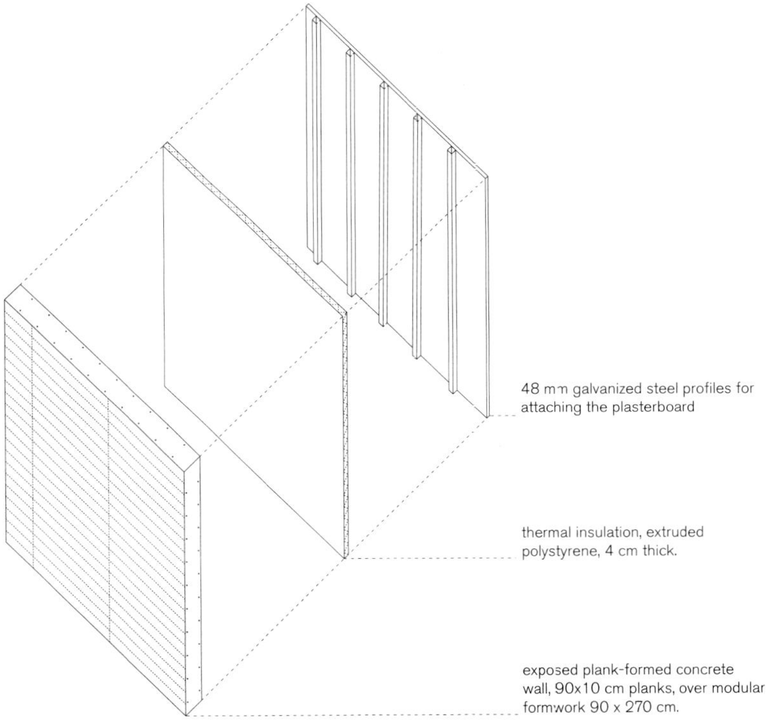
48 mm galvanized steel profiles for attaching the plasterboard
thermal insulation, extruded polystyrene, 4 cm thick.
exposed plank-formed concrete wall, 90x10 cm planks, over modular formwork 90 x 270 cm.

In the purest Semperian sense, a wall would be an element that, aside from being the visible boundary of a specific space, acquires value in its surface condition, regardless the thickness. By the action of dressing, the rank of "wall" can be conferred to a mass by any form of sheathing or paneling or even coating it, in what has been called the "dressing principle". The once indoor practice of dressing is translated in U onto the outer side of the spatial boundary in a smooth surface of metal mesh that takes some pride in showing its thinness. To some extent, following on the same idea of what is needed in order to wall in a built mass, one might think that the texture operations seen in S are to be considered the abstract dressing or dressing by absence of the concrete mass.

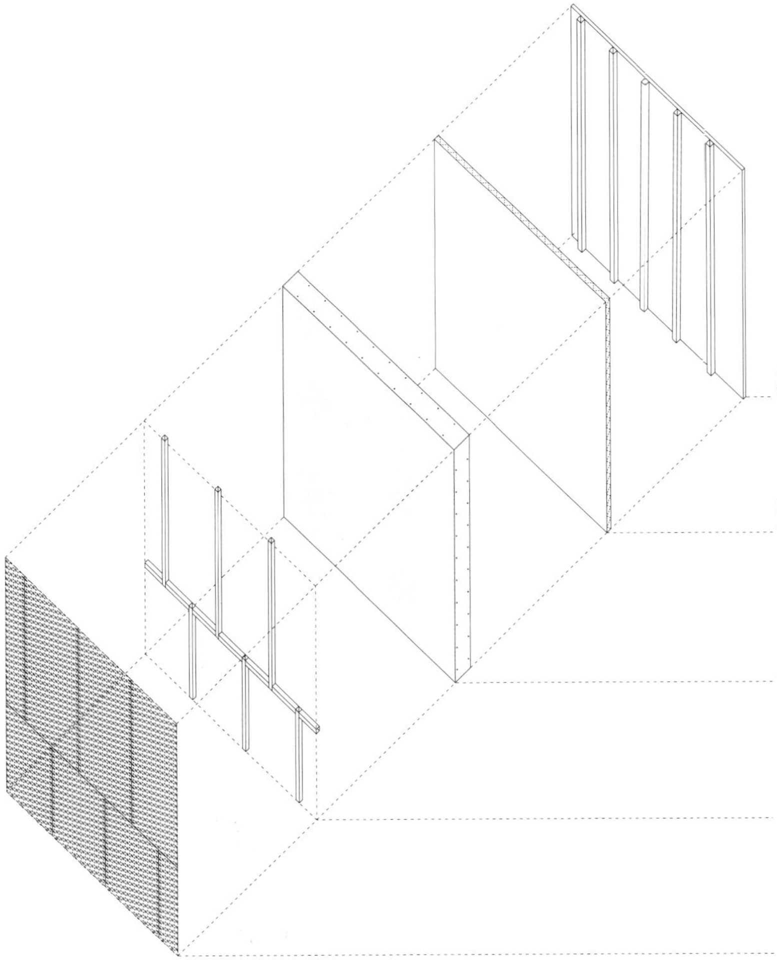

48 mm galvanized steel profiles for attaching the plasterboard
heat insulation, extruded polystyrene, 4 cm thick.
concrete wall with smooth finish.
substructure in anodized aluminum tube 40.40.1.5, gold, anchored to the concrete wall
expanded sheet metal mesh, Ambasciata model, gold color, by Italfin cut for modules of 66, 99 and 132 cm width and variable height, held to the substructure with rivets

The multiplication of layers of the V envelope, along with the richness that arises from the qualities of the material, adds depth to the flatness. Each layer has its mission, including the transition layers necessary for the implementation in the adjustment between base irregularities and the smoothness of the final layer, collaborating in the idea of building depth with thin elements – a kind of thickness without density.

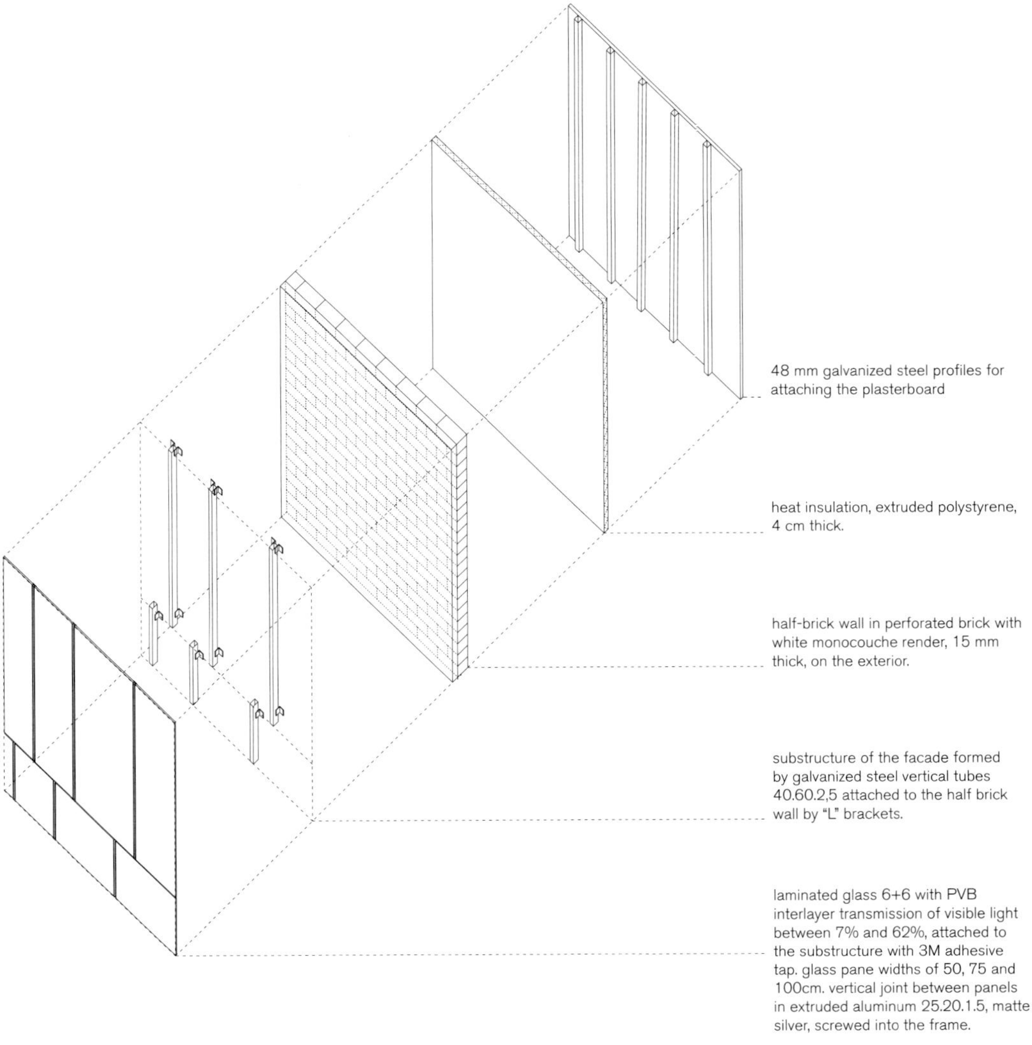
48 mm galvanized steel profiles for attaching the plasterboard
heat insulation, extruded polystyrene, 4 cm thick.
half-brick wall in perforated brick with white monocouche render, 15 mm thick, on the exterior.
substructure of the facade formed by galvanized steel vertical tubes 40.60.2,5 attached to the half brick wall by "L" brackets.
laminated glass 6+6 with PVB interlayer transmission of visible light between 7% and 62%, attached to the substructure with 3M adhesive tap. glass pane widths of 50, 75 and 100cm. vertical joint between panels in extruded aluminum 25.20.1.5, matte silver, screwed into the frame.

1. parapet cap in galvanized steel sheet, 1.5% interior slope
2. exposed board-formed concrete wall, 90x10 cm boards, over modular formwork
3. draining concrete floor Tennisquick, thk=10cm.
4. gravel over a layer of felt
5. heat insulation, extruded polystyrene (such as Roofmate), thk=4cm. over a waterproof layer plus 2 geotextile fabric layers
6. lightweight concrete with expanded clay aggregate, thk=10cm, to form slopes, screed finish
7. hollow-core slab, 30+5cm
8. heat insulation, projected polyurethane foam thk=4cm
9. grey terrazzo tile, 60x40 cm, staggered
10. bonding mortar
11. screed mortar
12. double hollow brick wall
16. plasterboard drop ceiling, in exam rooms
19. courtyard finish, gravel layer 10cm., white Macael 20mm., over a layer of felt
24. hidden profile, as support for the window frame
25. flat construction joint, coinciding with the horizontal cut of the slab
26. Nervometal sheet on the slab edge to create the construction joint
43. operable window frame, Technal Unicity model, with Climalit glass 6+6/12/8

S patios are clad in dark blue ceramic tiles arranged in lines with a third of a piece displacement from the one below, and that certain offset or displacement of the vertical joints results in a spiral effect, a textured surface that expands away from the static sense of a grid.
The offset of a third has a remote precedent in the so-called "Egyptian third" which, although it has its reason for being in the thickness of the wall, results in skidding joints on its surface. Tracing this strategy for arranging the parts, there are good examples on the façade of the Swiss Pavilion by Le Corbusier in Paris but also in the outside pavement of the Miró Foundation in Mallorca by Rafael Moneo.
It may or may not make sense here, but talking about tiles always makes me think of the mosaic with moon by Jorn Utzon at the entrance to his home in Mallorca (Porto Petro), where the lesson is that in order to avoid smaller pieces than a half or a third at the edges, the solution is to "third" the previous one.

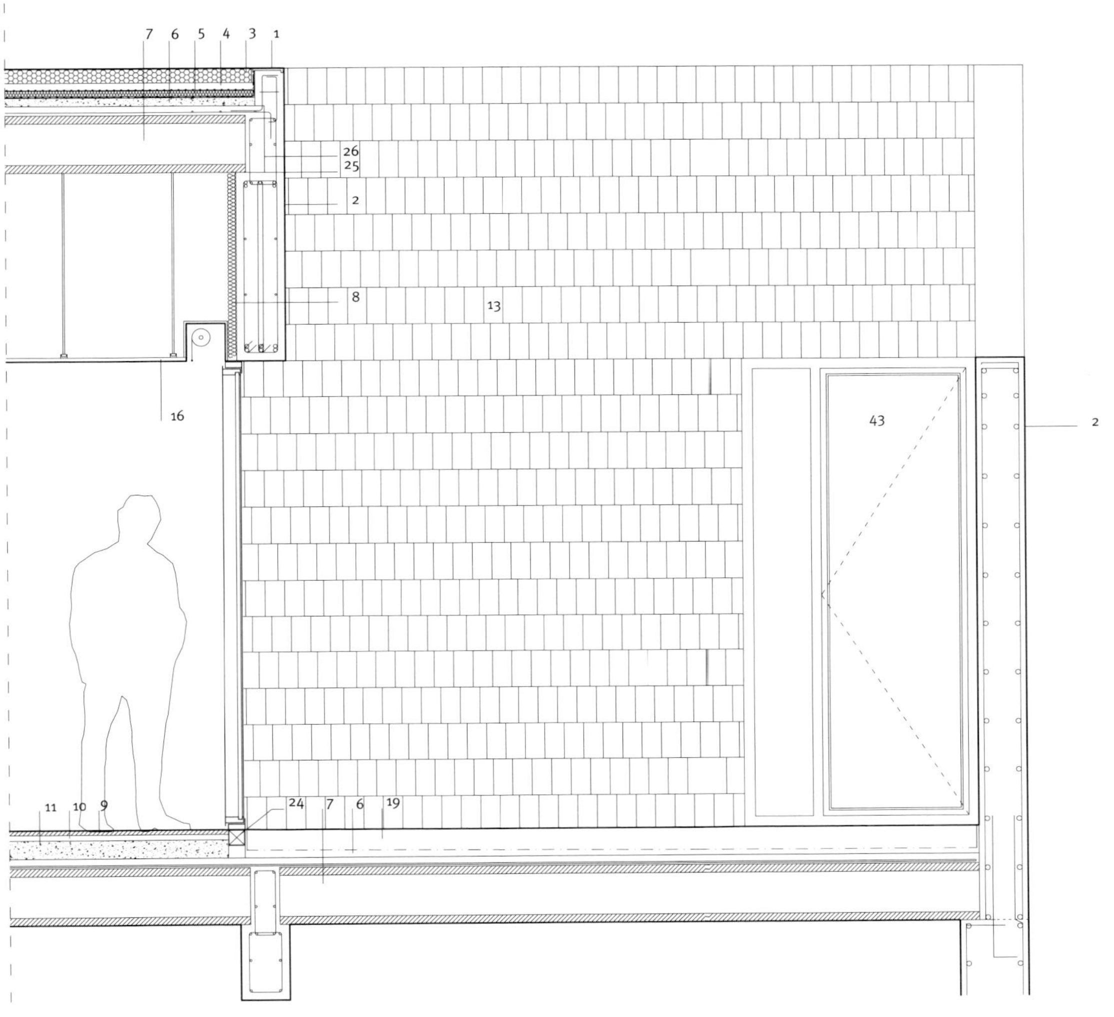
7
6
5
4
3
1
26
25
2
8
13
16
43
2
24
7
6
19
11
10
9

1. parapet cap in galvanized steel sheet, 1.5% interior slope
2. exposed board-formed concrete wall, 90x10 cm boards, over modular formwork
3. draining concrete Tennisquick, thk=10cm.
4. gravel over a layer of felt
5. heat insulation, extruded polystyrene (such as Roofmate), thk=4cm. over a waterproof layer plus 2 geotextile fabric layers
6. lightweight concrete with expanded clay aggregate, thk=10cm, to form slopes, screed finish
7. hollow-core slab, 30+5cm
8. heat insulation, projected polyurethane foam thk=4cm
9. grey terrazzo tile, 60x40 cm, staggered
10. bonding mortar
11. screed mortar
16. plasterboard drop ceiling, in exam rooms
17. half-brick closure in perforated brick
18. stadip protect glass, climalit 66.2/8/8, in common areas climalit glass 4+4/8/4, in exam rooms
19. courtyard finish, gravel layer 10cm., white Macael 20mm., over a layer of felt
24. hidden profile, as support for the window frame
25. flat construction joint, coinciding with the horizontal cut of the slab
26. Nervometal sheet on the slab edge to create the construction joint
29. white ceramic tiles, 10x20 cm, laid vertical, staggered
30. concrete wall over modular formwork
31. substructure in anodized aluminum tube 40.40.1.5, gold, anchored to the concrete wall
32. expanded sheet metal mesh, Ambasciata model, gold color, by Italfin
41. galvanized sheet metal finish, 1 cm thick, black lacquer
43. operable window frame, Technal Unicity model, with Climalit glass 6+6/12/8

"Action of one" defines the potential of an entity, an item, or an action that is repeated and multiplied to generate a sequence of events. Tile surfaces are not framed, seeking a balance between the finite or infinite of the layout – basic ceramic tiles reflecting the surroundings and blurring presences.

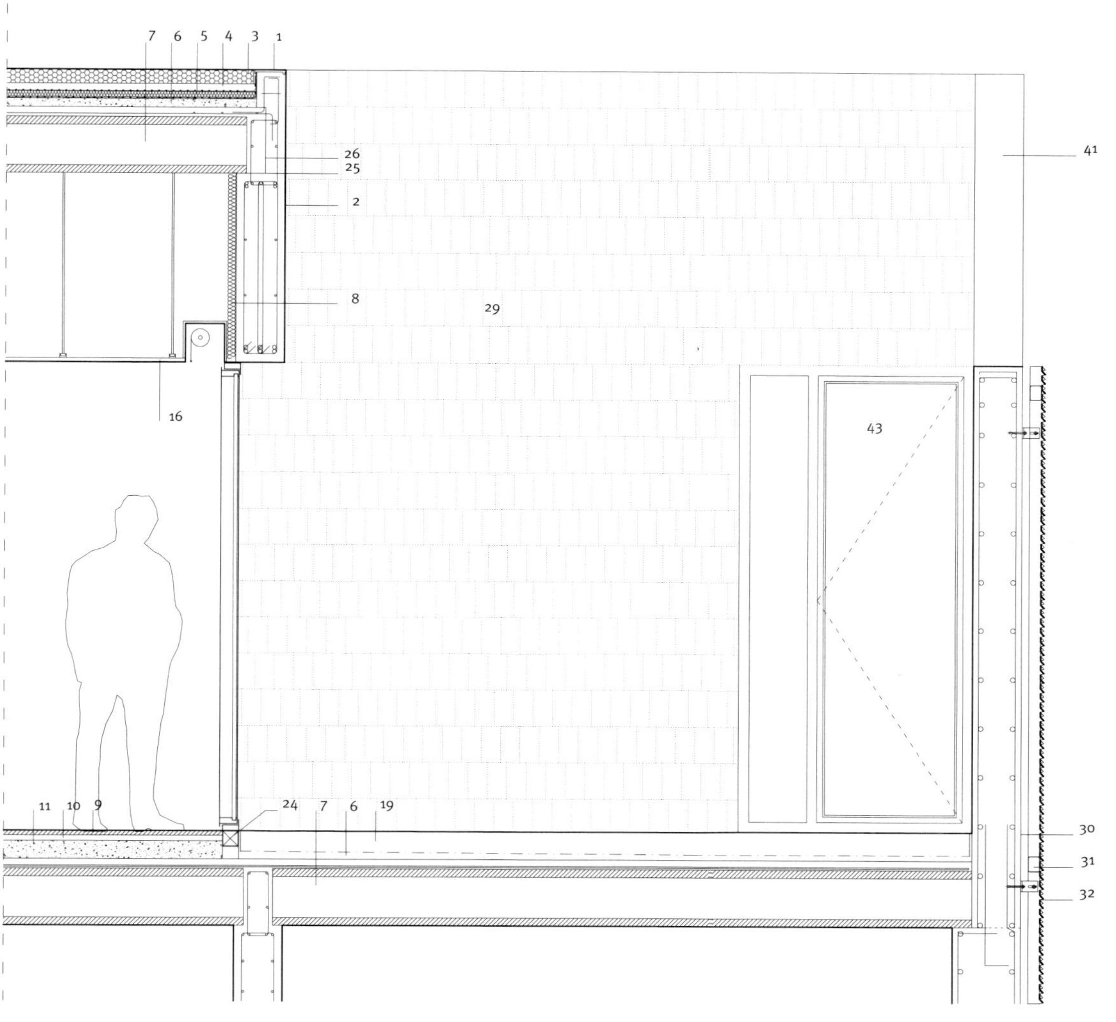
7
6
5
4
3
1
26
25
2
8
29
41
16
43
11
10
9
24
7
6
19
30
31
32

1. parapet cap in galvanized steel sheet, 1.5% interior slope
3. draining concrete floor Tennisquick, thk=10cm.
4. gravel over a layer of felt
6. lightweight concrete with expanded clay aggregate, thk=10cm, to form slopes, screed finish
7. hollow-core slab, 30+5cm
8. heat insulation, projected polyurethane foam thk=4cm
9. grey terrazzo tile, 60x40 cm, staggered
10. bonding mortar
14. white monocouche render, 15 mm thick
16. plasterboard drop ceiling, in exam rooms
17. half-brick closure in perforated brick
19. courtyard finish, gravel layer 10cm., white Macael 20mm., over a layer of felt
25. flat construction joint, coinciding with the horizontal cut of the slab
33. screed mortar
35. substructure. steel tube frame 40.40.4 treated at the plant and with two layers of enamel on site.
36. galvanized steel sheet, thk=1mm. anchored to the tube substructure 40.40.4
37. polycarbonate honeycomb, model DANPALON MULTICELL 16 ice grey
38. exposed board-formed concrete wall, 10 cm boards, over modular formwork
39. façade finish. laminated glass 6+6 with PVB interlayer
40. glass substructure, steel tube 40.60.2,5 galvanized fixed to the half-brick wall
42. trench for the meeting between the façades formed from folded steel sheet, 5 mm thick
43. operable window frame, Technal Unicity model, with Climalit glass 6+6/12/8

V patios are cladded with polycarbonate panels which, for practical reasons, exist in the construction market in two different widths. In the territory of construction "to divide in equal parts" is almost an entelechy. As modulation is closely tied with contingency, the issue is to make things look like they are modulated; if no part is evidently larger or smaller than others our distracted minds read them as equal.

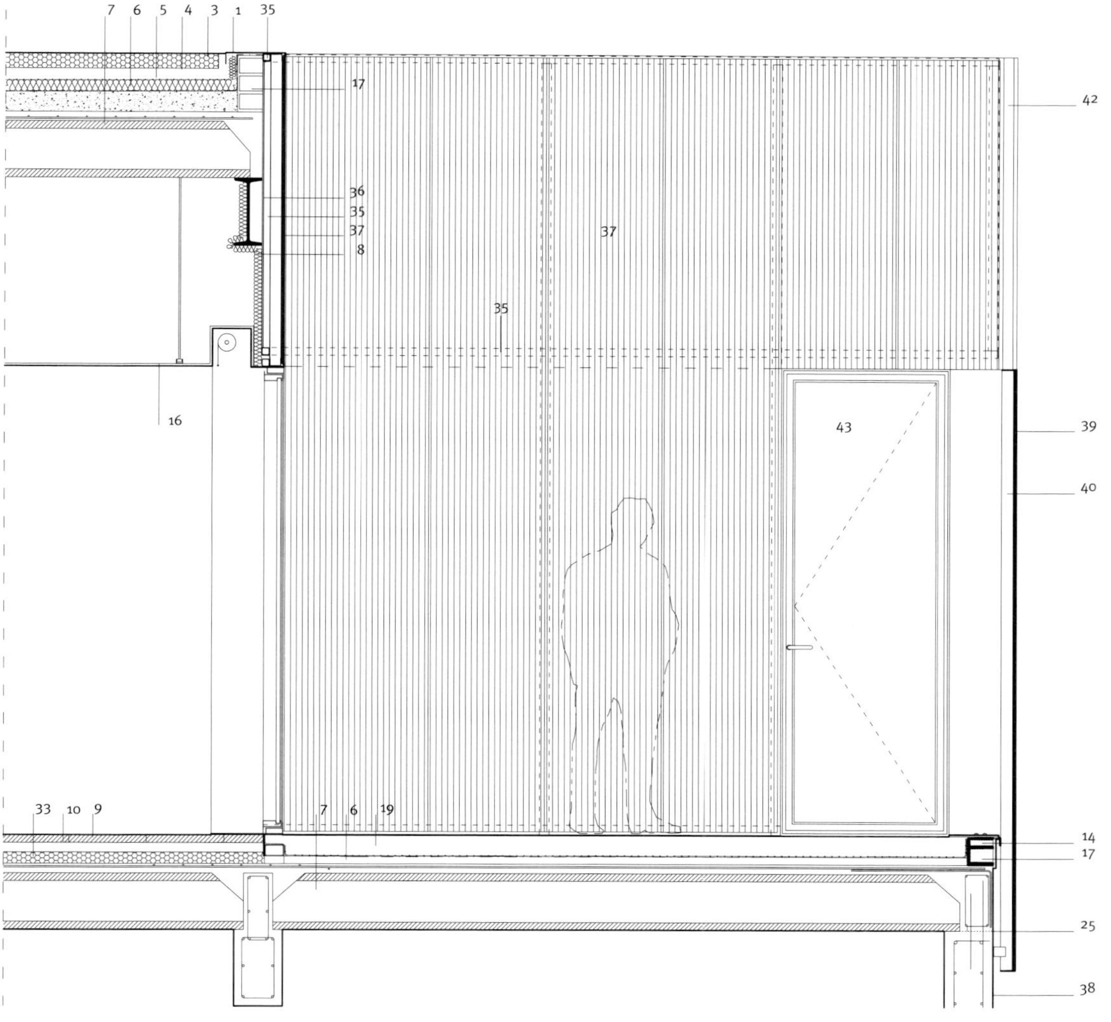
7
6
5
4
3
1
35
17
42
36
35
37
8
37
35
16
43
39
40
33
10
9
7
6
19
14
17
25
38

Actually, the reason modulation is so hard to address has to do with the width of construction; yet an even bigger question comes with the width, which might be called "the edge problem" or "problema al canto" in Spanish.

Carlos Ferrater enjoys explaining how the "problema al canto", which is a well known Spanish saying, is an expression born in the language of carpenters; in putting two boards together edge by edge, whether flushed or angled, the board's thickness and whether or not it will be exposed play an important role in the type of connection.

The question here is how to incorporate the width of materials into the abstract order of a project without betraying it, and how to recalibrate the parameters. For example in Musac, as in many other buildings by Mansilla-Tuñon, we identify the rule of "no parts are folded"; there are no bending corners. Materials and building components get cut and flushed, but they are never bent or wrapped. Following the same edge problem in giving width to the surface that defines a volume, a difference can be established between things that work from the inside-out and others from the outside-in (system from within or system from without). An internal system or spatial logic rules, for example, in the Serpentine pavilion by Toyo Ito, where in bending the thickness of the structural shell from roof to wall the internal continuity is preserved, and discontinuities in the pattern manifest on the outside. The opposite case happens, for example, in the Spanish pavilion for Aichi Expo by FOA, where the external forces rule, and the intention is in preserving the formal integrity of the box with the ceramic pattern in perfect continuity from side to side; exceptions and adjustments are solved in the interior.

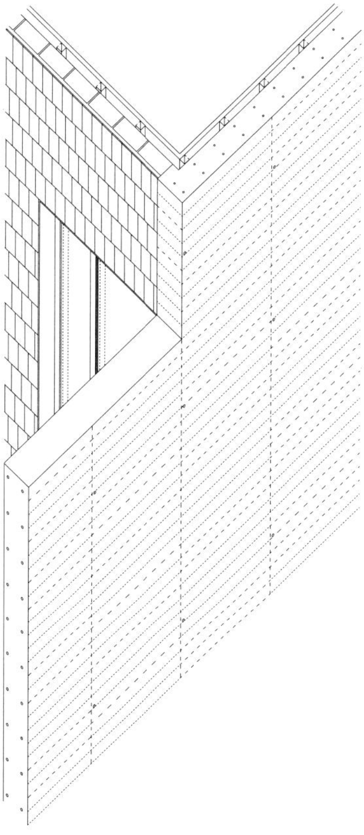

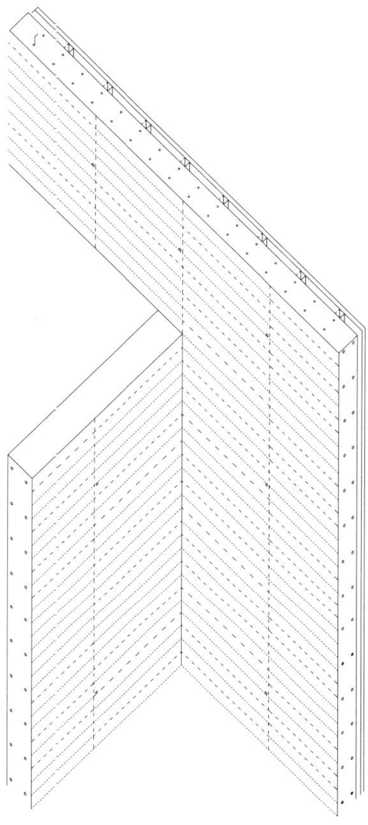

The high degree of flatness of the U envelope brings up the idea of smoothness. Smoothness is evenness, the absence of wrinkles, and also clean, bright and shining. It is paradoxical that something so thin can look so stiff, seem so strained. The absence of frame and the continuity in the pattern of the mesh collaborate in this golden surface tension, standing in front of a concrete volume as a mask, concealing the figure it is hiding.

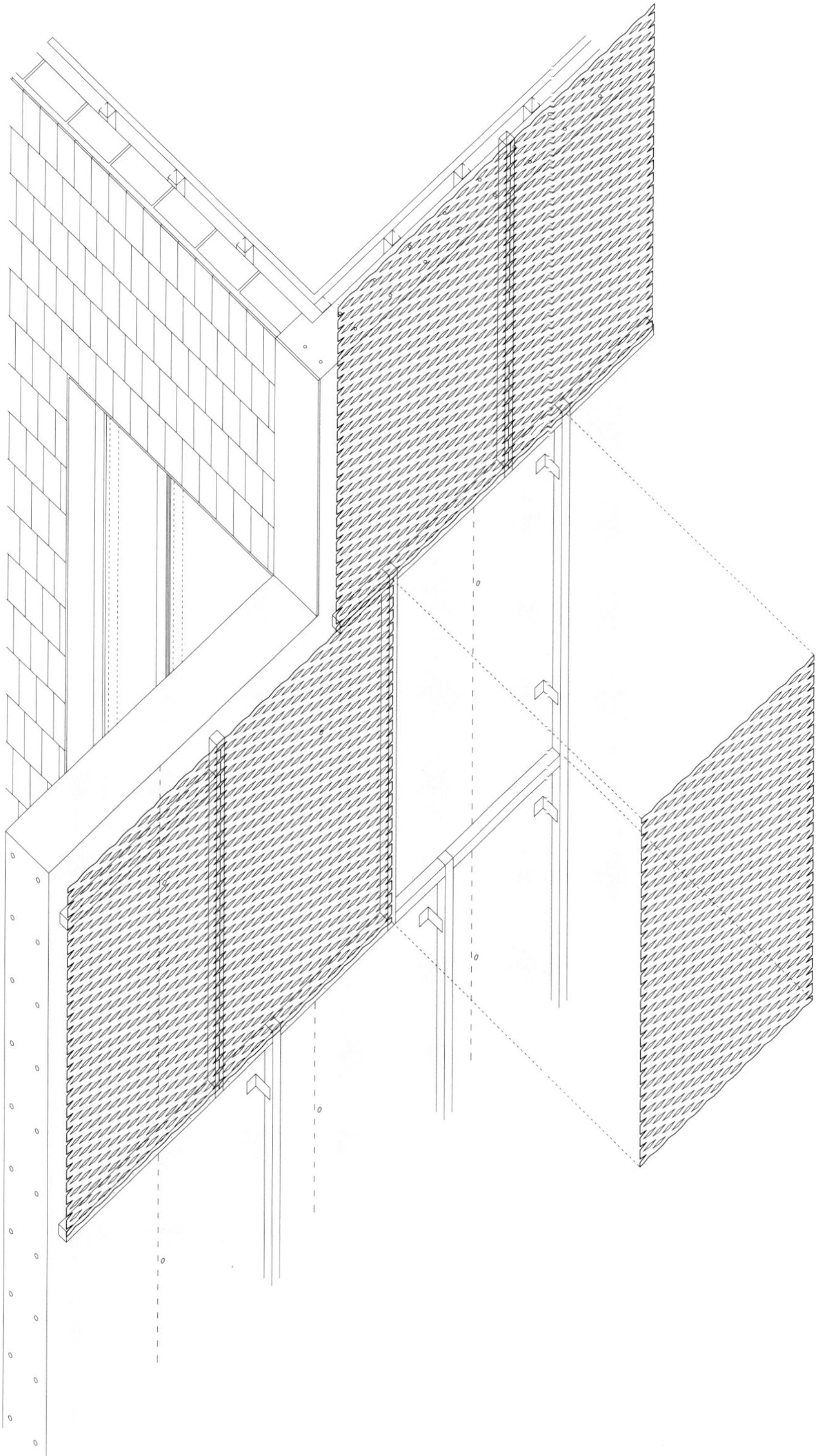

1. metal substructure 40.40.4
2. polycarbonate panel, model DANPALON MULTICELL 16 ice grey
3. polycarbonate lateral clip
4. painted steel plate, 10 mm thick
5. L form, folded steel sheet, 5 mm thick, painted
6. 6 + 6 laminated glass
7. metal substructure for glass panels 40.60.3 attached to a half-brick wall
8. lacquered aluminum omega profile, 1.5 mm thick (glass fixing)
9. polycarbonate panel clip profile
10. reveal, folded steel sheet, 5 mm thick
11. perforated steel sheet, painted, 3 mm thick

In 3x1 there are no typical details, but only typical intentions. In general, all solutions for concavity in a project are often solved similarly, and the conditions of convexity too. The difficulty comes when the two worlds of the concave and convex meet, and the same built plane has to respond to each of the two conditions at each of the faces.
When V patios are sitting by the outer perimeter skin, they are crystalline enclosures from the outside and polycarbonate cladding from the inside. Exceptions in the way things meet multiply, and developing complex corner details is necessary for the sole purpose of not looking complex. "As much nothing as possible" said Alejandro de la Sota.

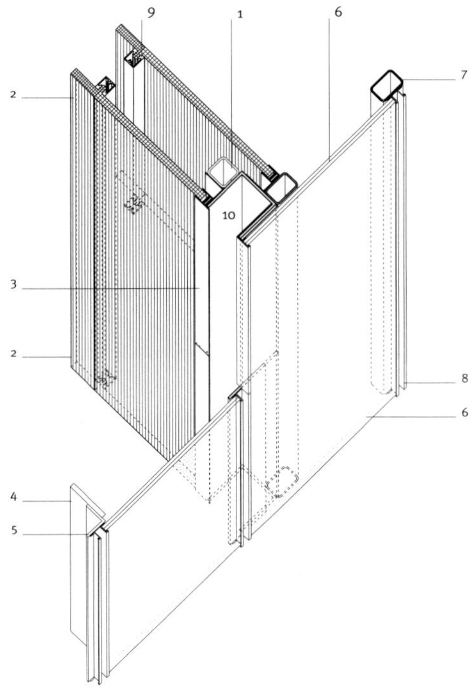
9
1
6
7
2
10
3
2
8
6
4
5

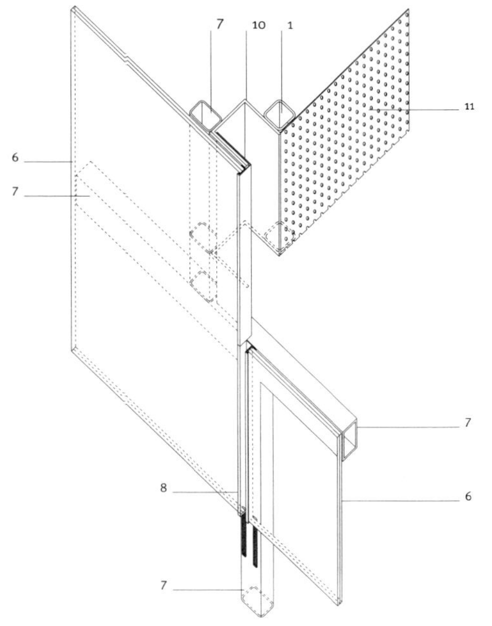
7
10
1
11
6
7
7
8
6
7

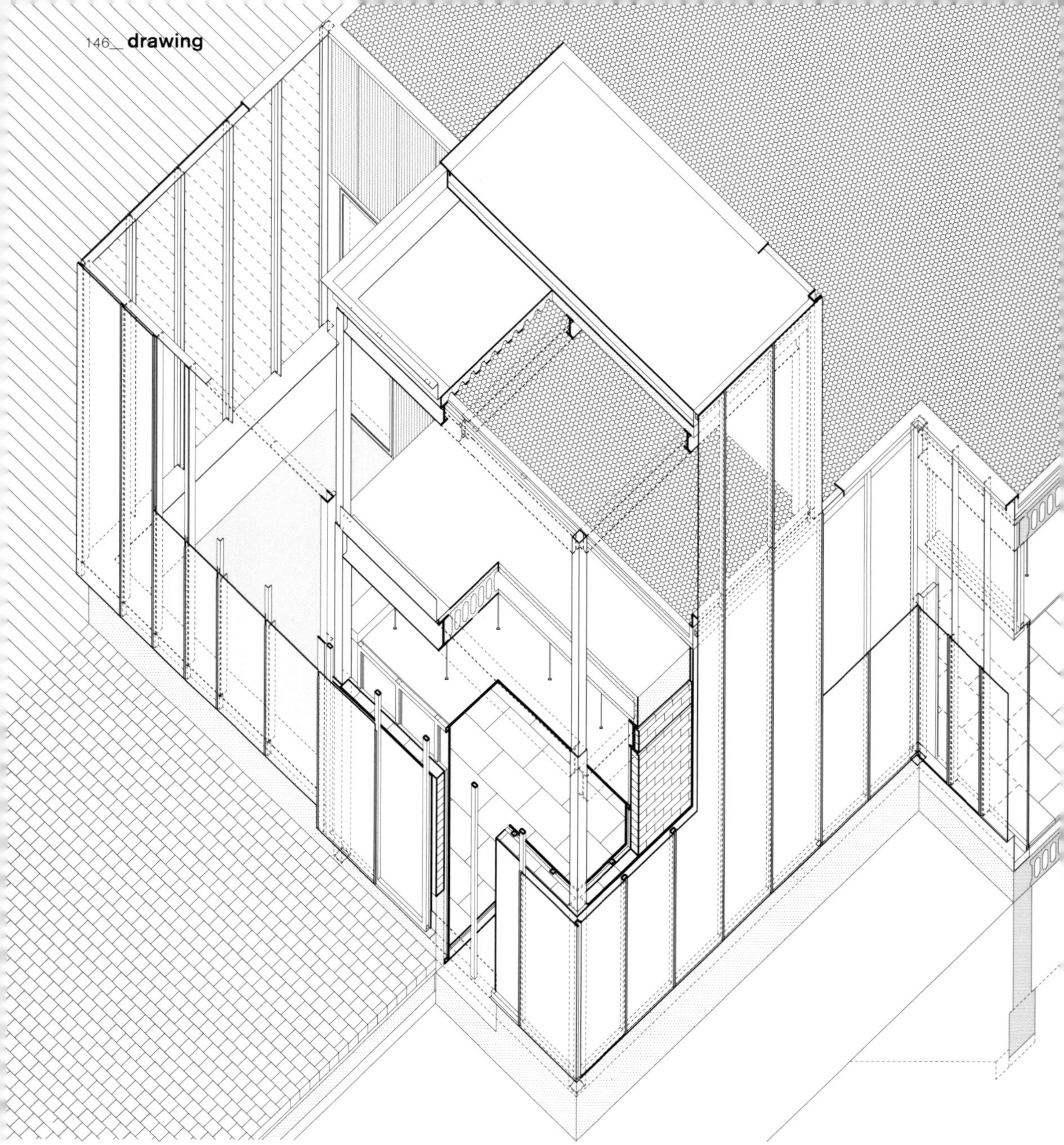

This is our own cost efficiency rule of thumb: "the more the architect draws, the better cheap looks".

(pag. 146_147)

After building 3x1 we have had several opportunities to rehearse how its spatial and ordering strategies could be supported by other programs, in other contexts, at a different time. The best derivative comes with this project for a single family home in Medellín.
As was the case for the clinics, the most general intentions begin with the desire to establish a new link between ordinary and extraordinary, trying to enable the coexistence of day-to-day situations, such as the house program, with the unexpected.
We organized the program suggested by the client by following the criteria of the greatest common divisor. The unit is a rectangular module of 3.60 x 4.20m and all rooms are multiples of this spatial unit. The counterbalance to the programmed spaces is proposed as outdoor spaces that are the visual extension of rooms, following the same modular approach. Both interior and exterior cells are disposed in parallel bars with interstitial circulation spaces in a strict pattern of the rhythm "aba". A continuous enclosure includes interiors and exteriors in an overall figure, which again blurs its perimeter.

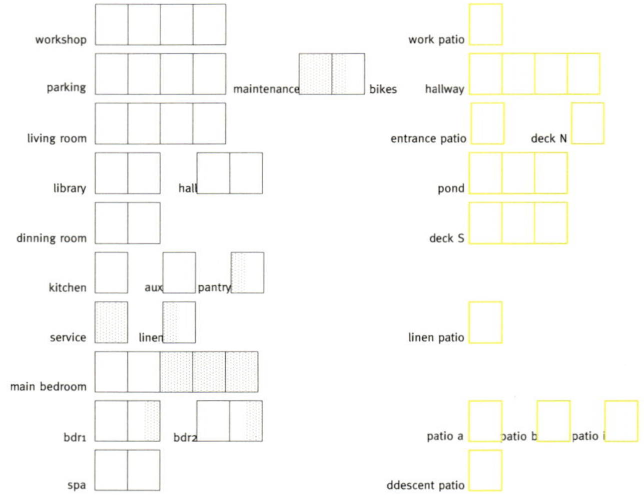
workshop
parking
maintenance
bikes
living room
library
hall
dinning room
kitchen
aux
pantry
service
linen
main bedroom
bdr1
bdr2
spa
work patio
hallway
entrance patio
deck N
pond
deck S
linen patio
patio a
ddescent patio

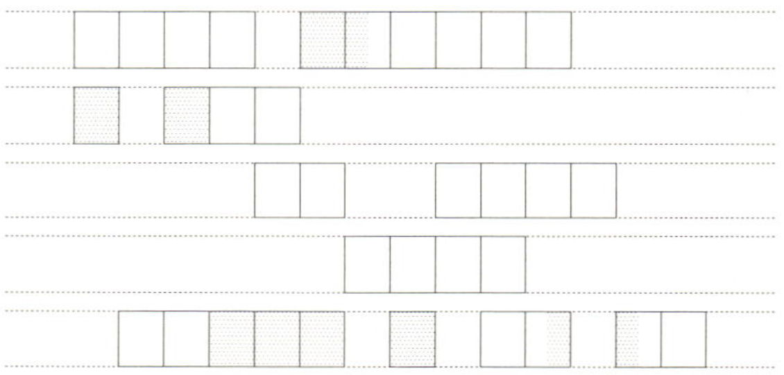

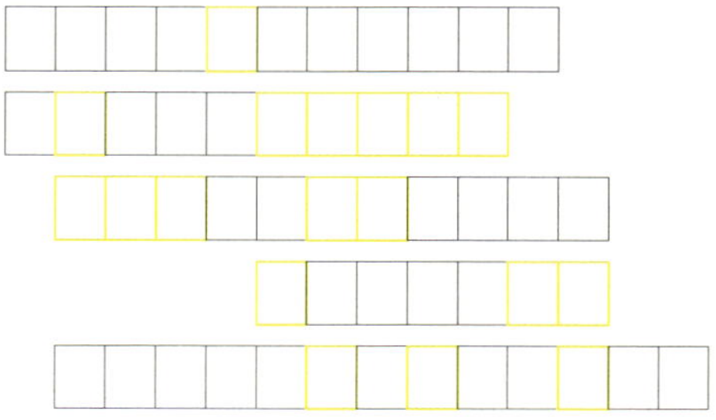

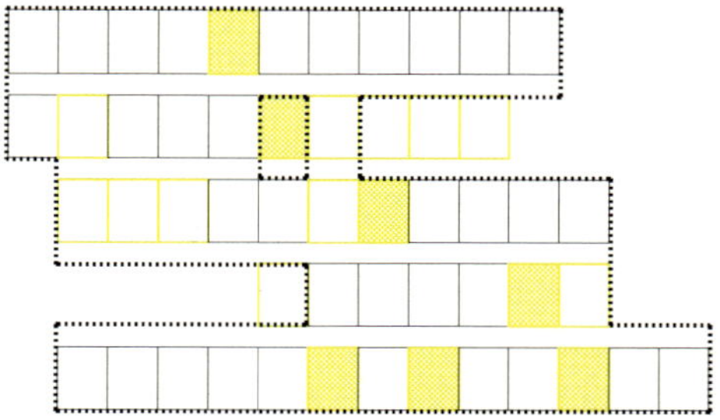

paved surface 836,41 m²

roofed surface 892,73 m²

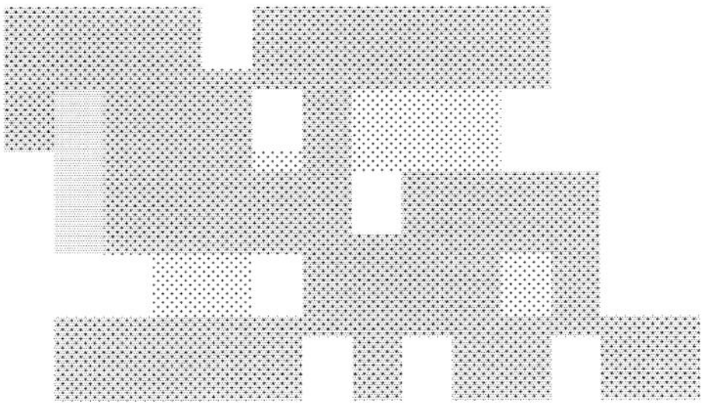

roofed + paved surface 933,88 m²

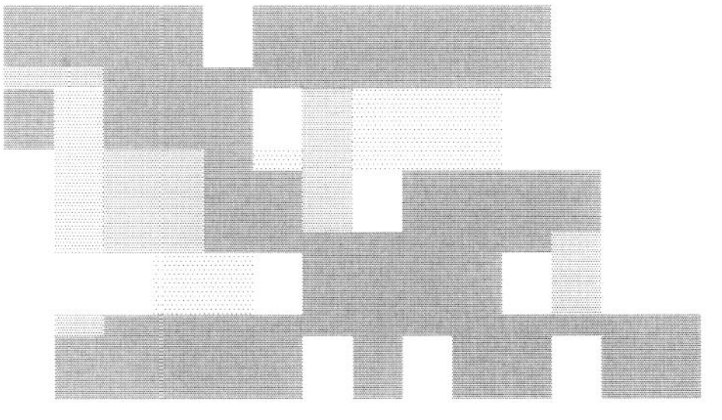

in-door surface 672,04 m²
out-door surface 261,84 m²
roofed and paved 123,31 m²
paved 41,07 m²
roofed 97,46 m²

opaque roof
translucent roof
transparent roof
permeable roof

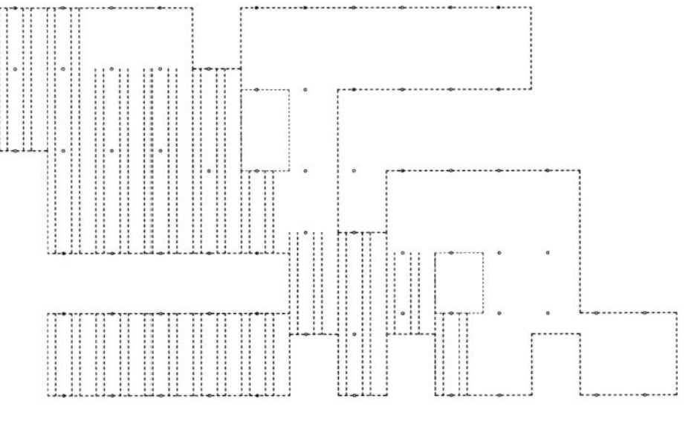

In plan, the stripes' disposition (programmatic bars) is by function: services on one side, daytime activities at the core and bedrooms on the other side. Perhaps now it is easier to understand how implied corridors are spatially incorporated into the rooms they cross, but they remain as visual corridors along the plan. On the other hand, the initial modular grid fades with diagonal connections that produce landslides of parts over others.

Going back to the role of the supporting structure in the construction of space, in this project, despite the structural evidence of vertical supports and metal trusses of the roof and its consistency with the spatial order, one could say that the structural elements are not exactly relevant to the spatial definition. Their contribution is more to be considered in the desire for material abstraction.

All spaces in the house are somehow equivalent allowing for layout flexibility and equating, for example, the spatial quality of the living room with the parking area, which could eventually become a gathering place.

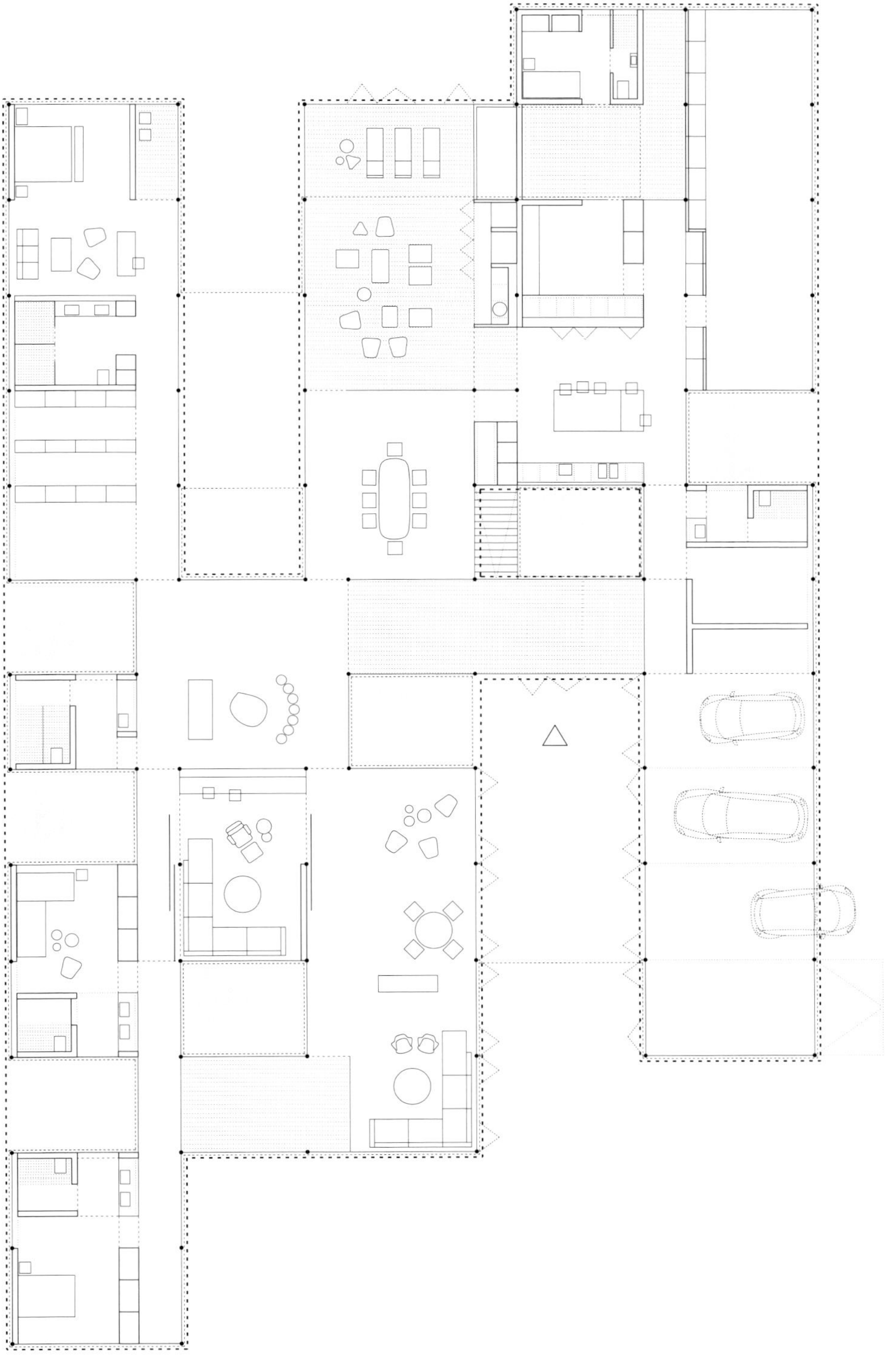

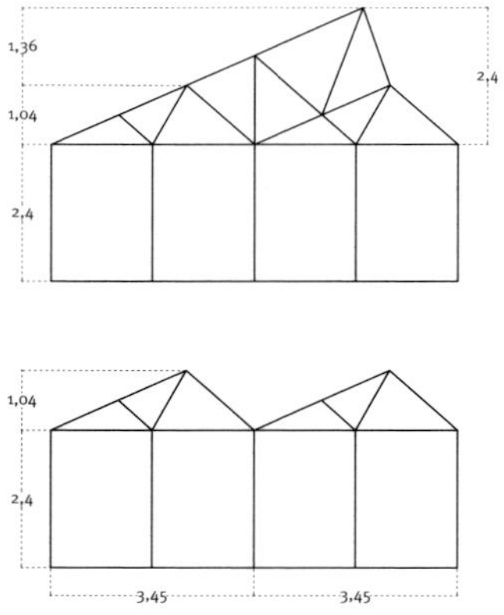

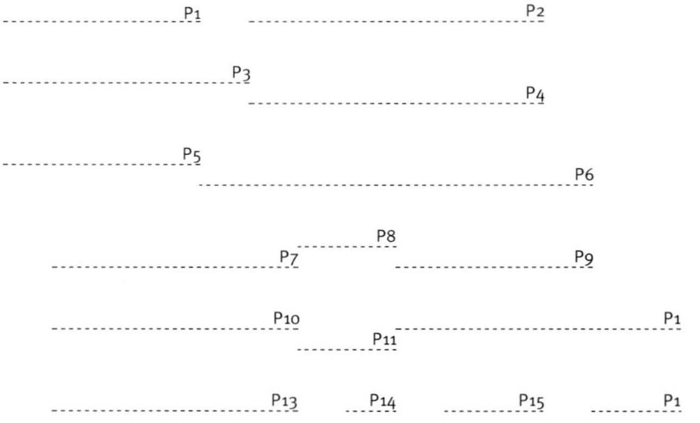

In addition to the floor plan strategy, this project incorporates a sectional movement, merging into the single folded plate what was understood volumetrically before (in the clinics) as two levels. This folded surface as roof has a syncopated rhythm of double and single pace according to the program and incorporates the interstitial spaces between the programmatic bars alternately to one side or the other, producing an unexpected transversal continuity of the roof skirts. There are single and double module structural trusses, with congruent slopes and geometries – i.e. the large contains the small.

It is again a field condition, an extensive matrix upon which a geometrical strategy is imposed by modulation of the program (interior and exterior spaces) in visual continuity. Light comes from above, recurrently this time through the sawtooth roof that acts as a light-directing layer.

In touching the ground, the house is gently placed at the front on a green lawn that abruptly becomes a reef. The palafitic condition creates an antigravity perception by flotation to the main floor and a new spatial opportunity underneath. Along with it comes the idea of the sixth façade (the belly), a reflective folded plane that blurs what it reflects.

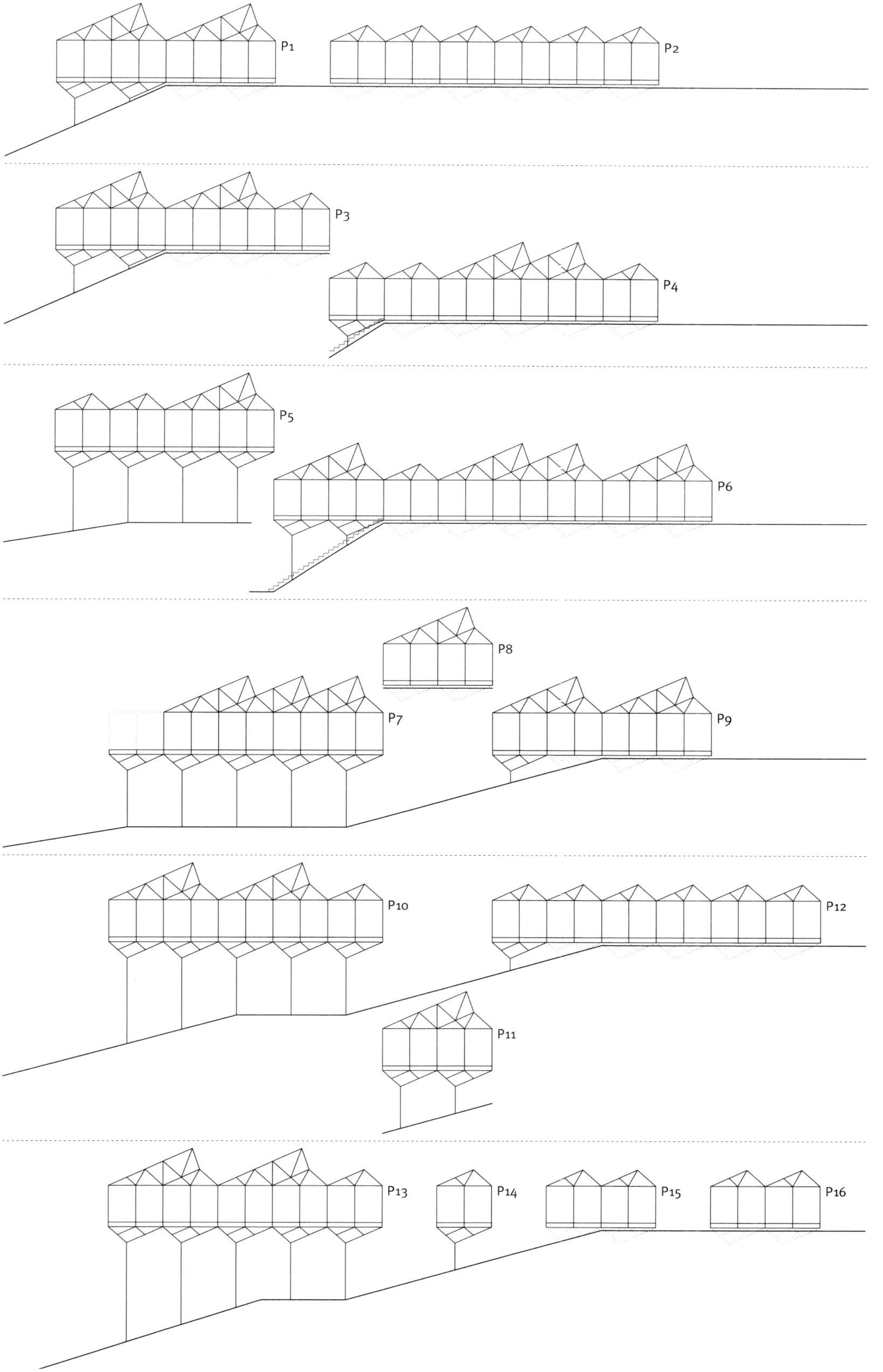
P1
P2
P3
P4
P5
P6
P8
P7
P9
P10
P12
P11
P13
P14
P15
P16

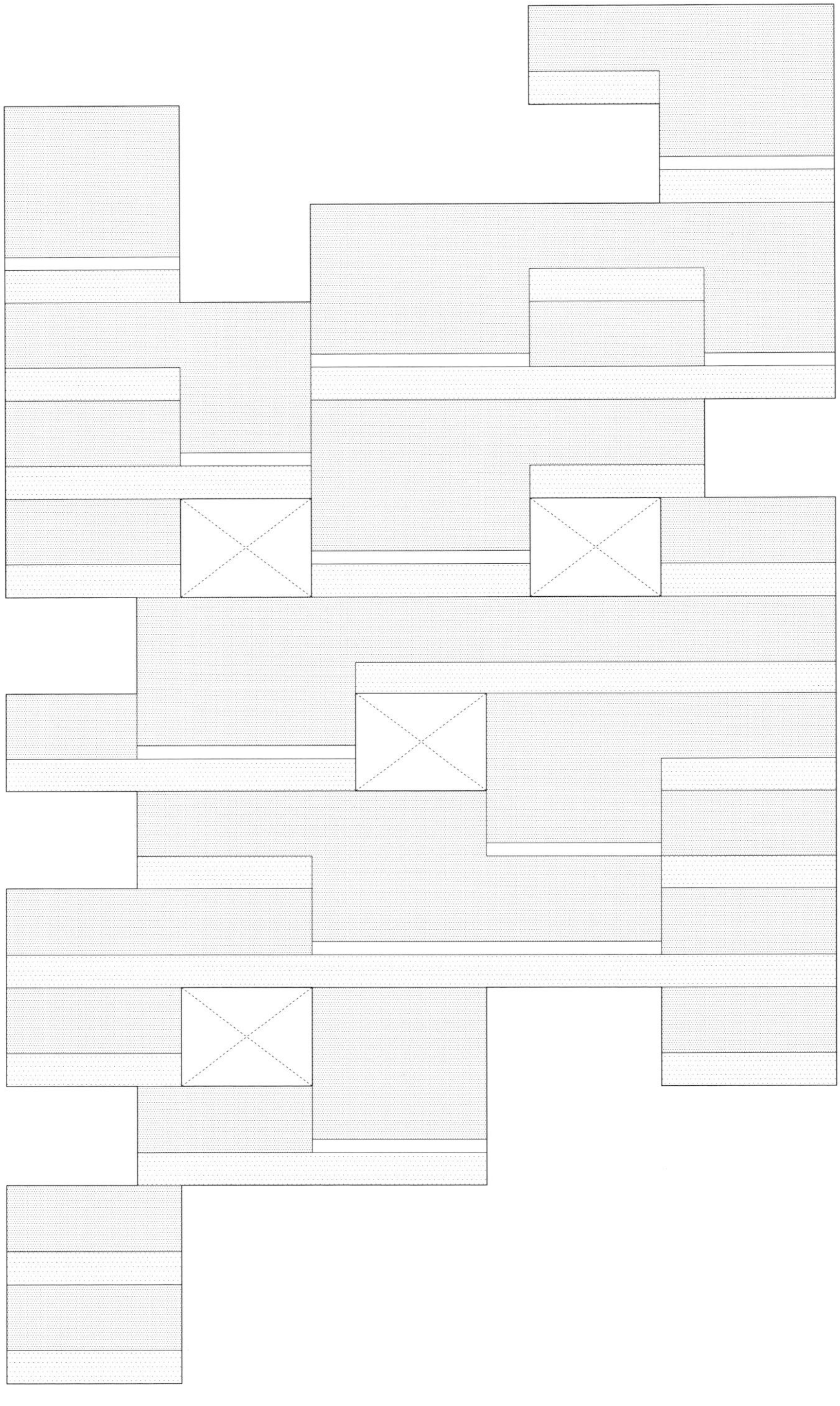

Fifth façade

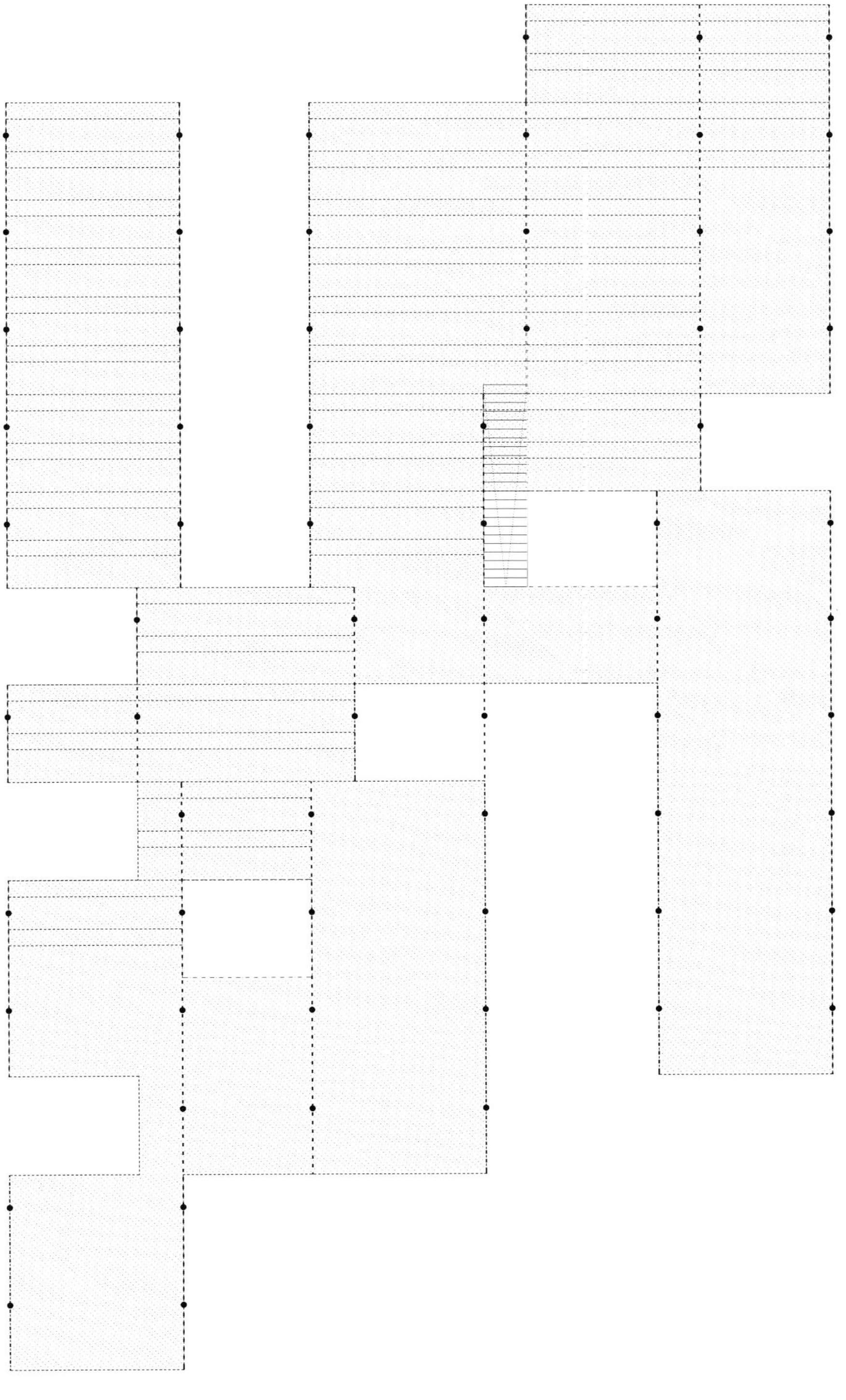

Sixth façade

The Pursuit of Rigor to Confront the Inexact

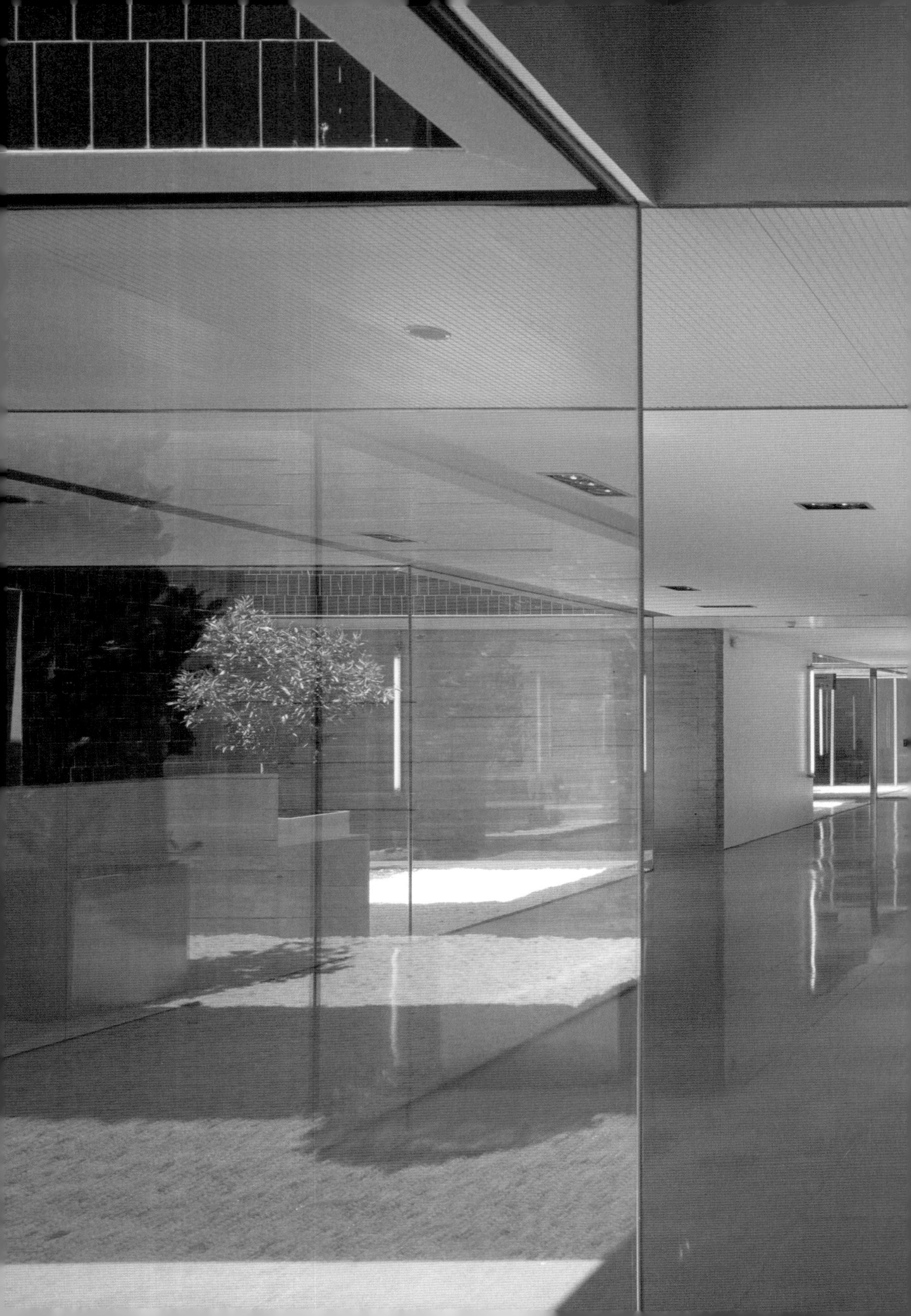

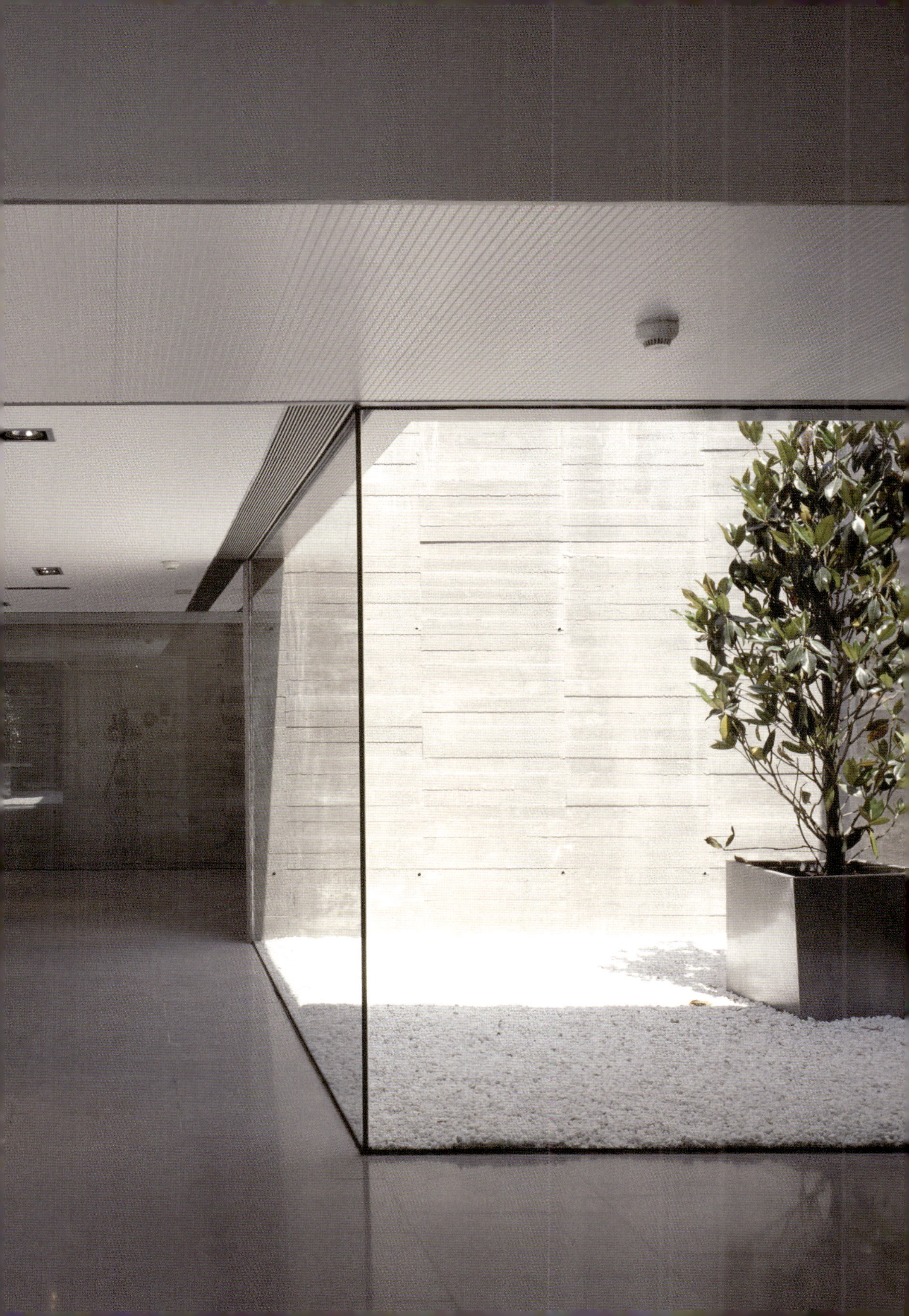

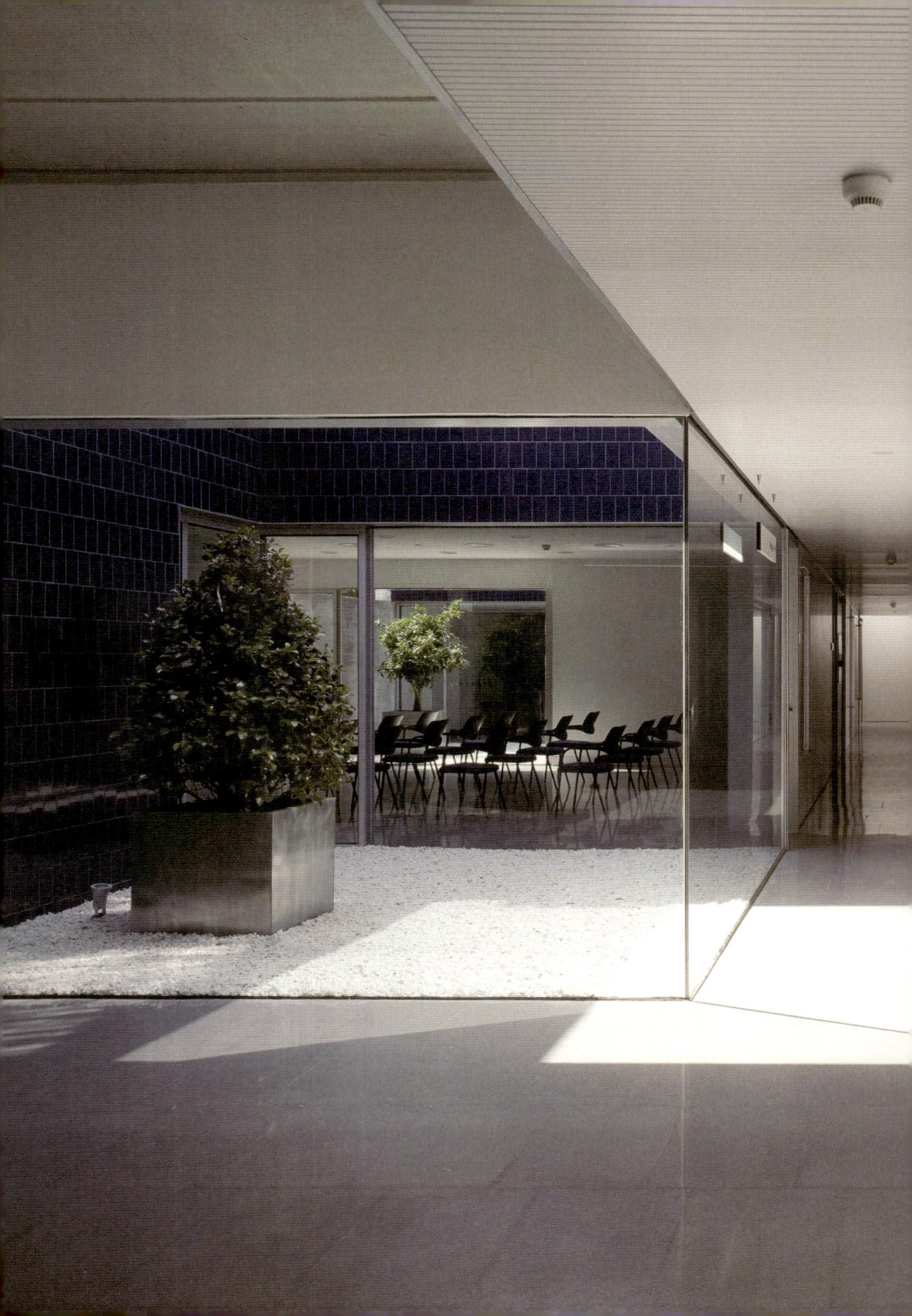

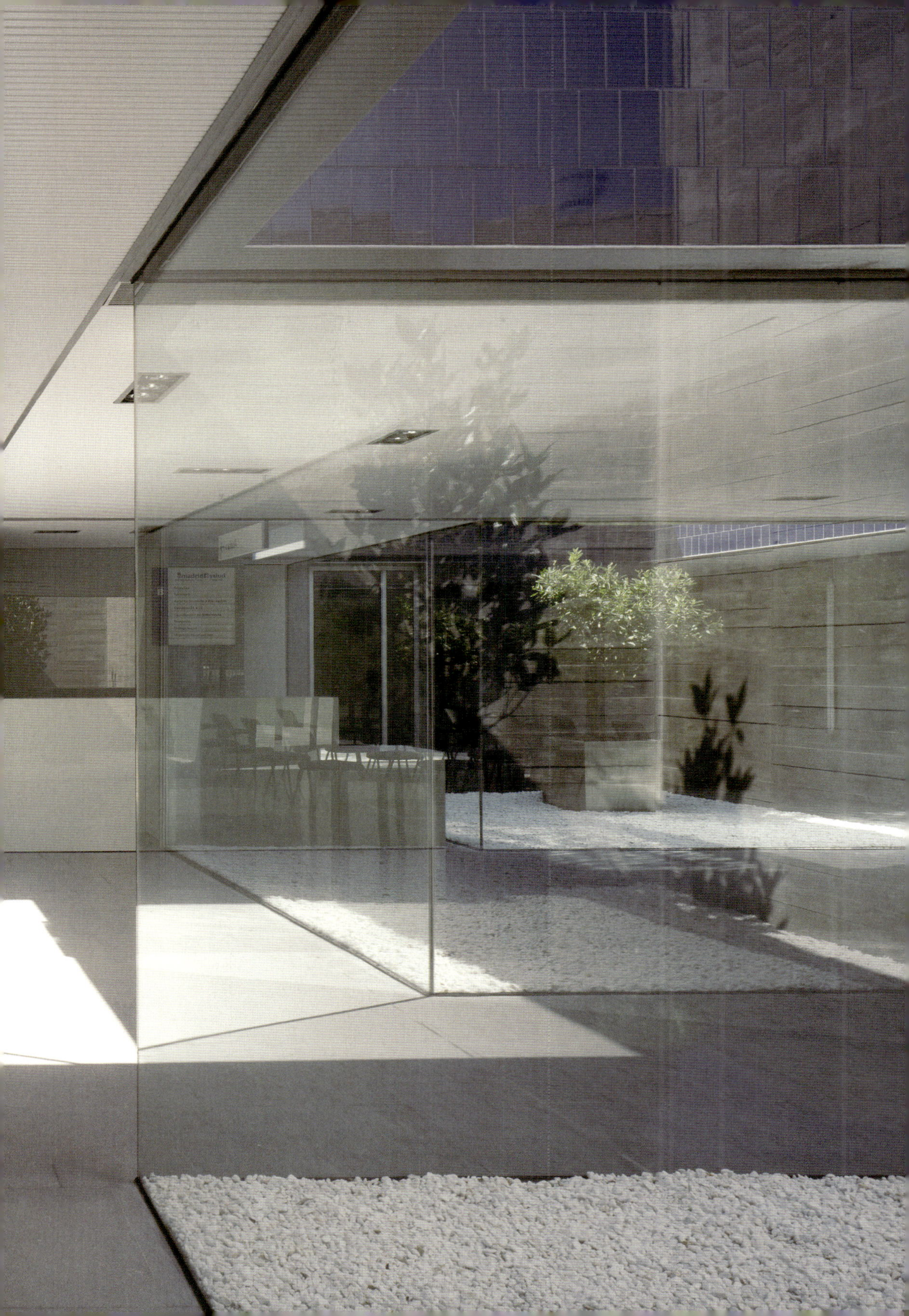

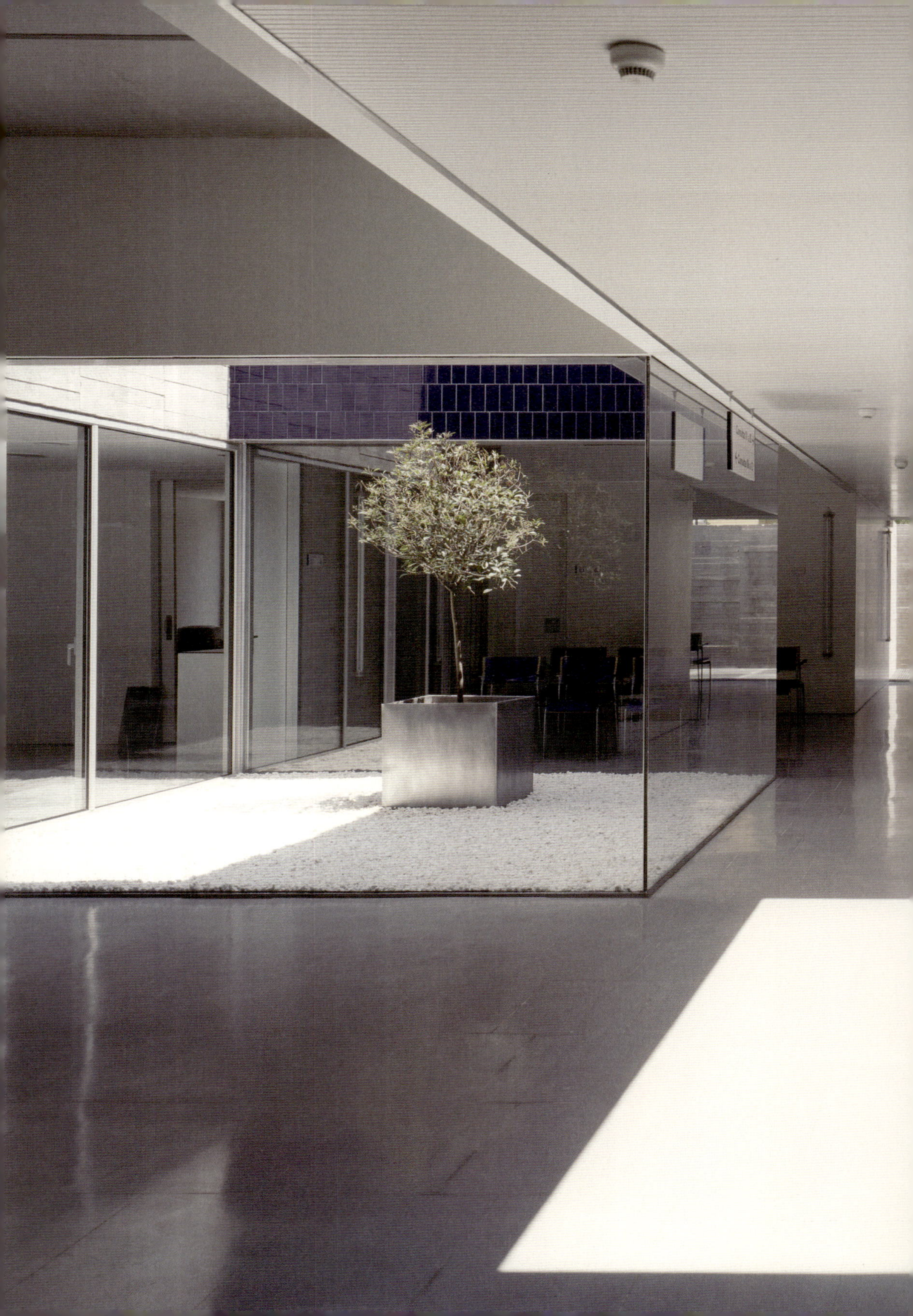

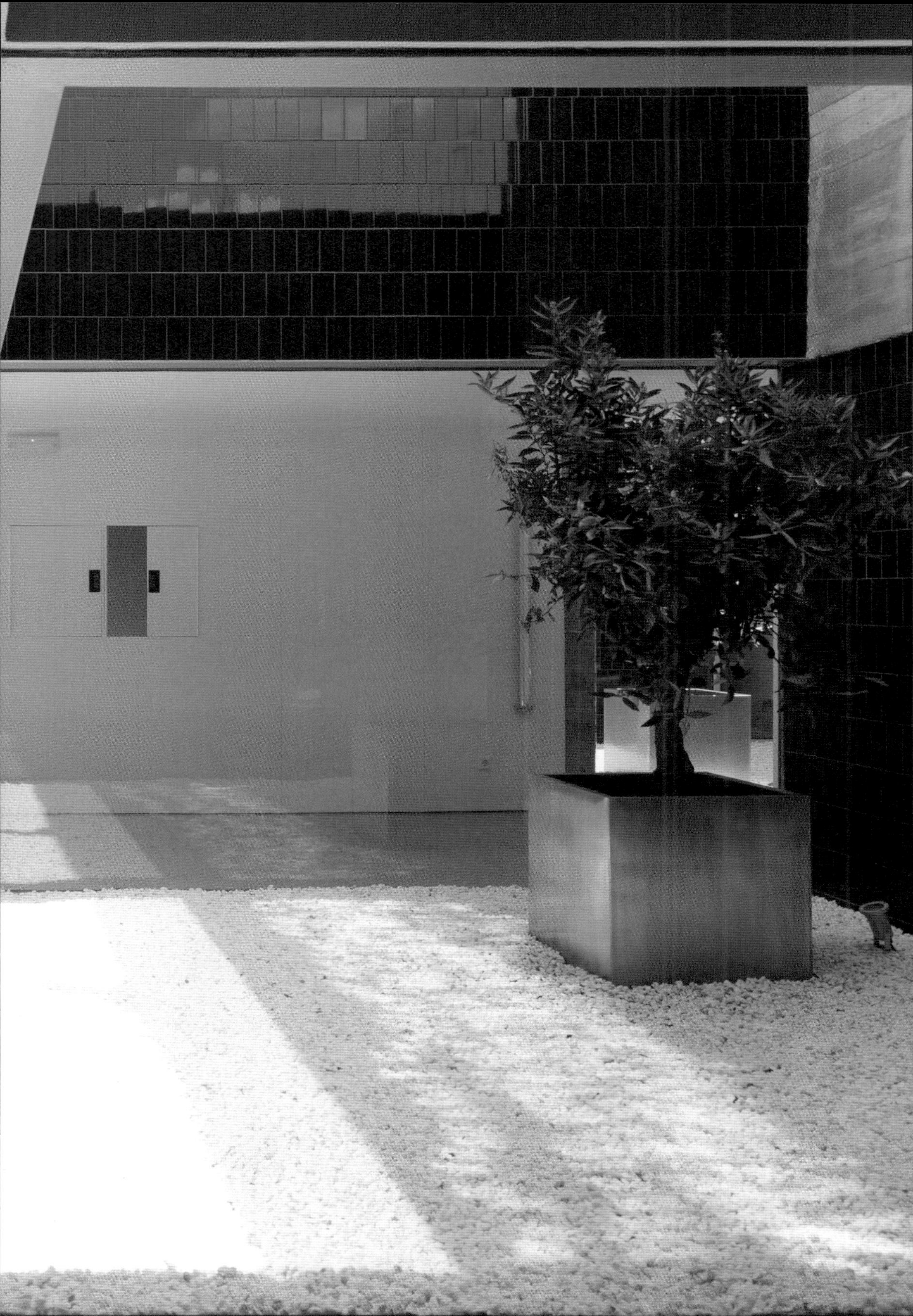

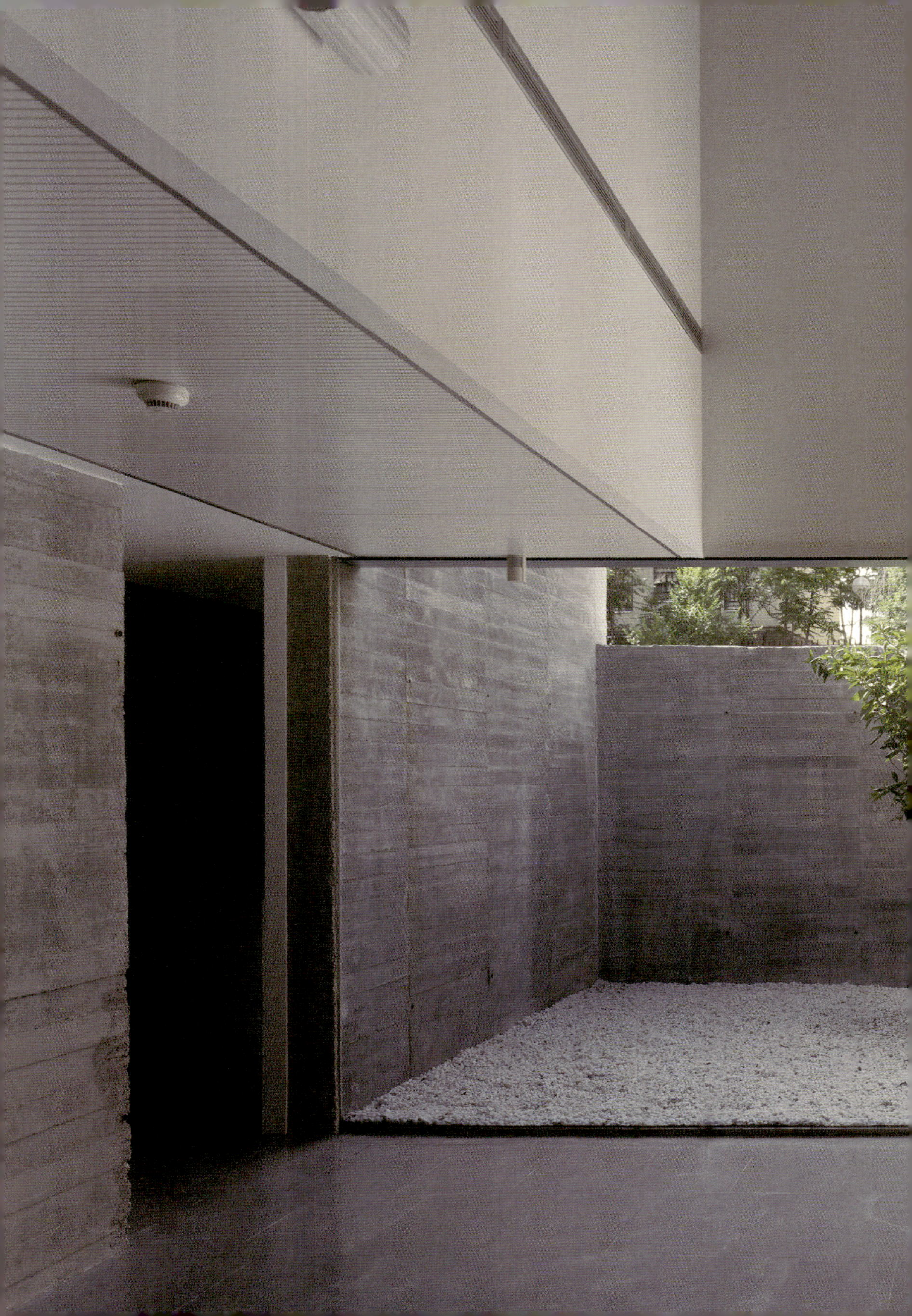

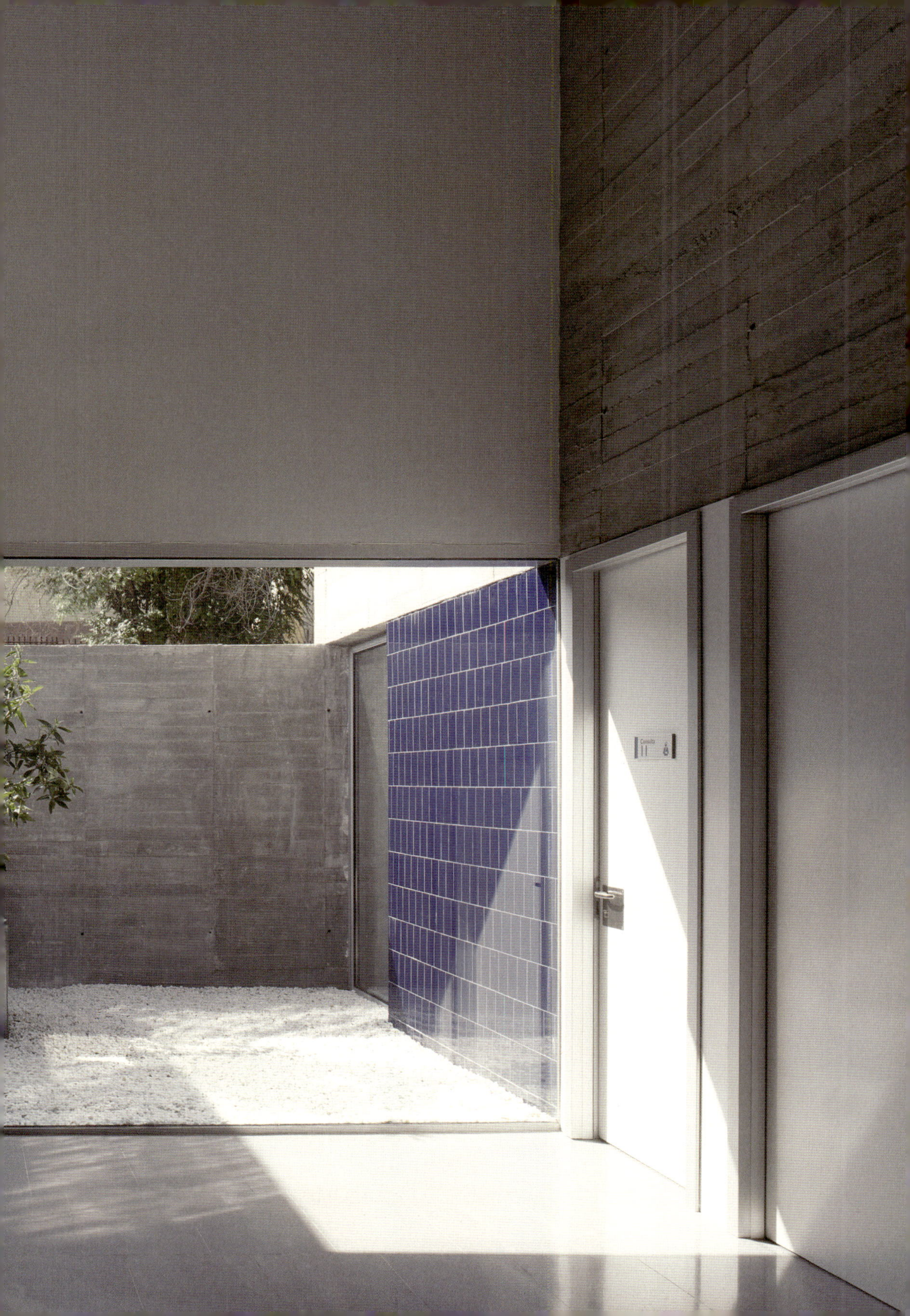

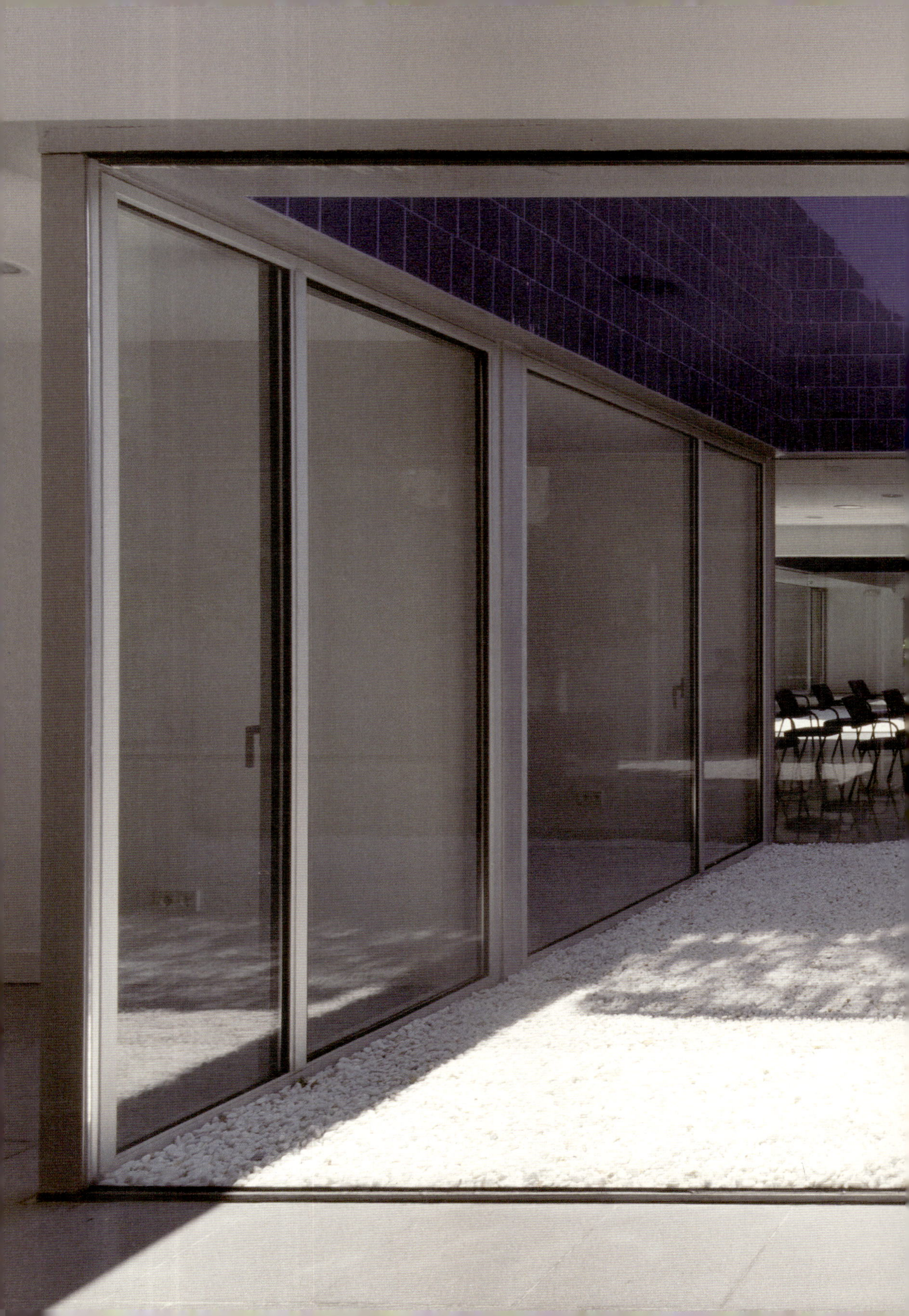

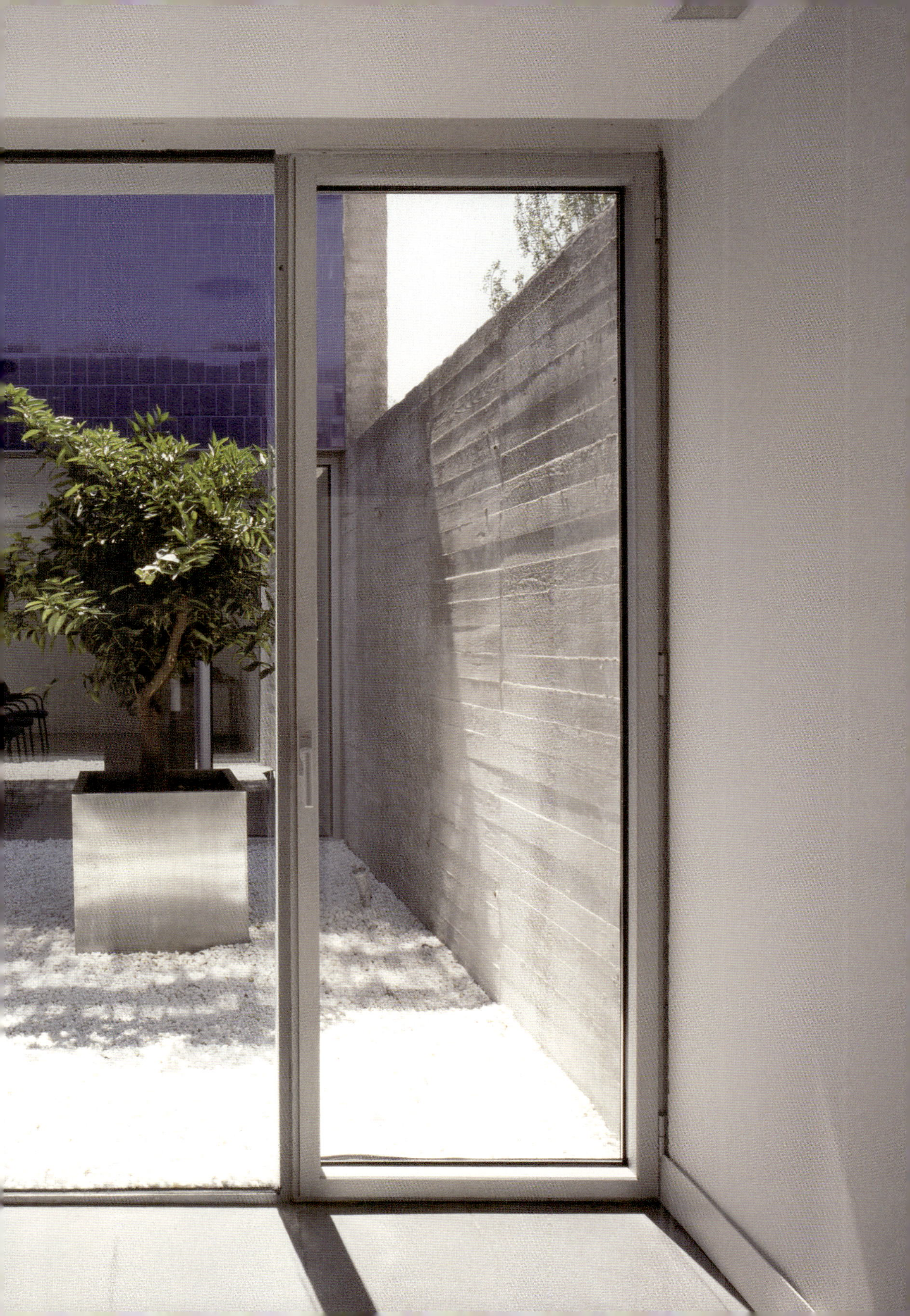

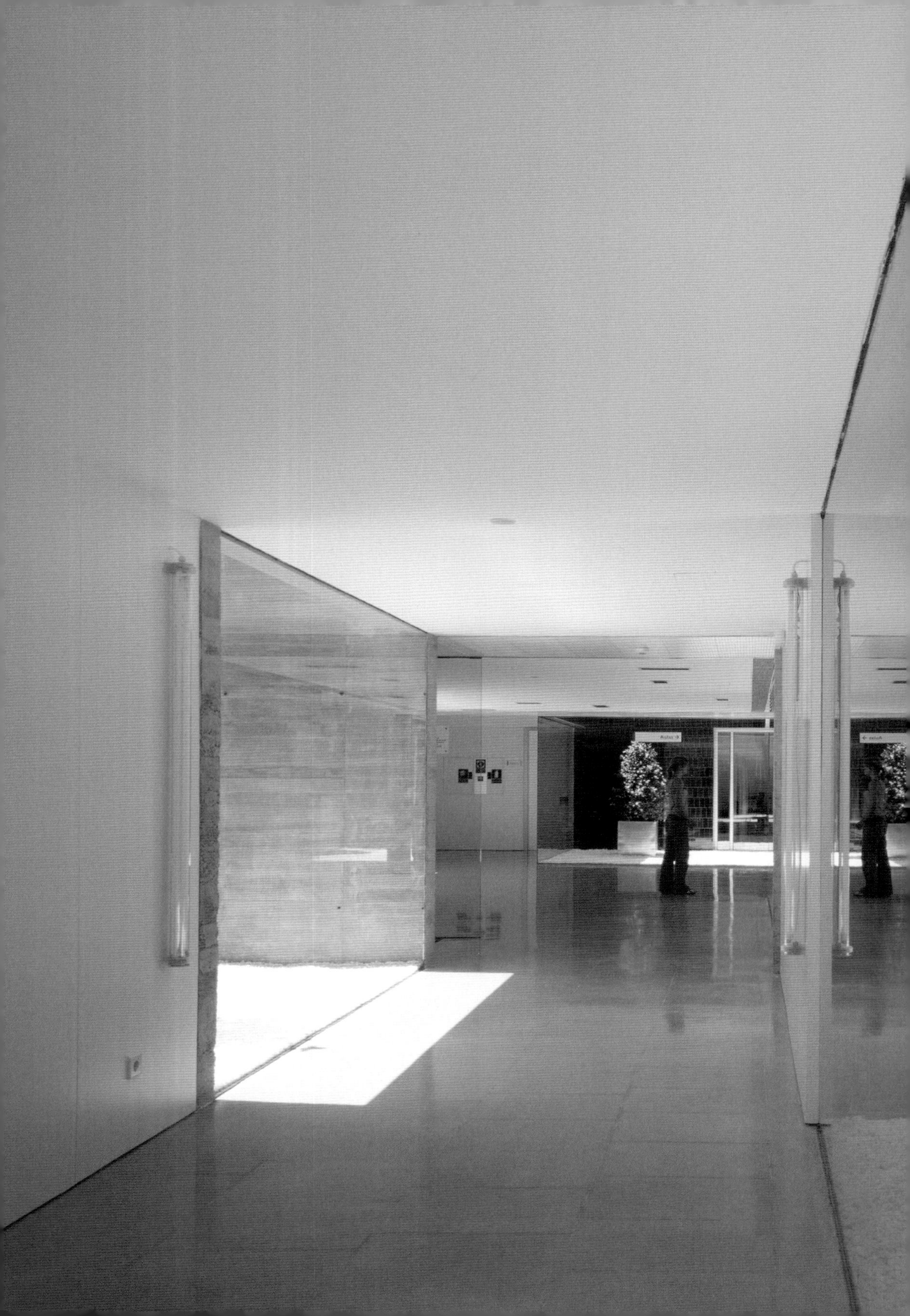

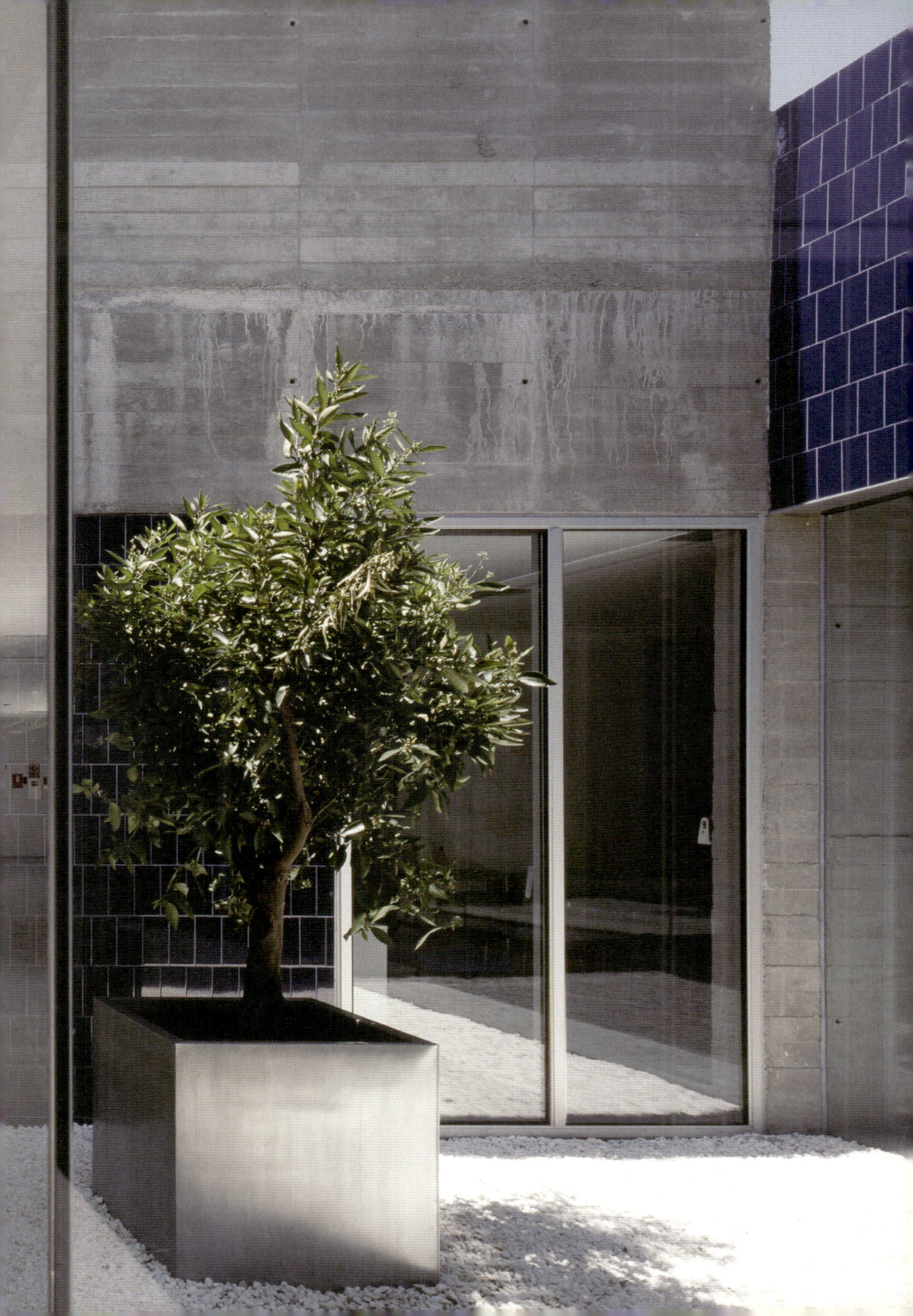

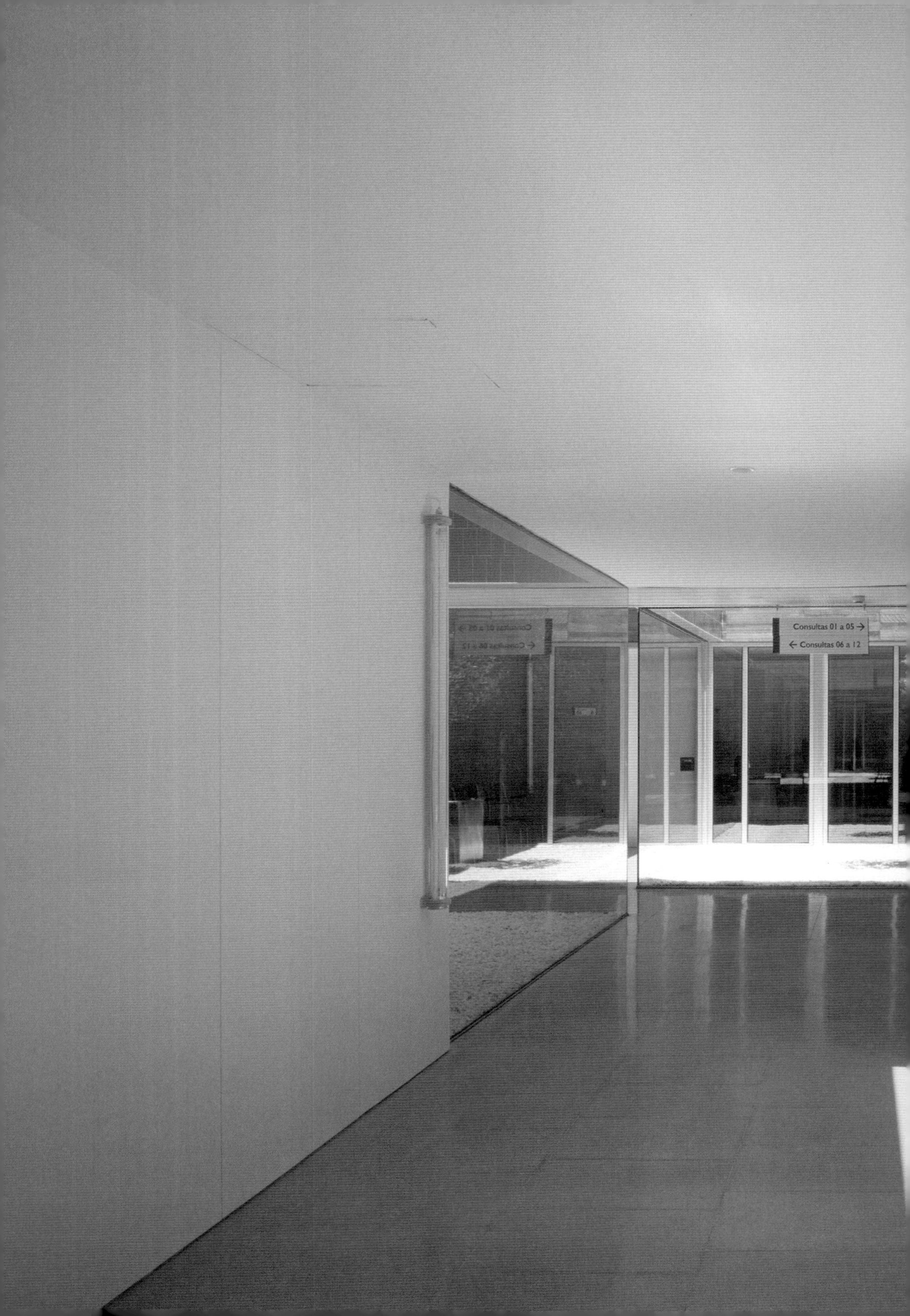

Consultas 01 a 05 →
← Consultas 06 a 12

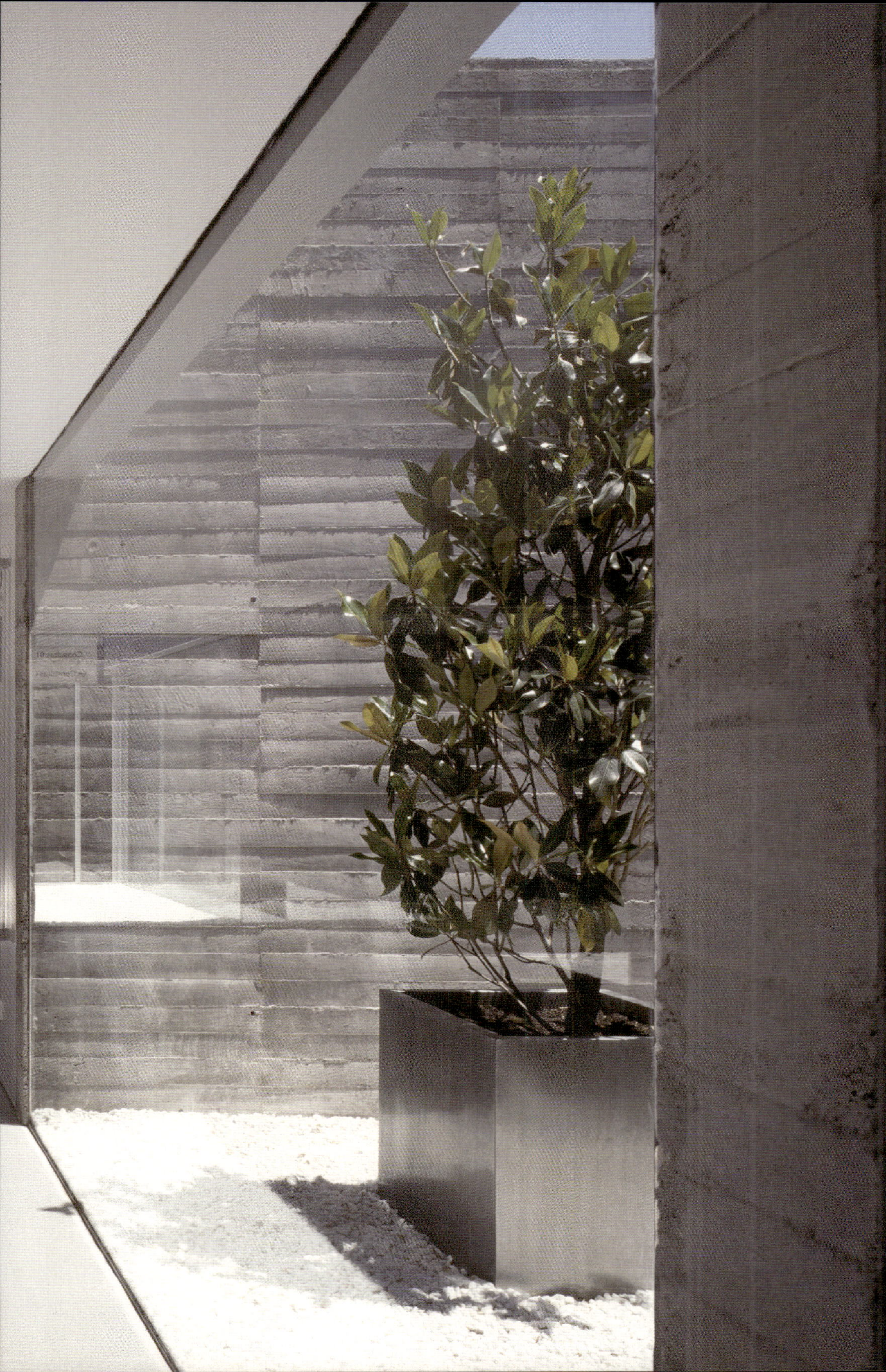

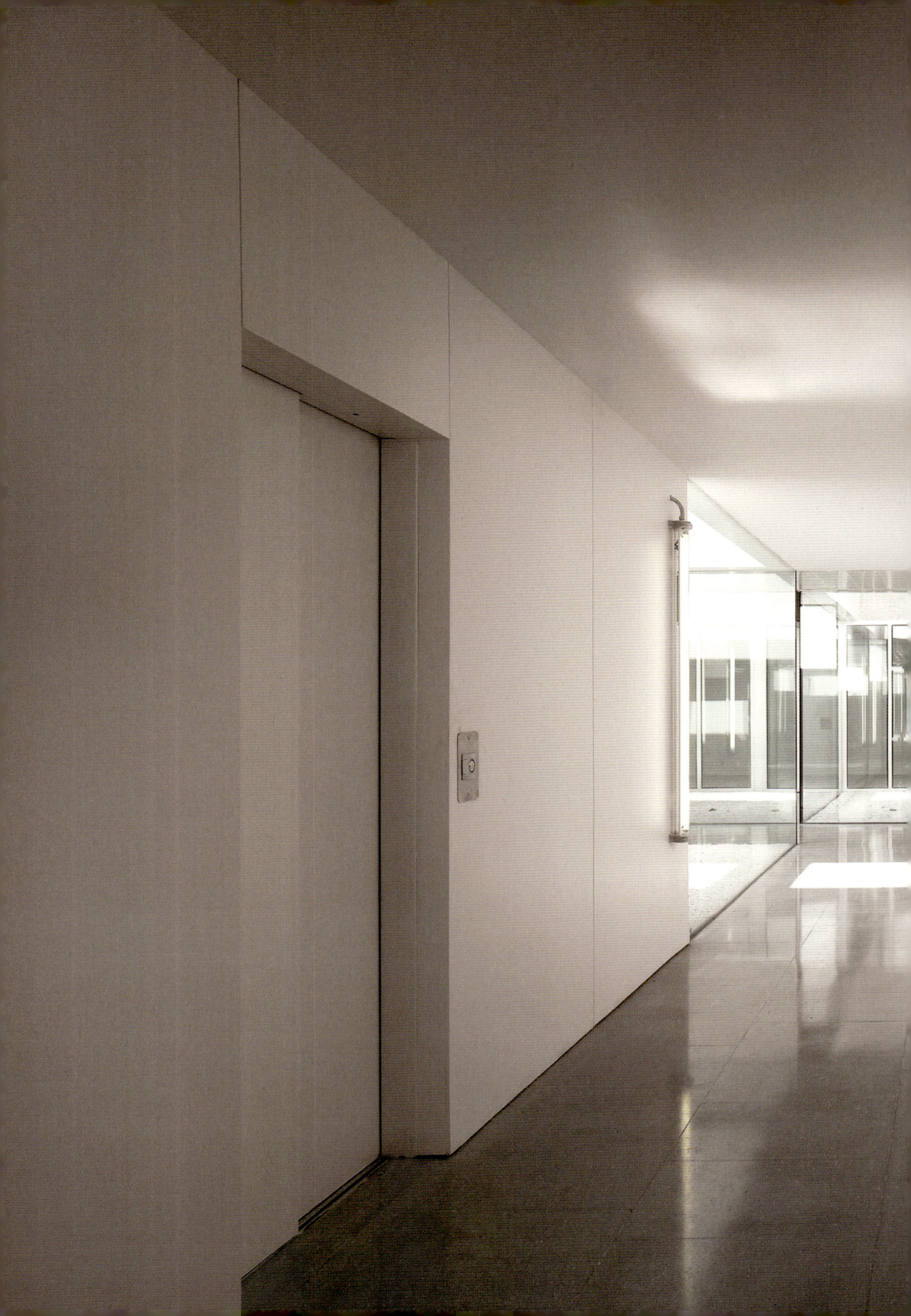

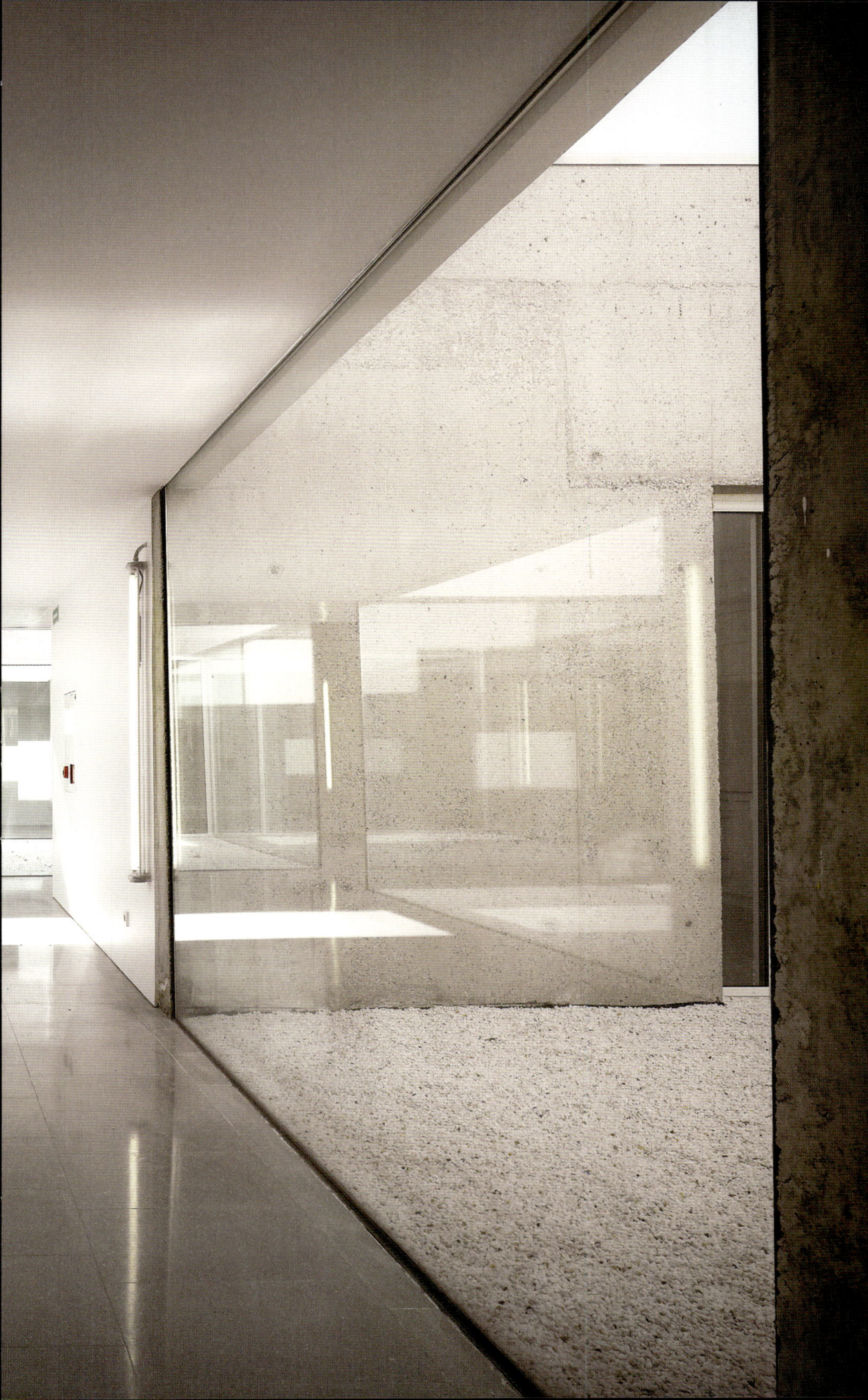

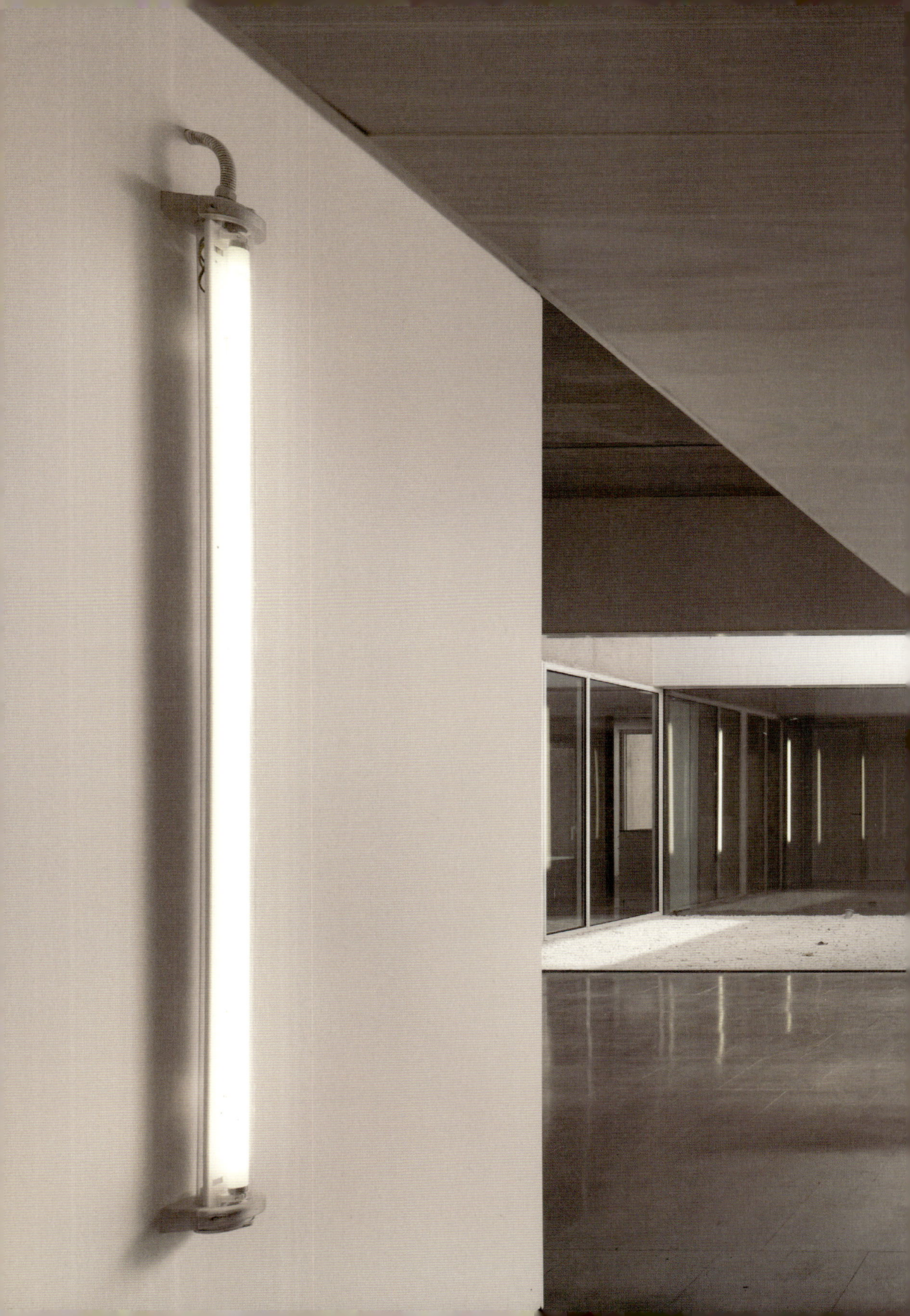

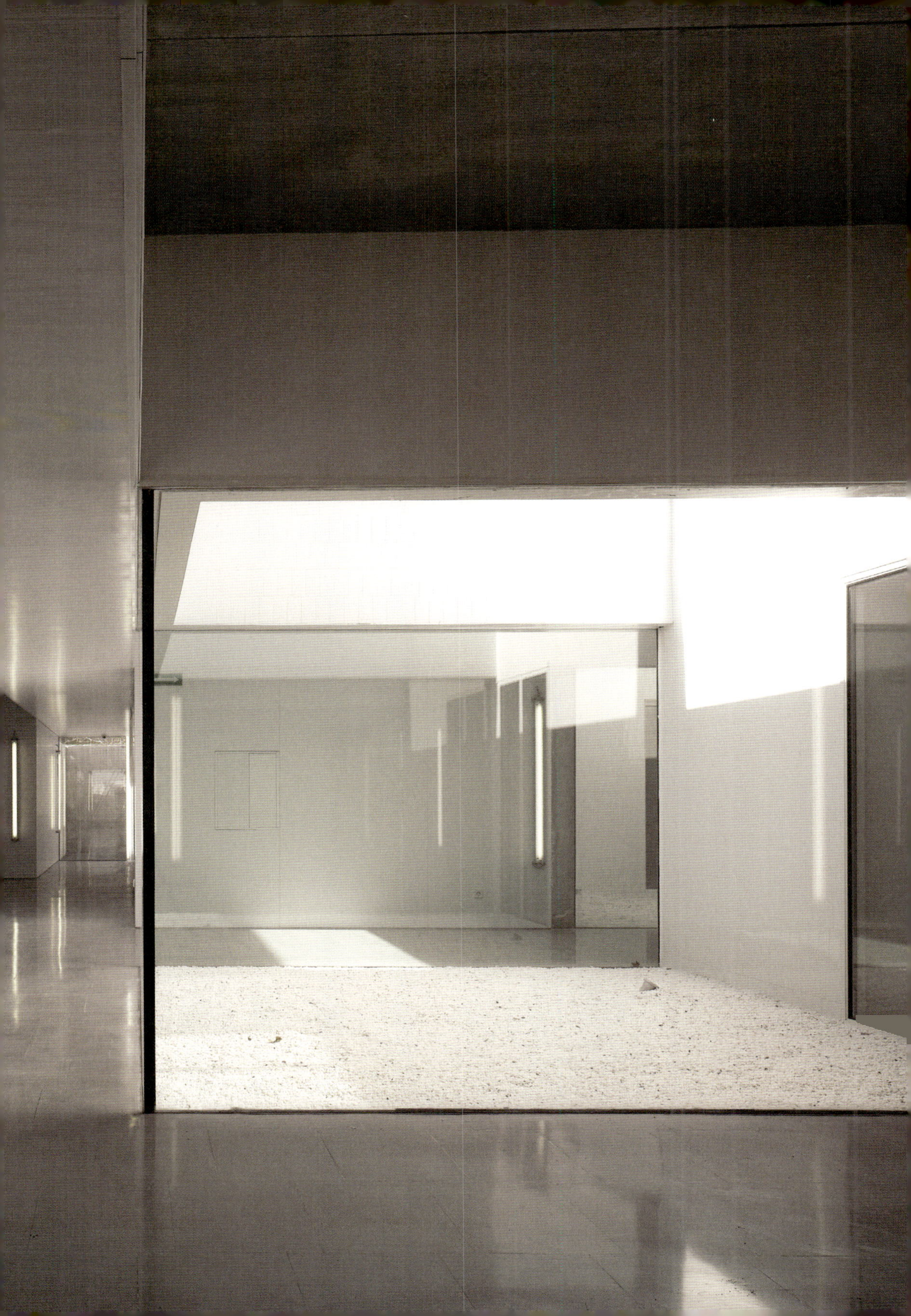

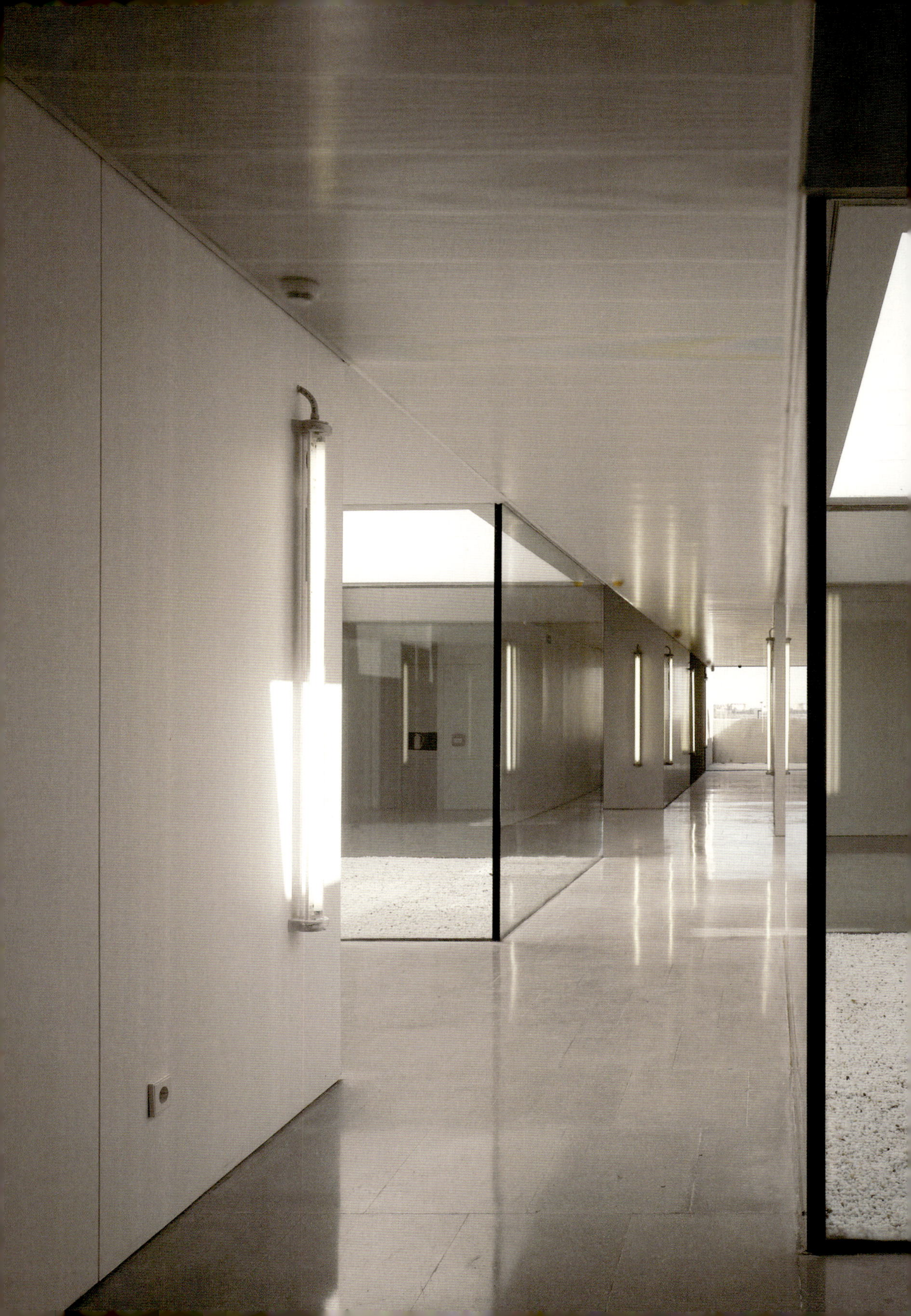

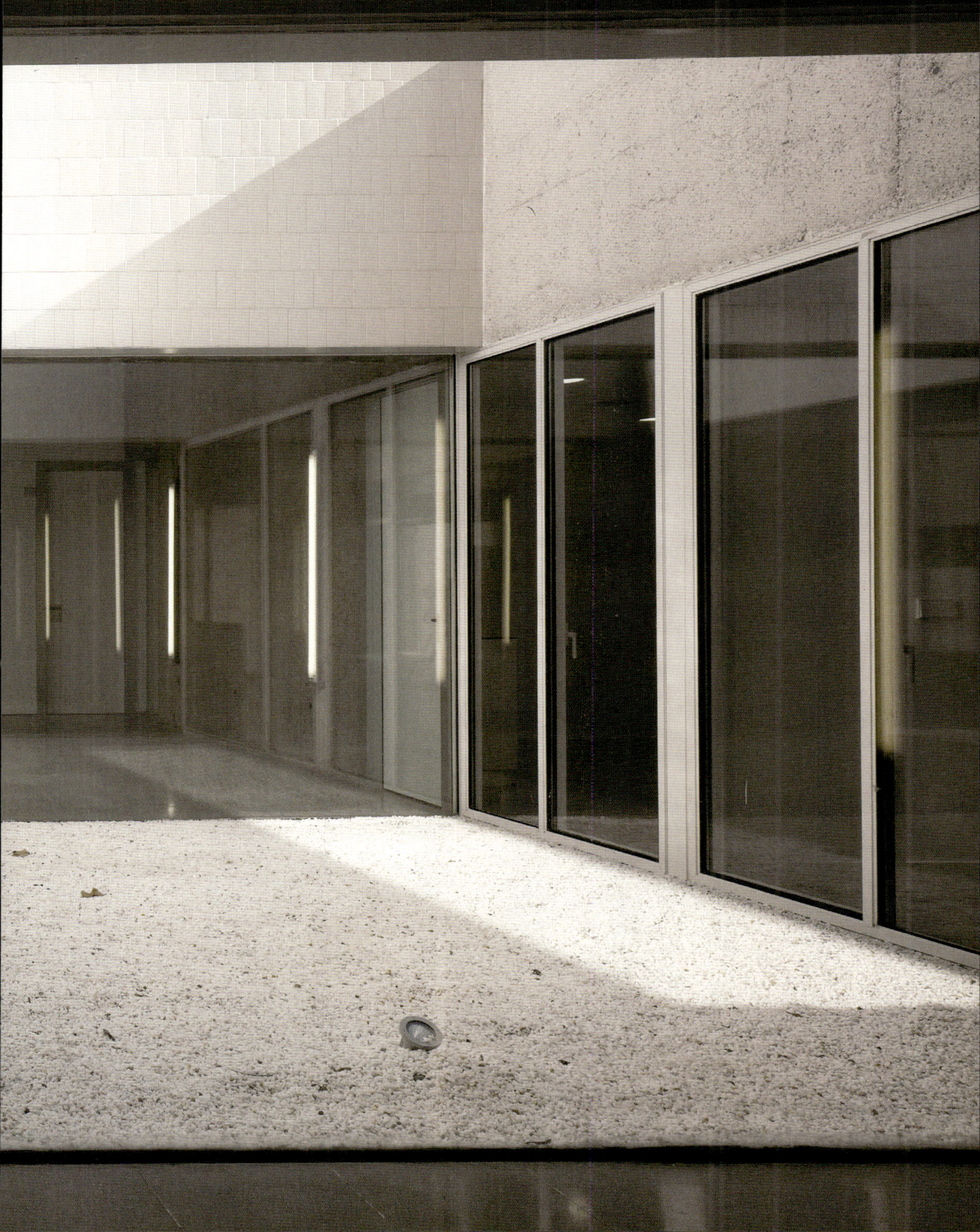

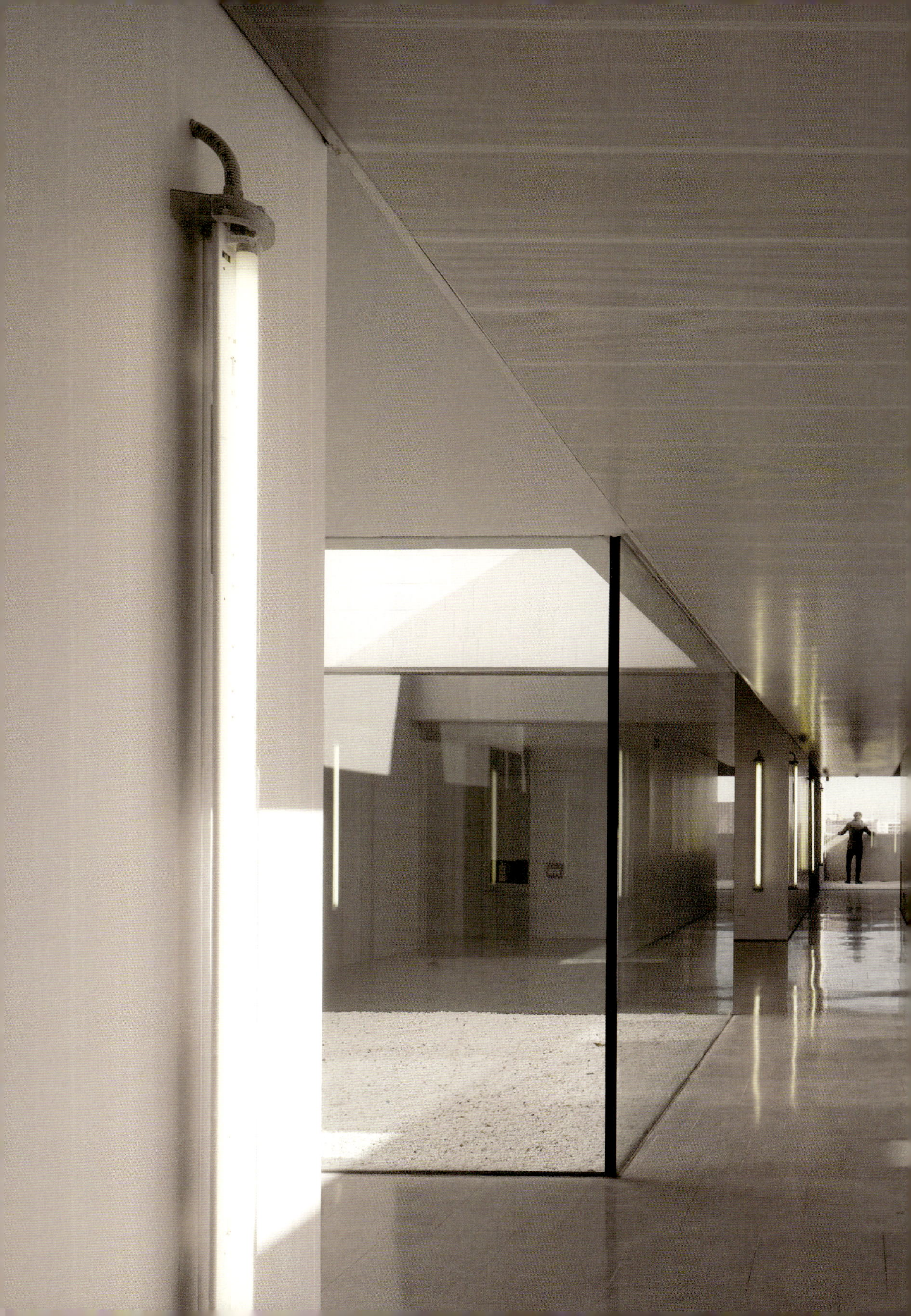

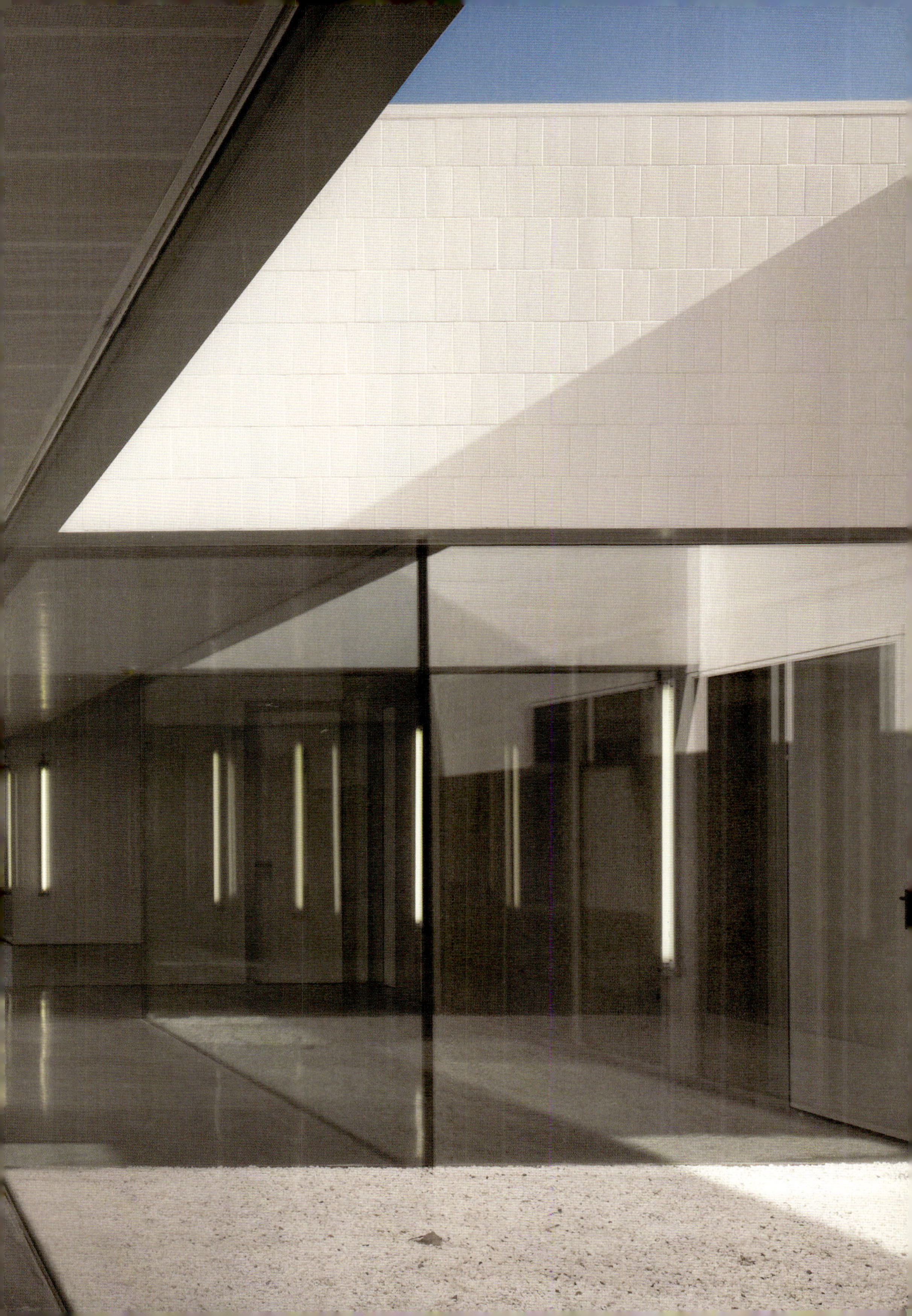

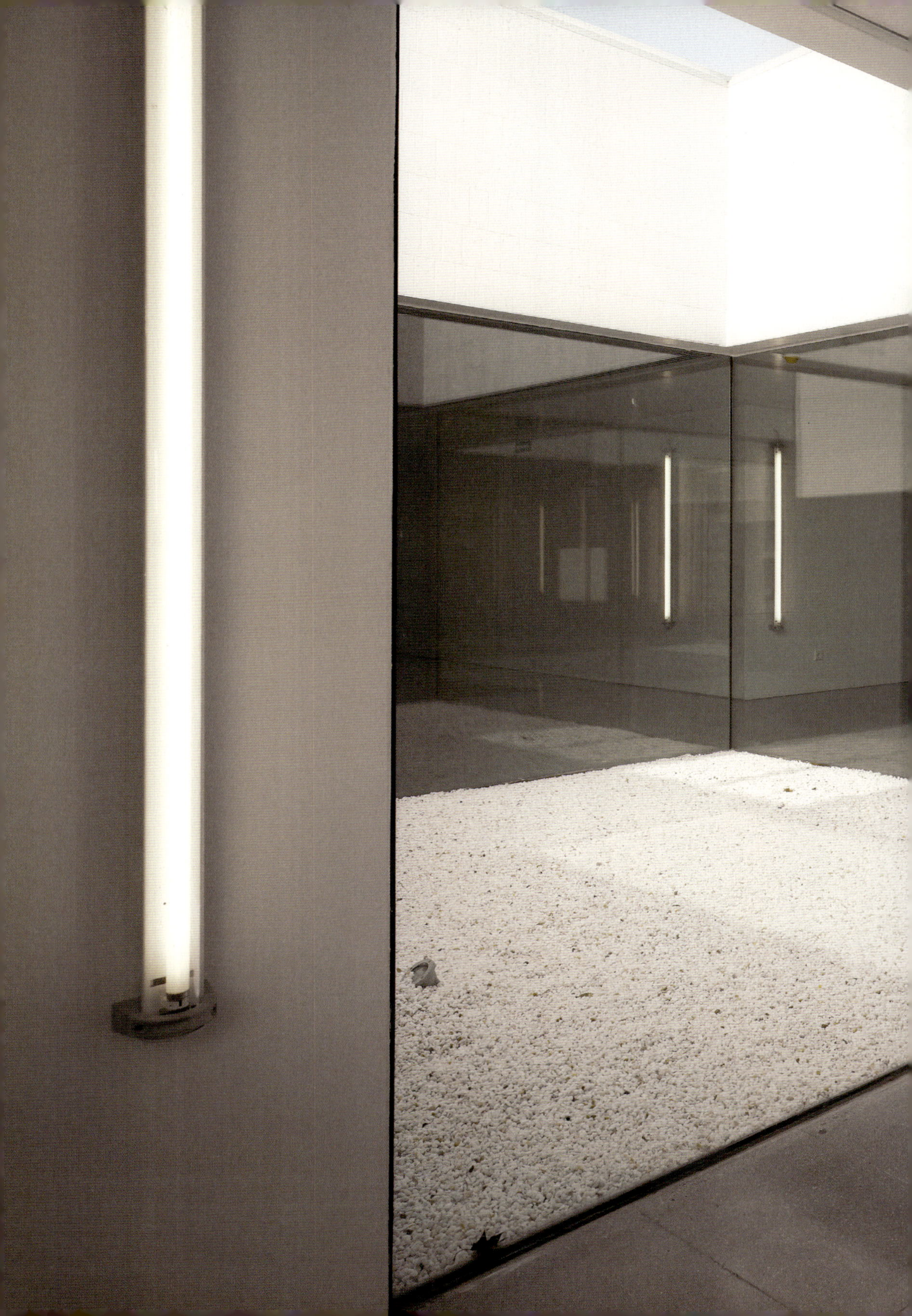

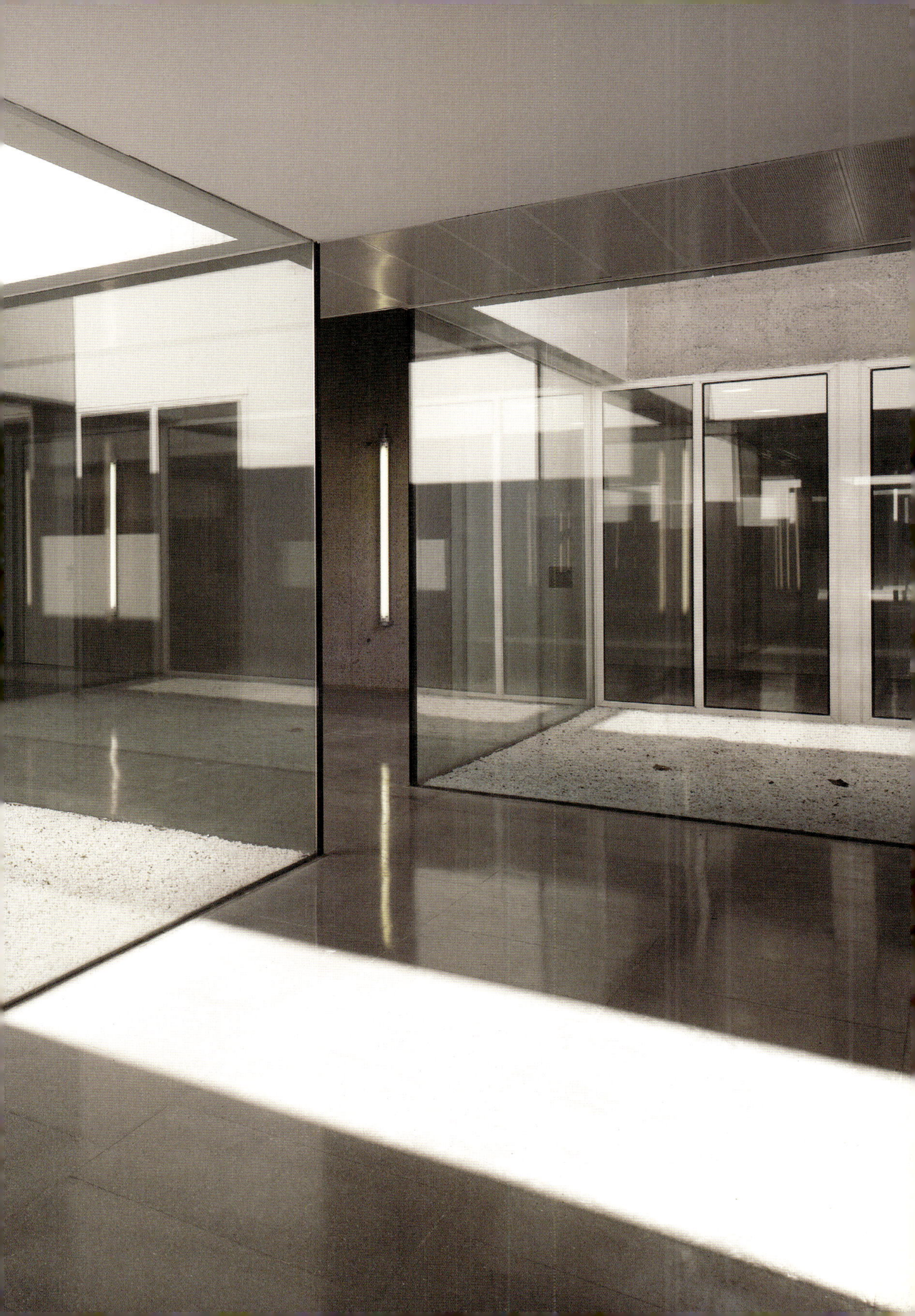

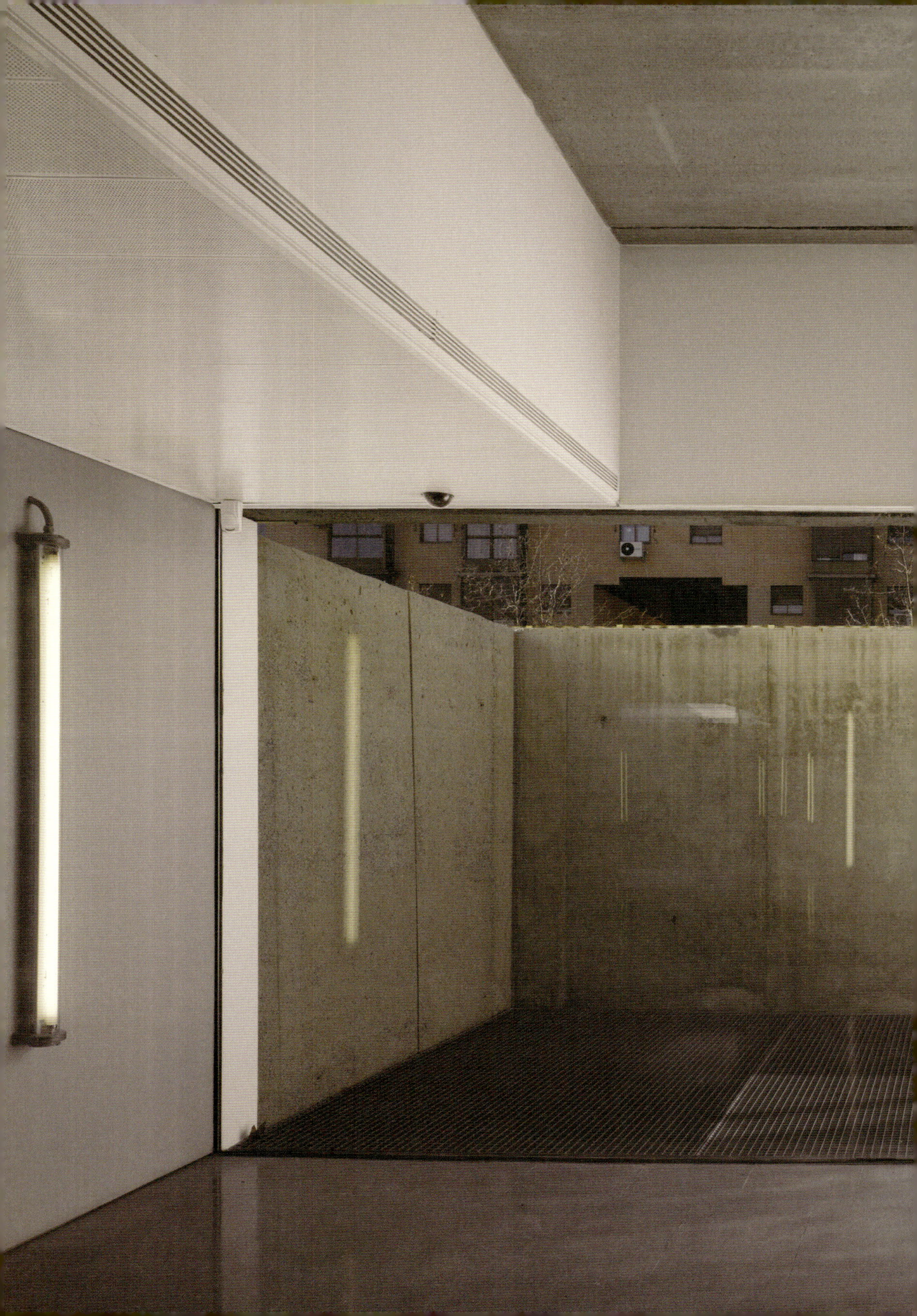

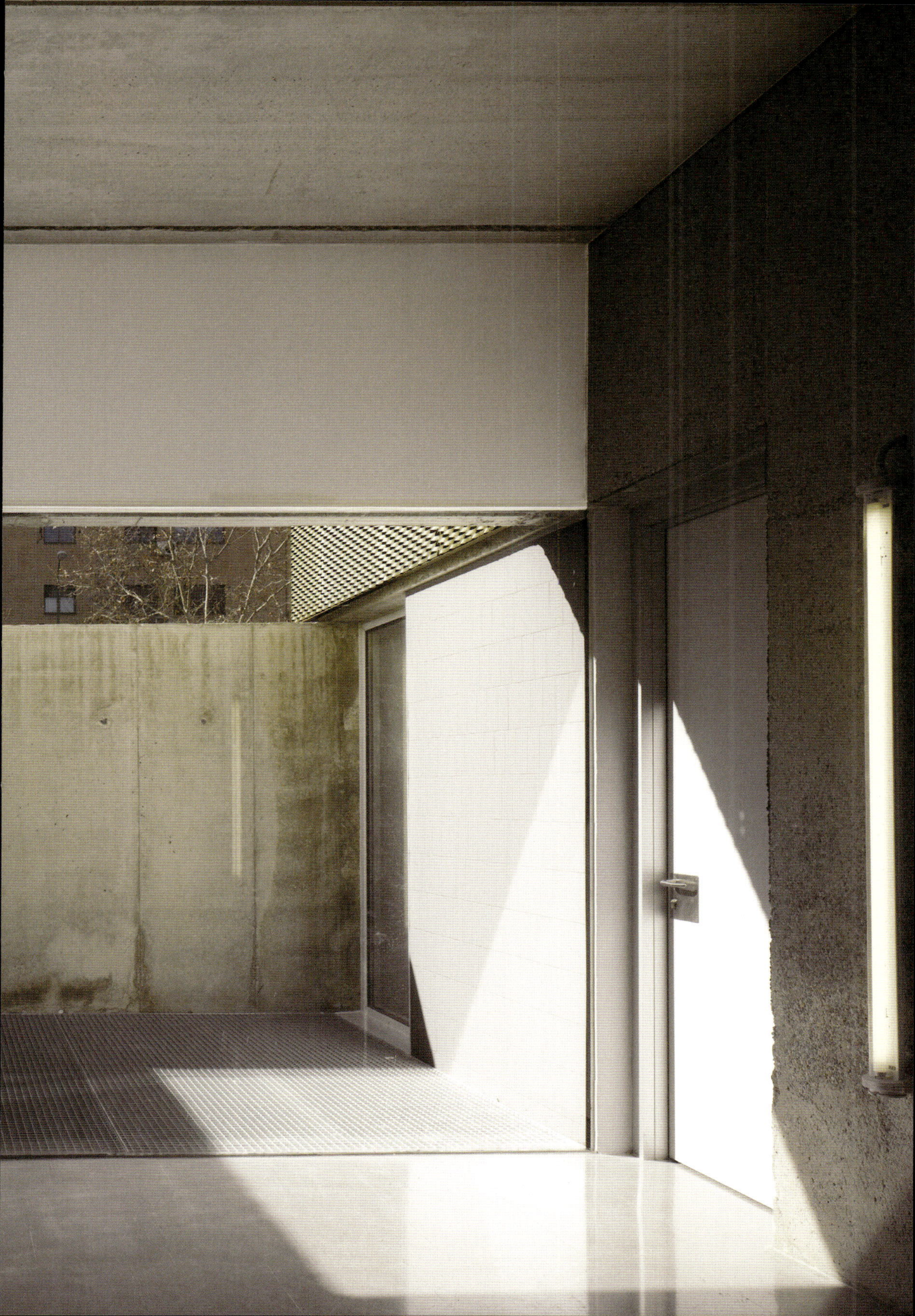

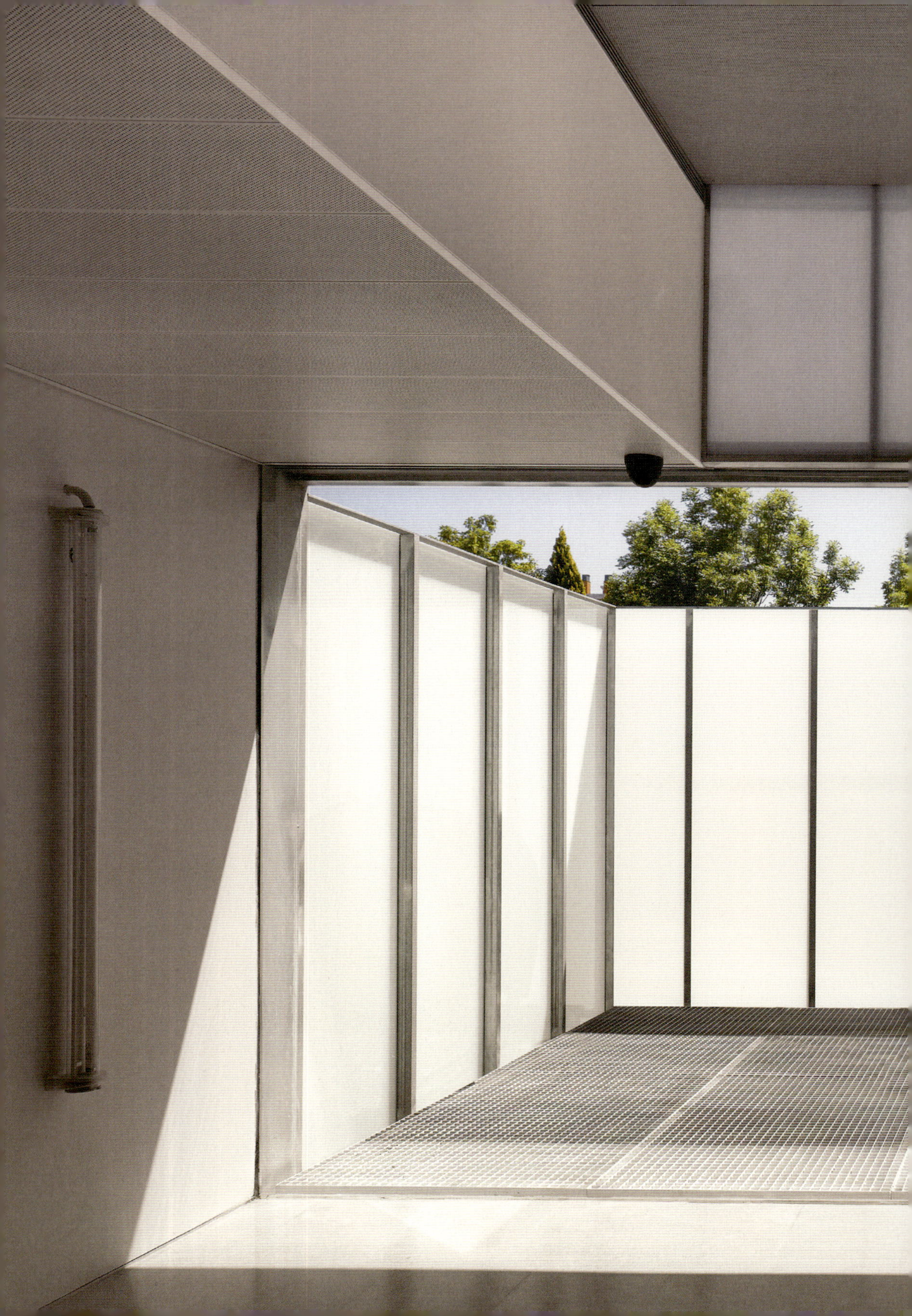

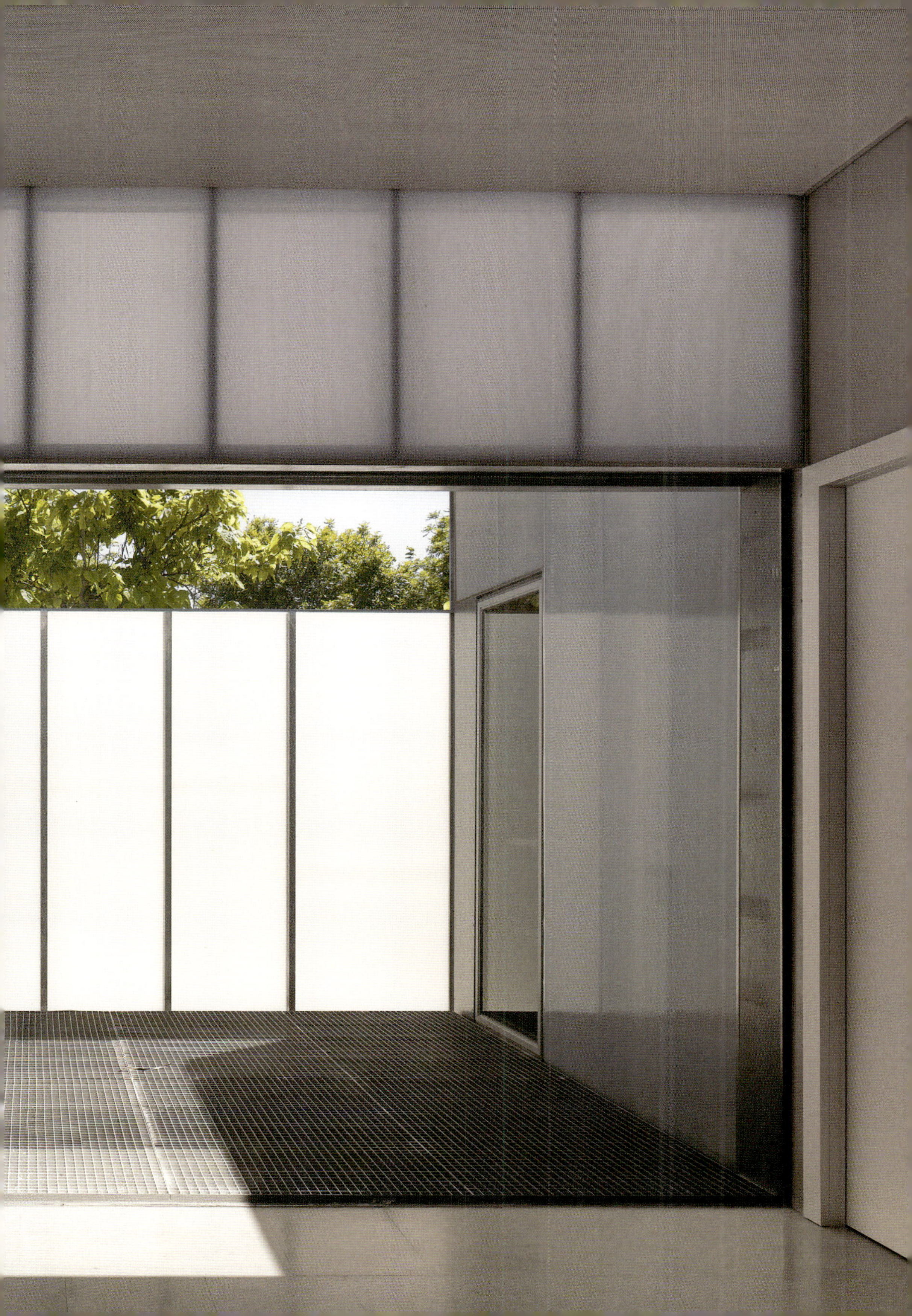

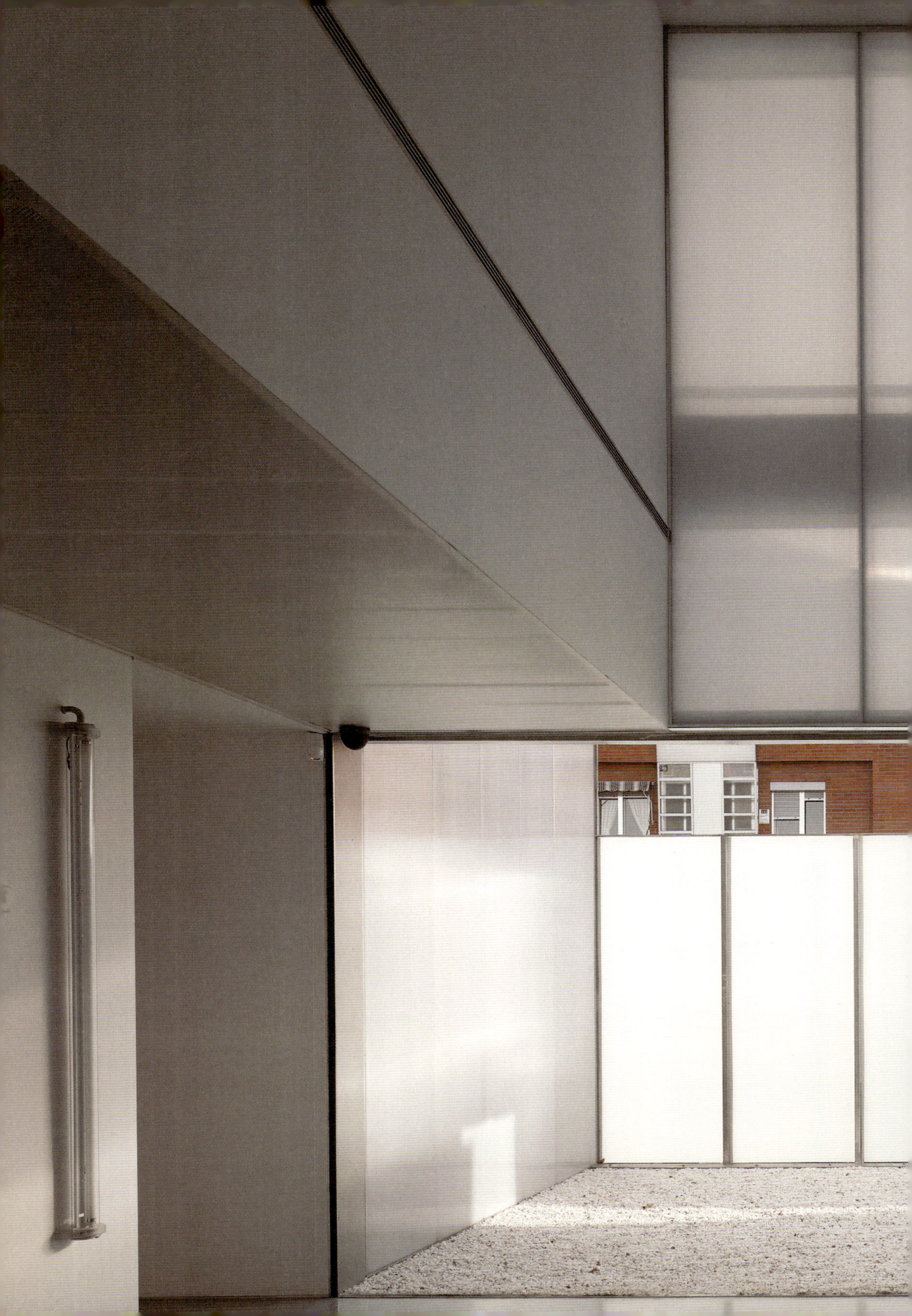

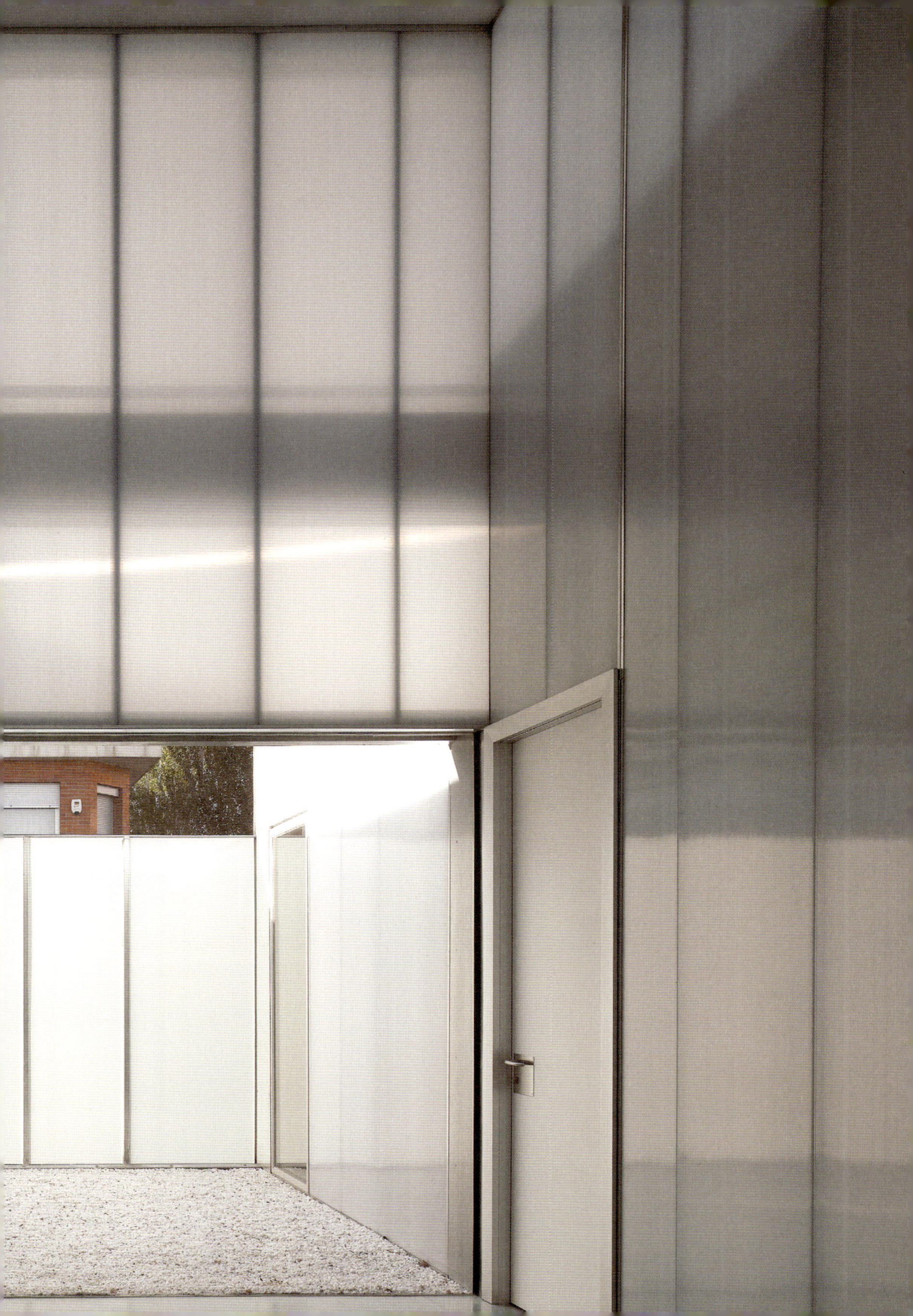

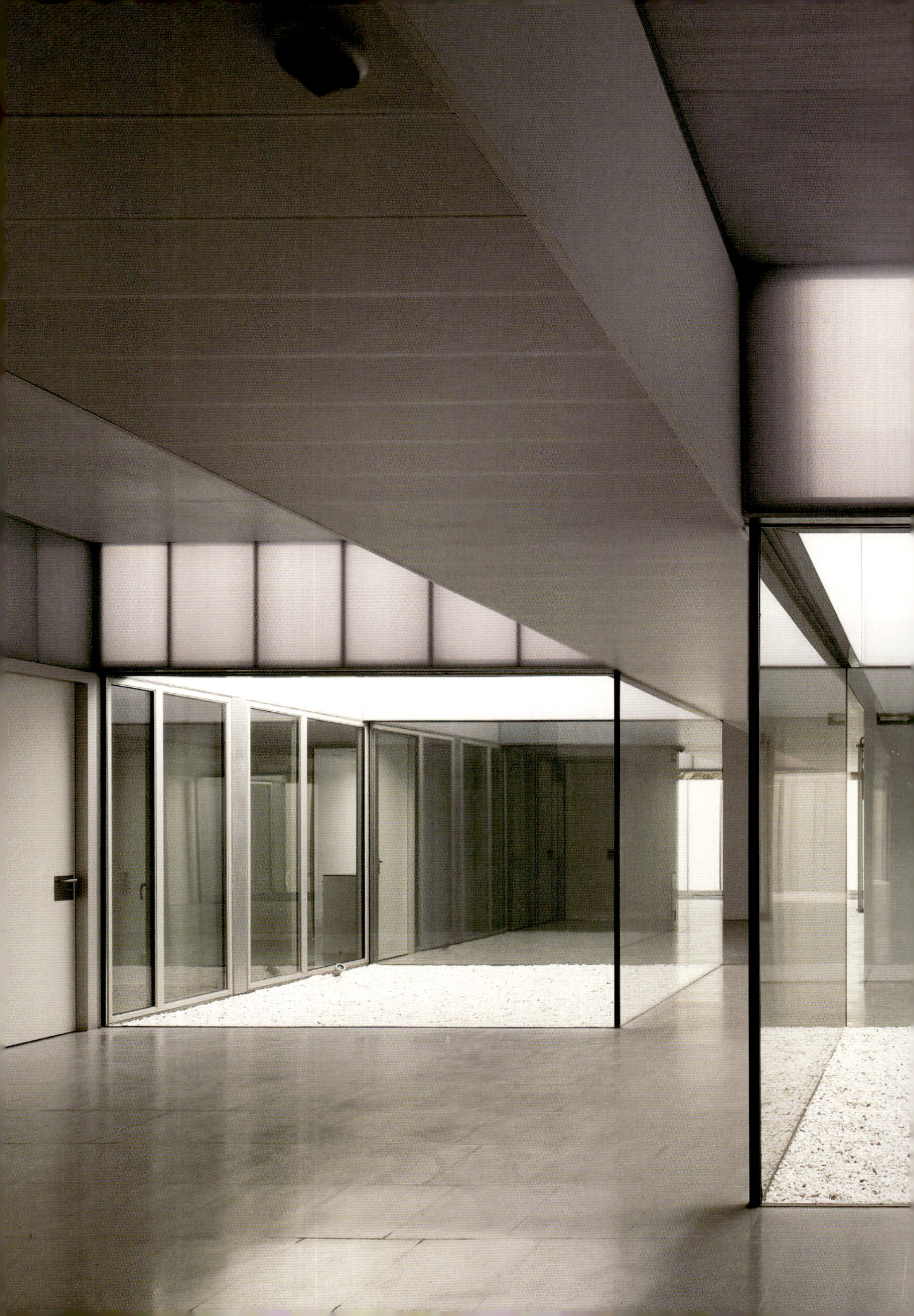

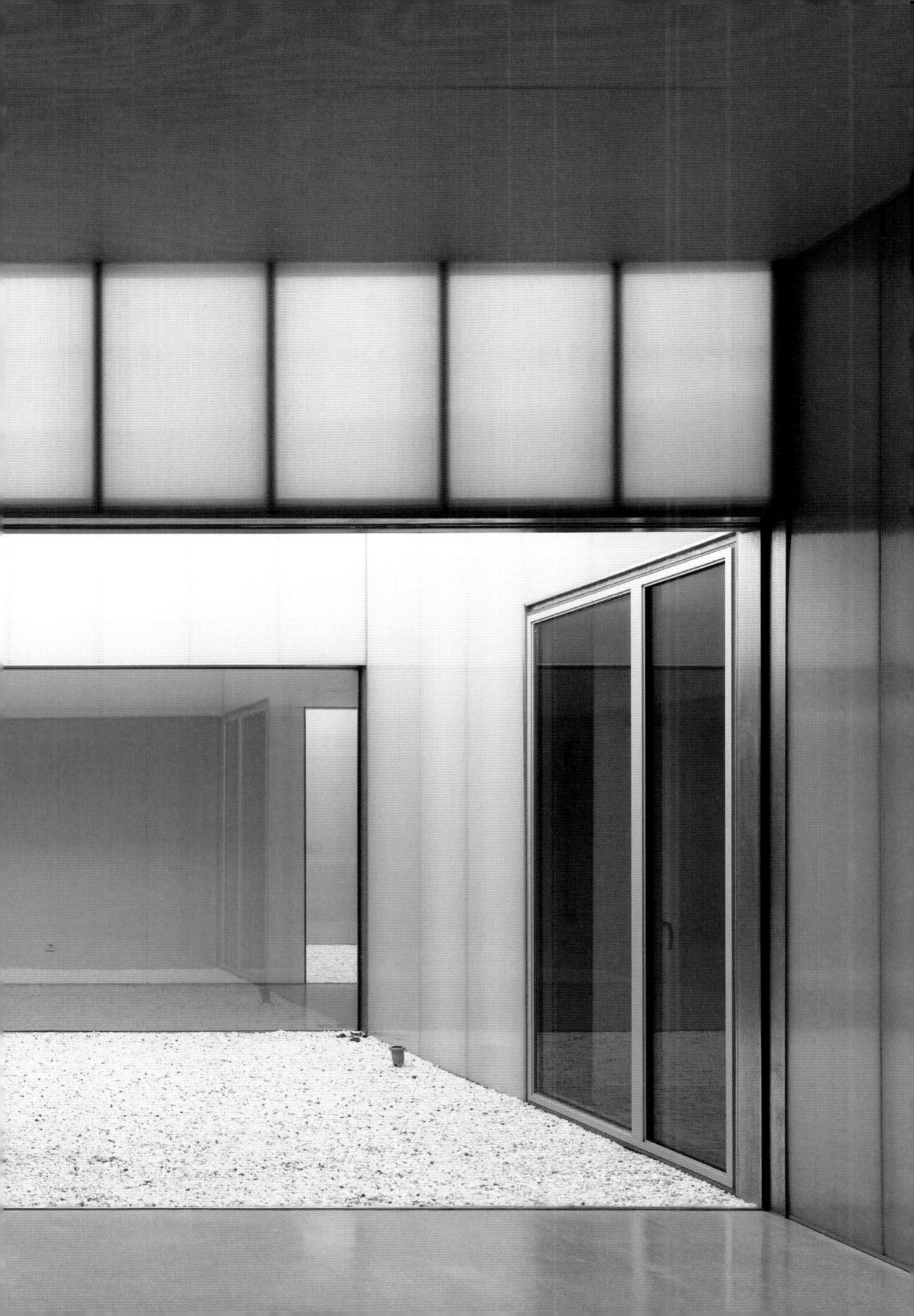

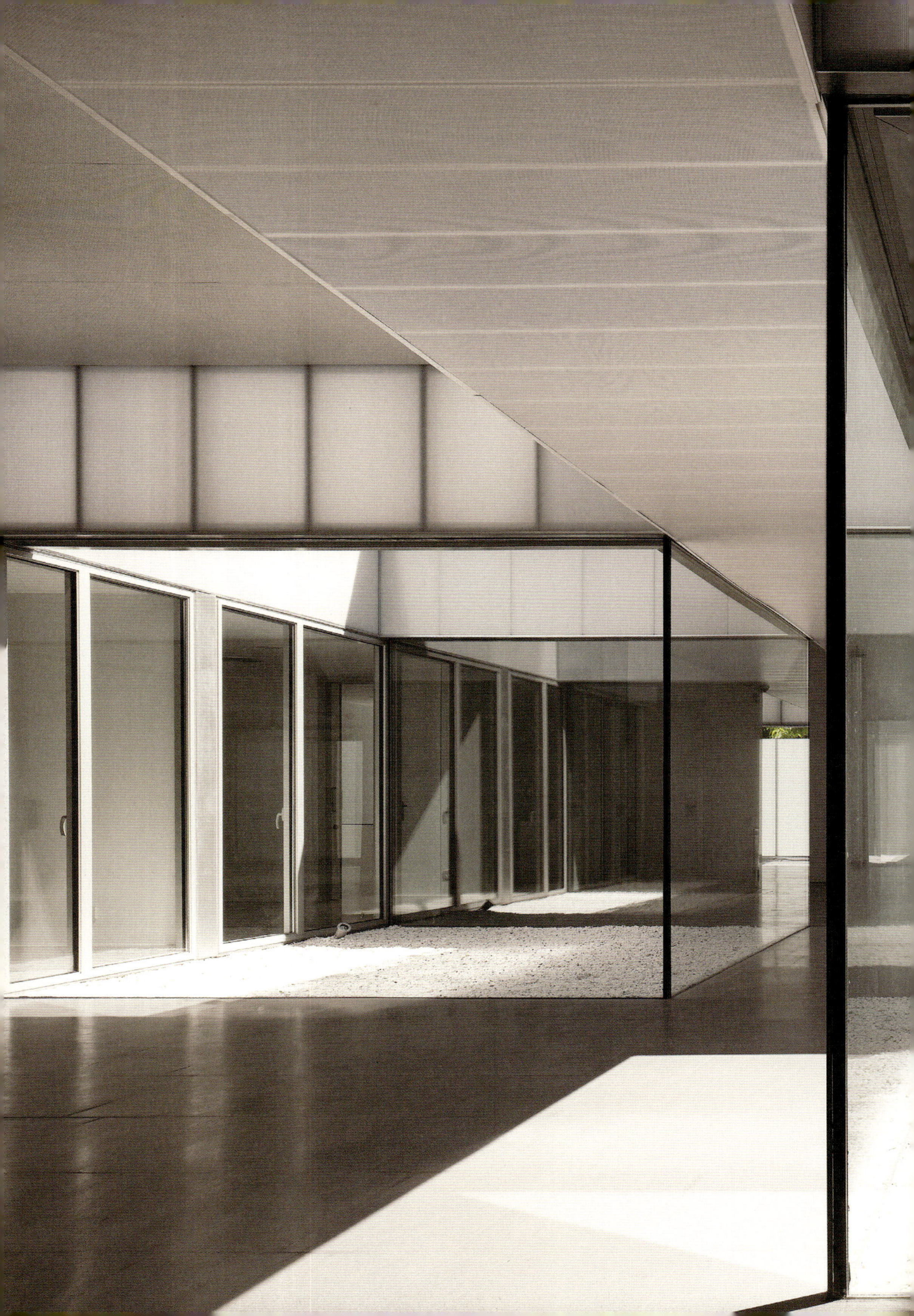

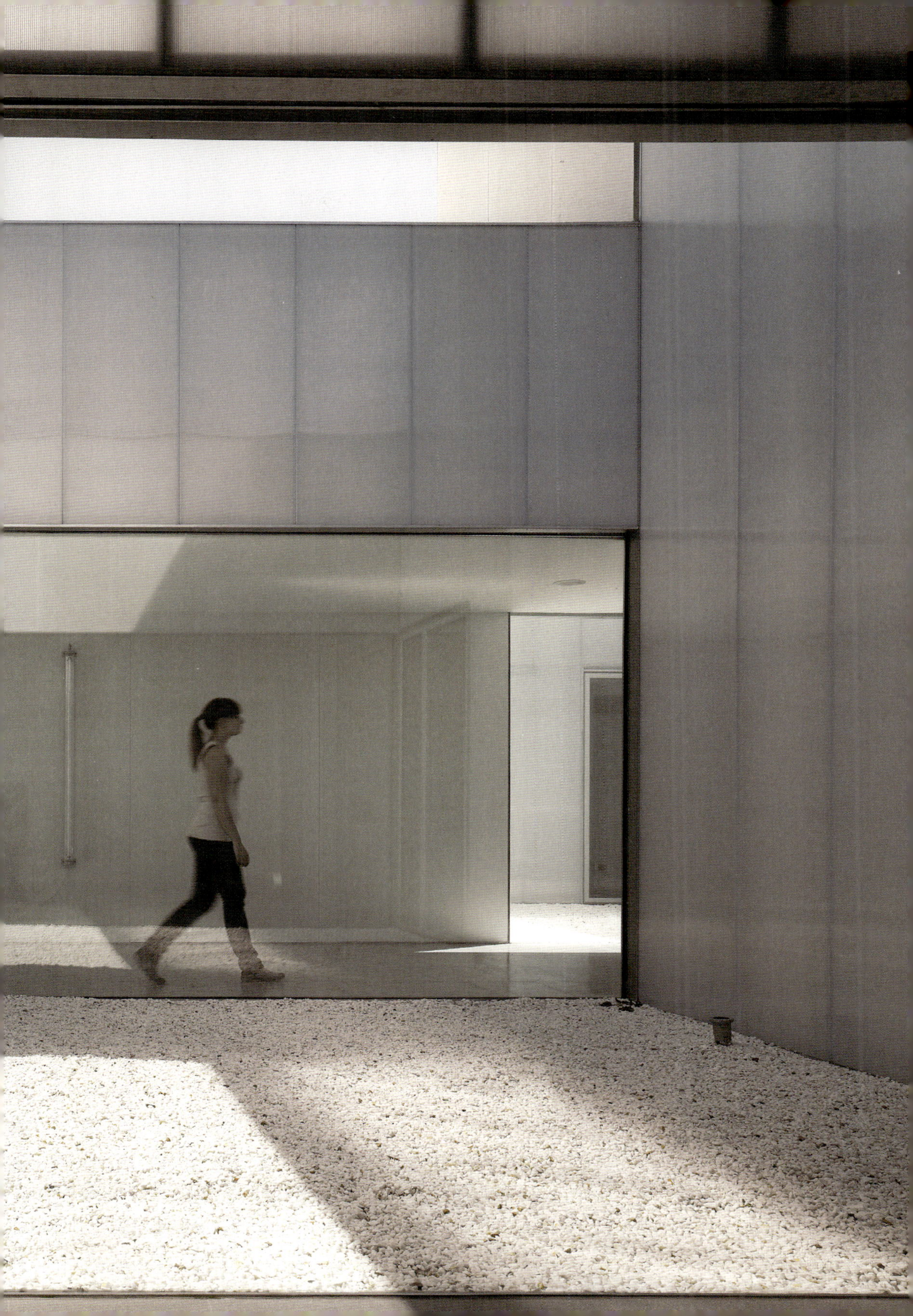

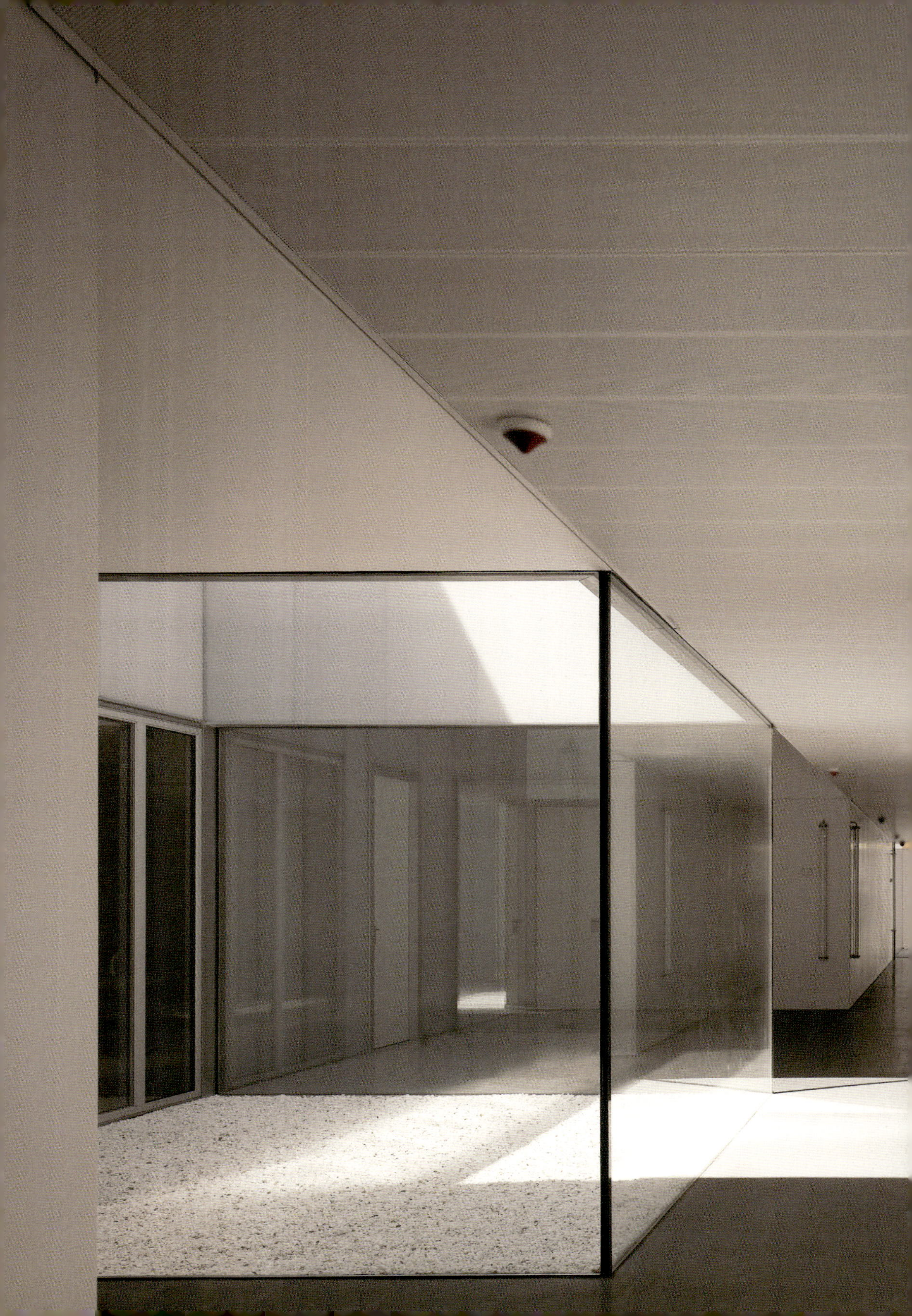

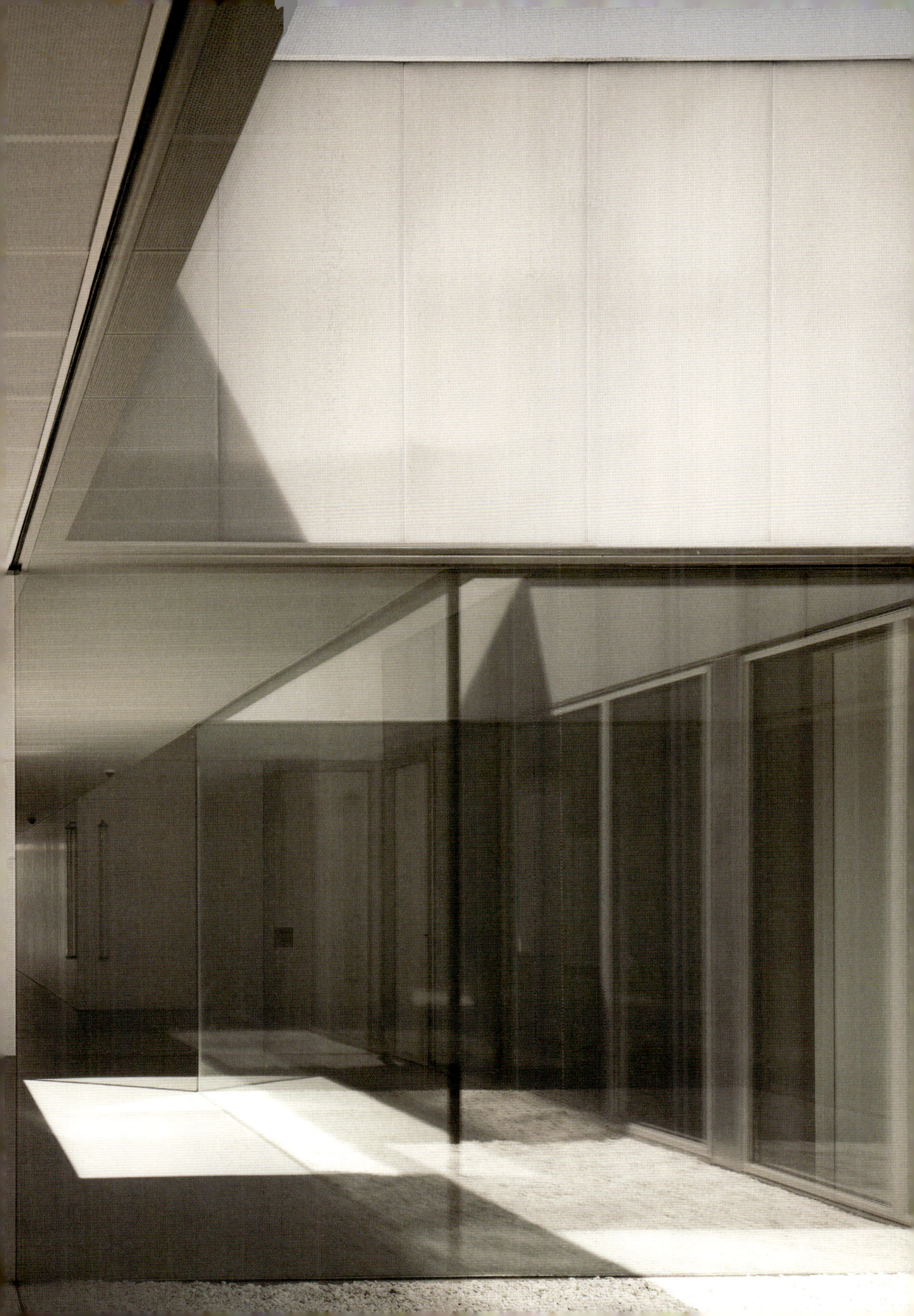

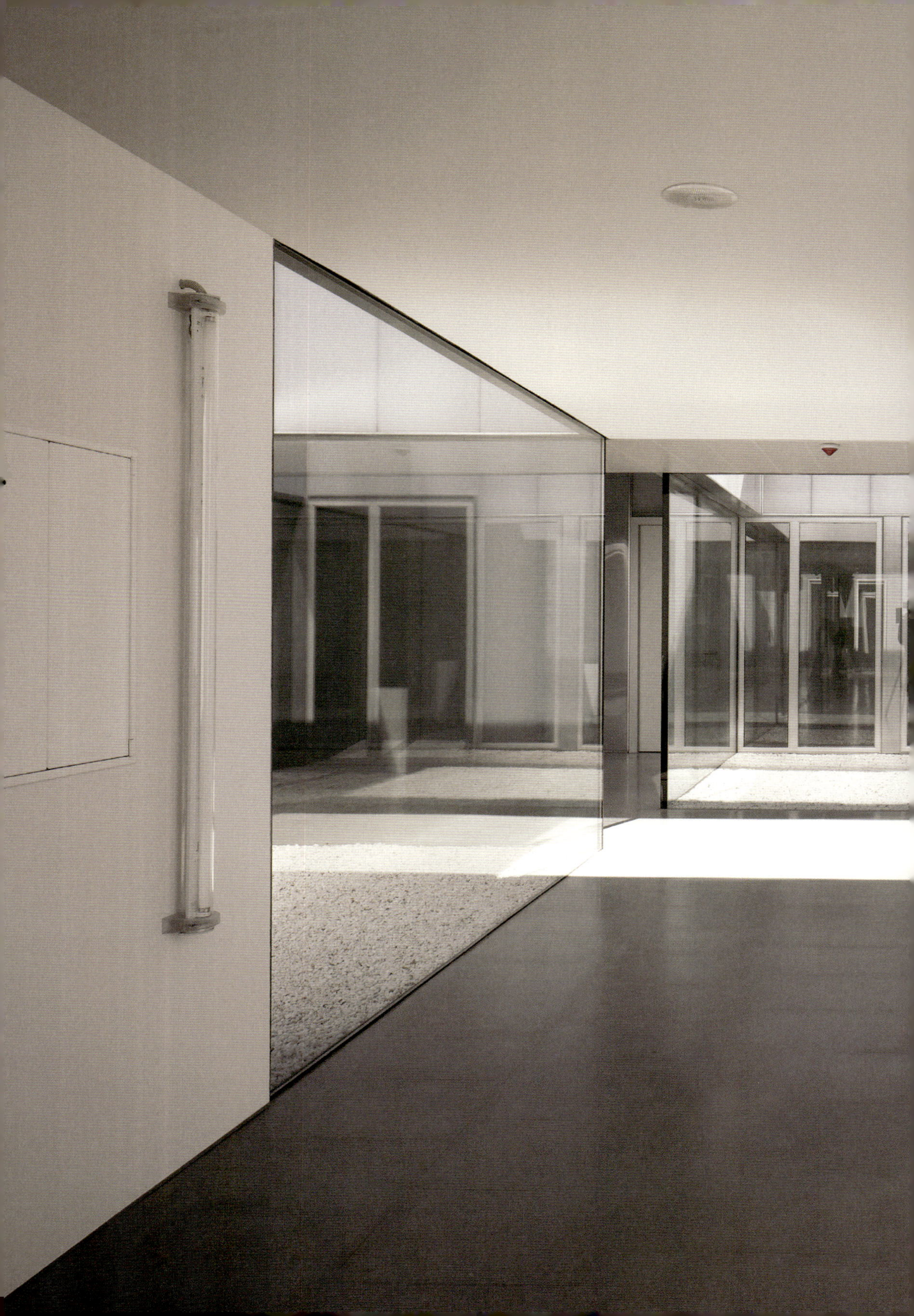

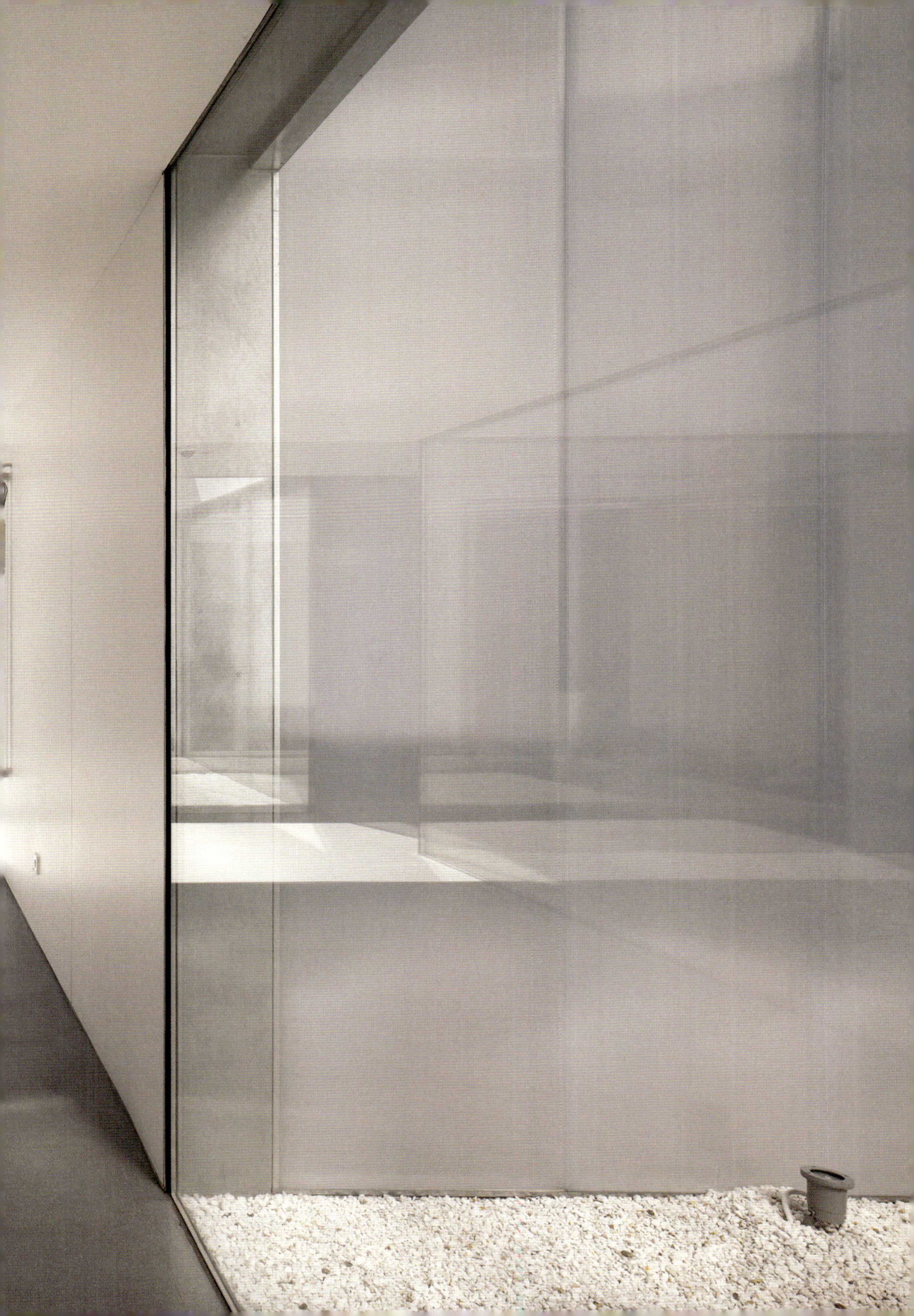

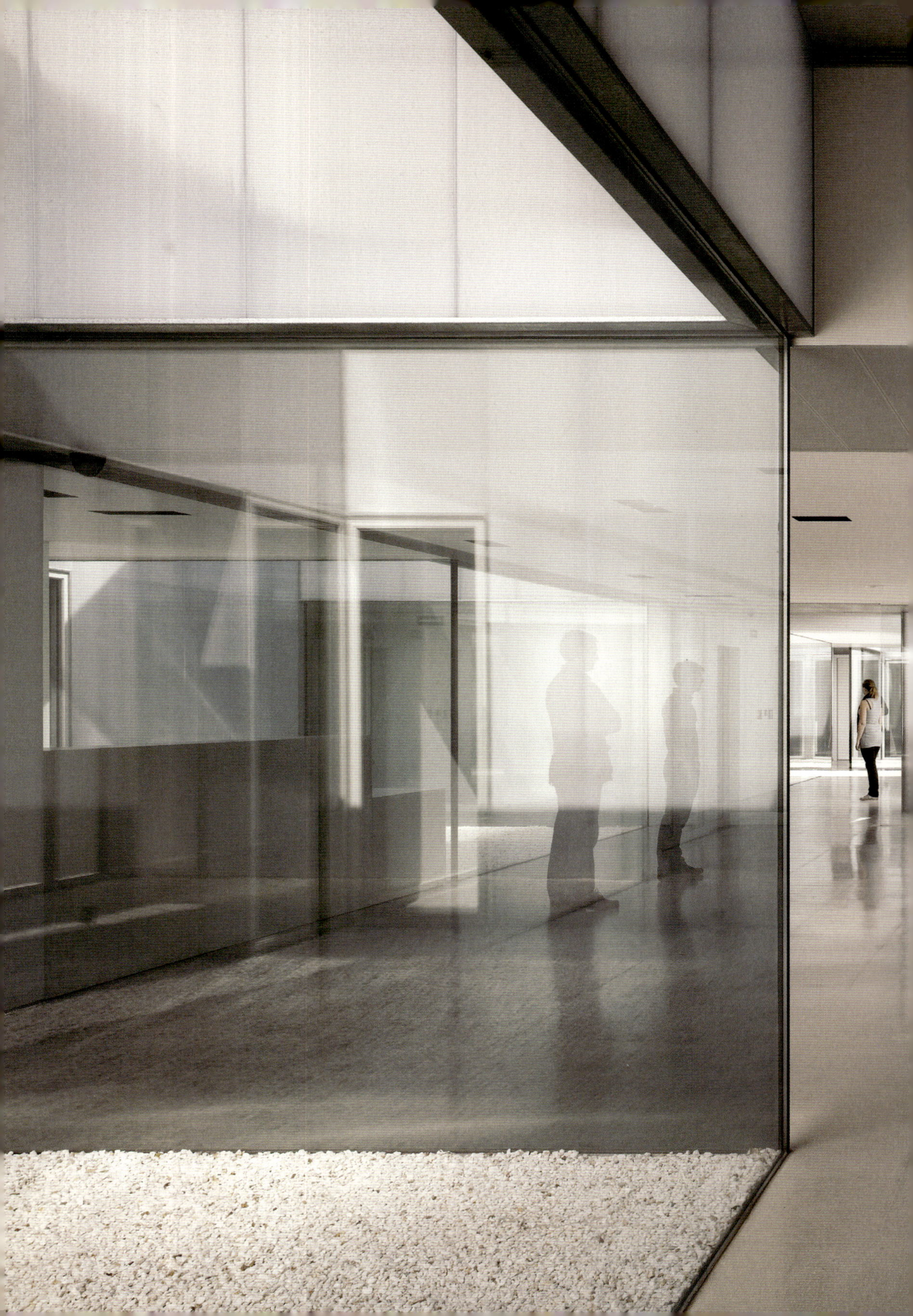

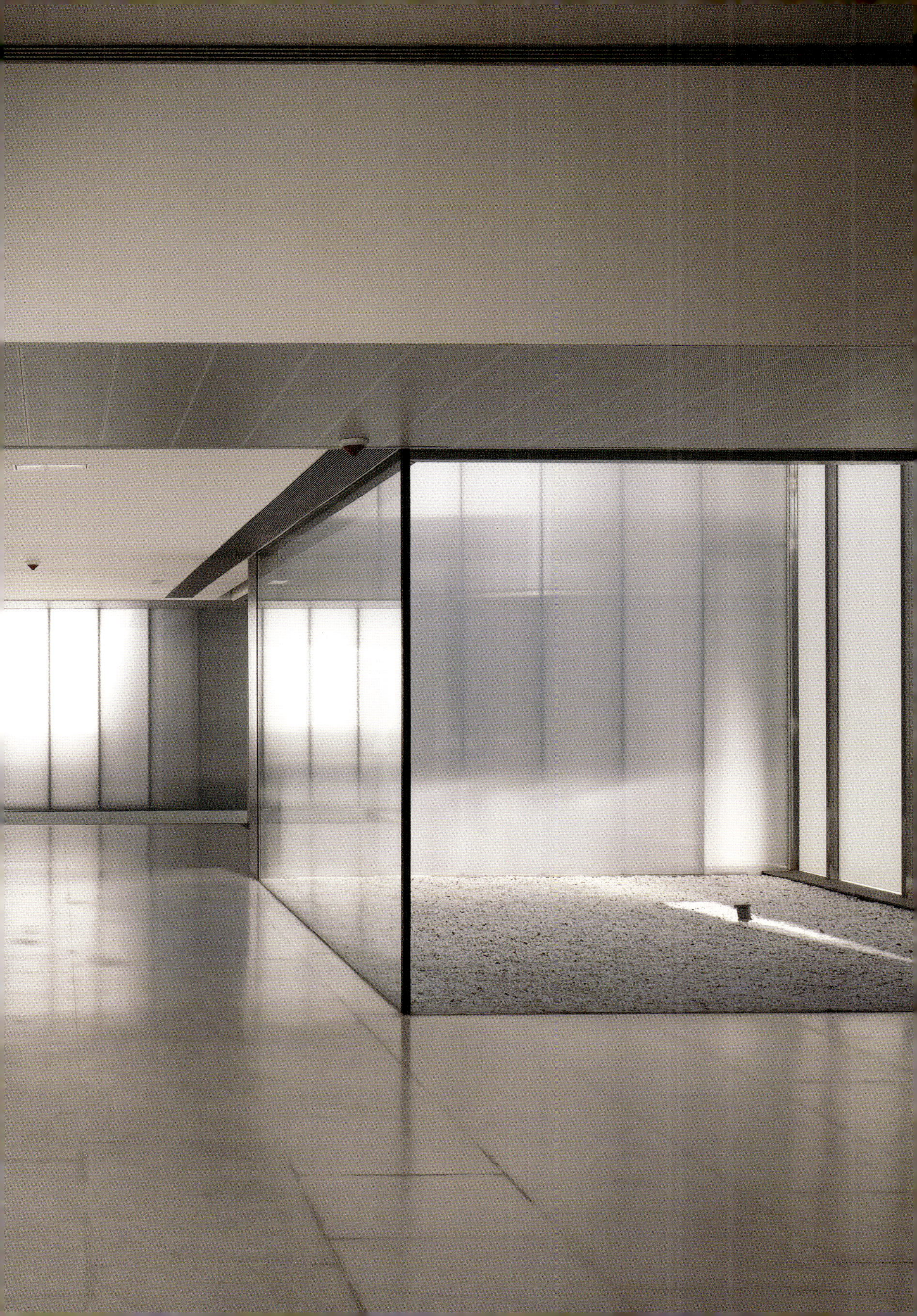

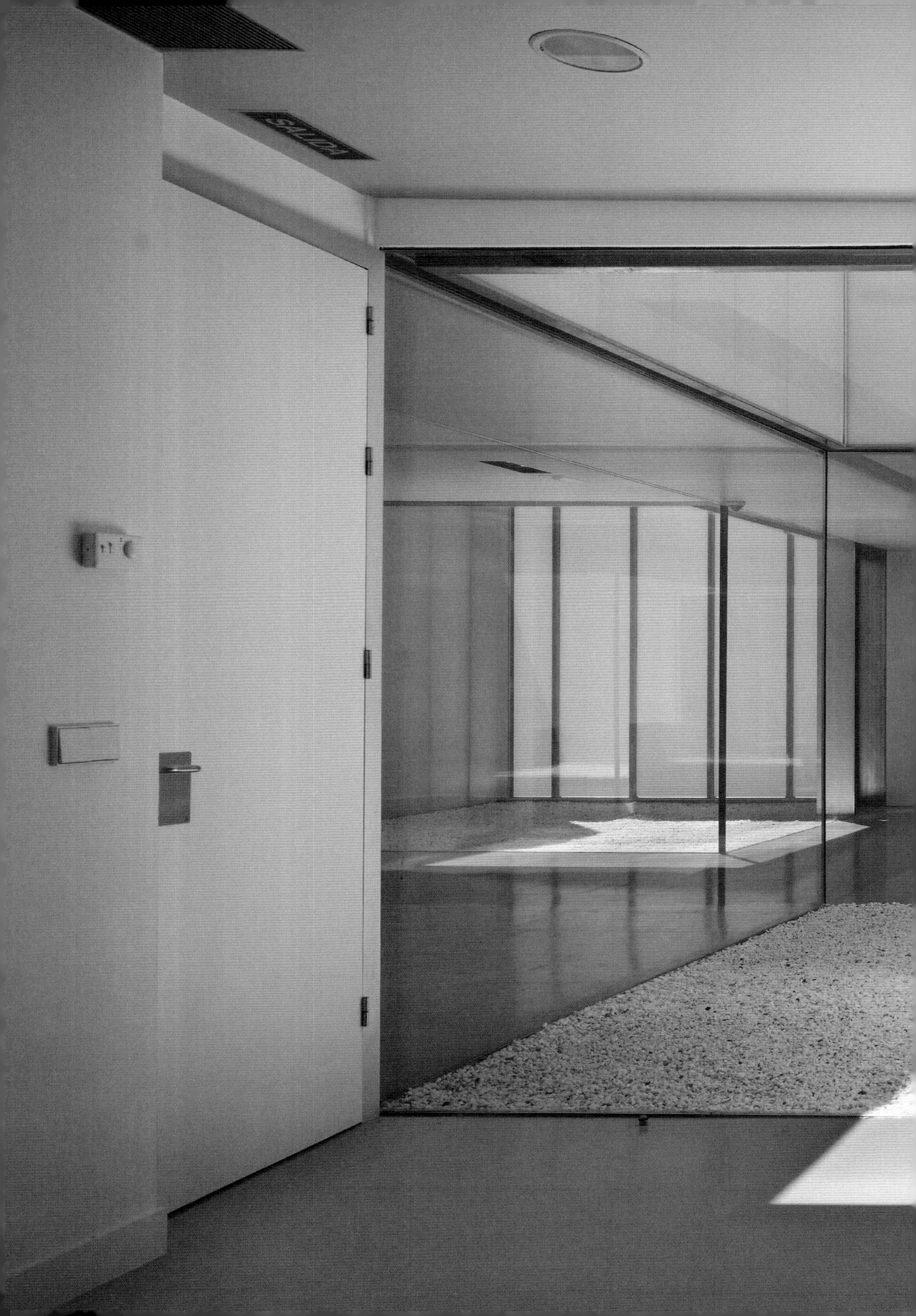
SALIDA

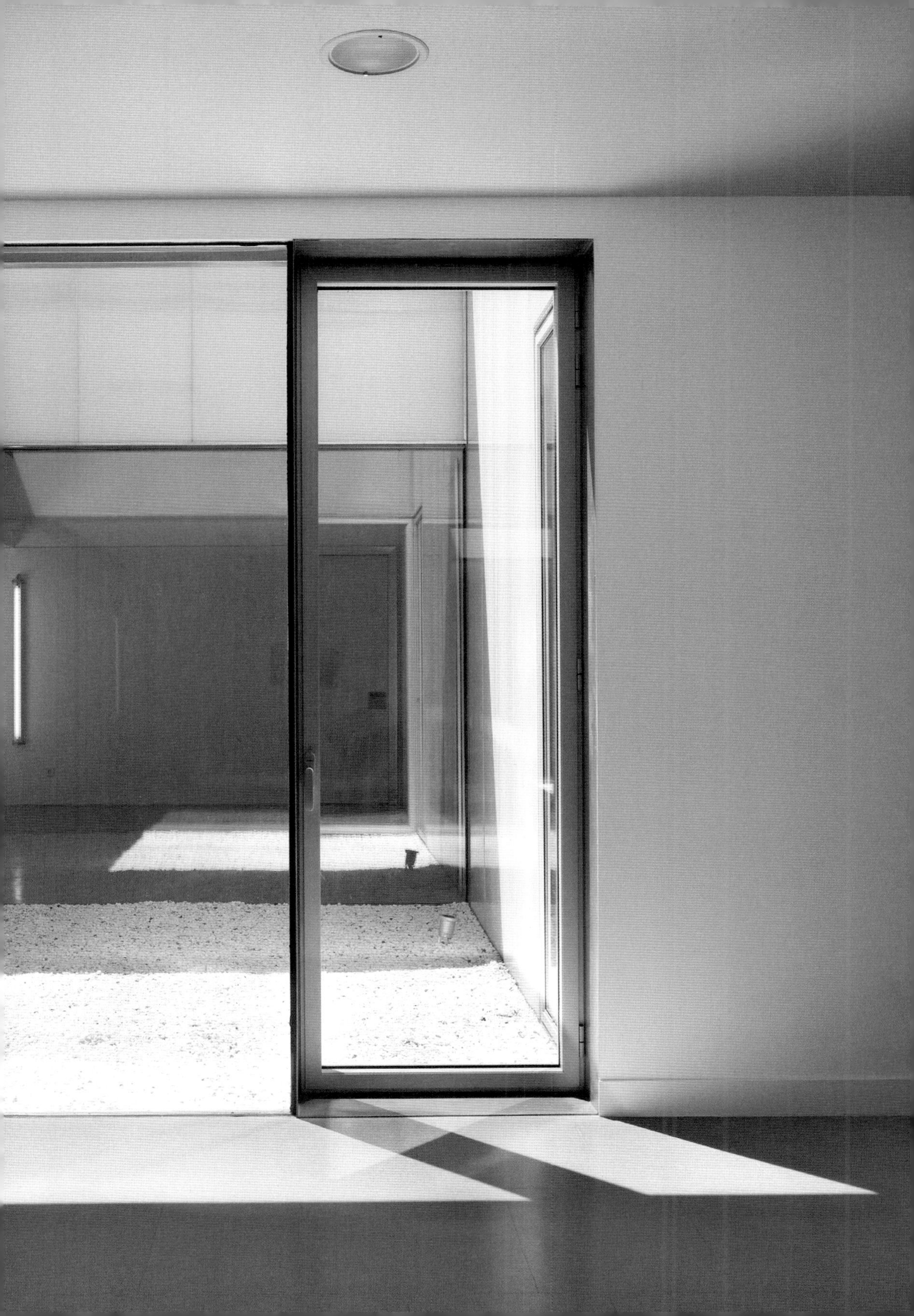

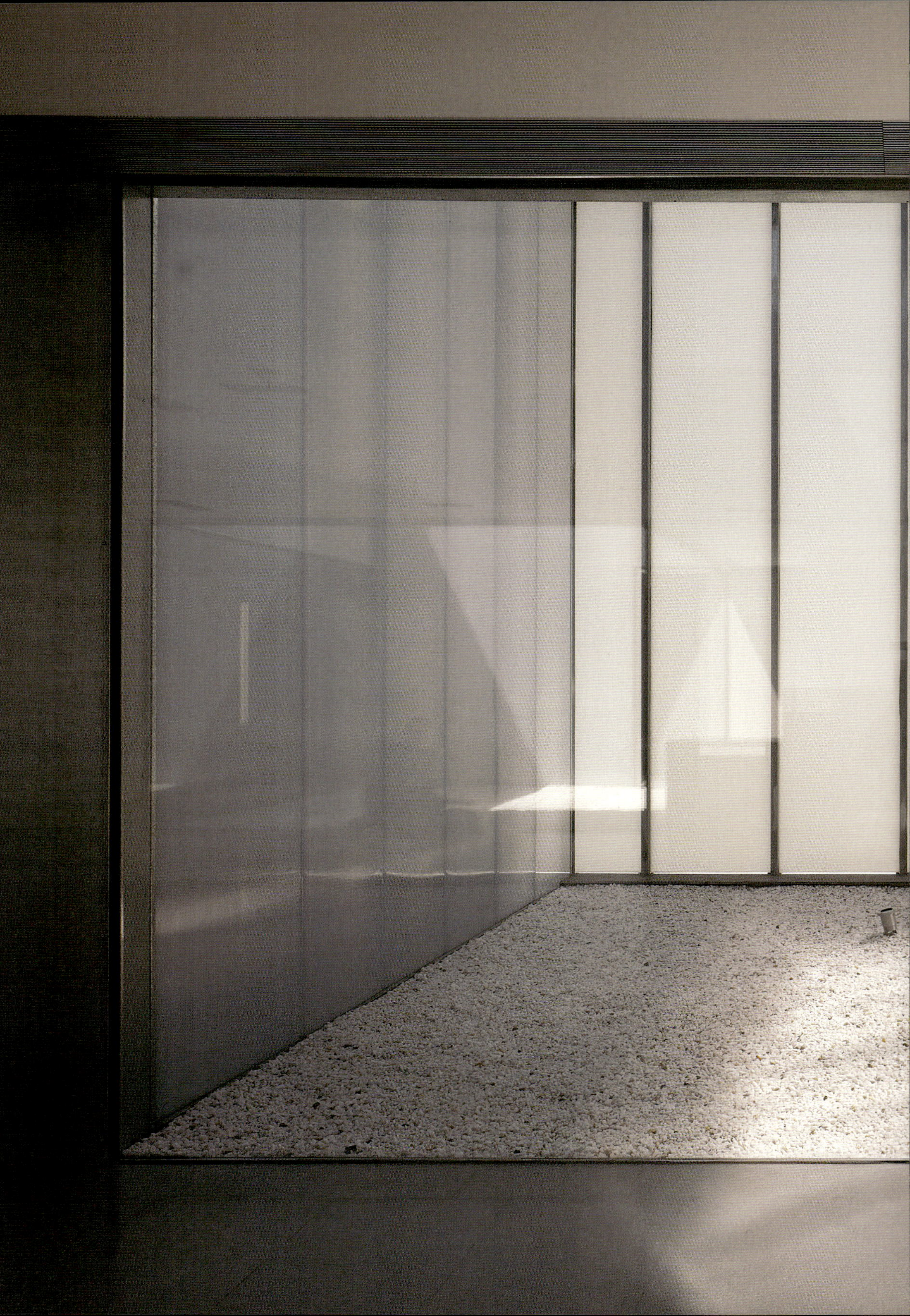

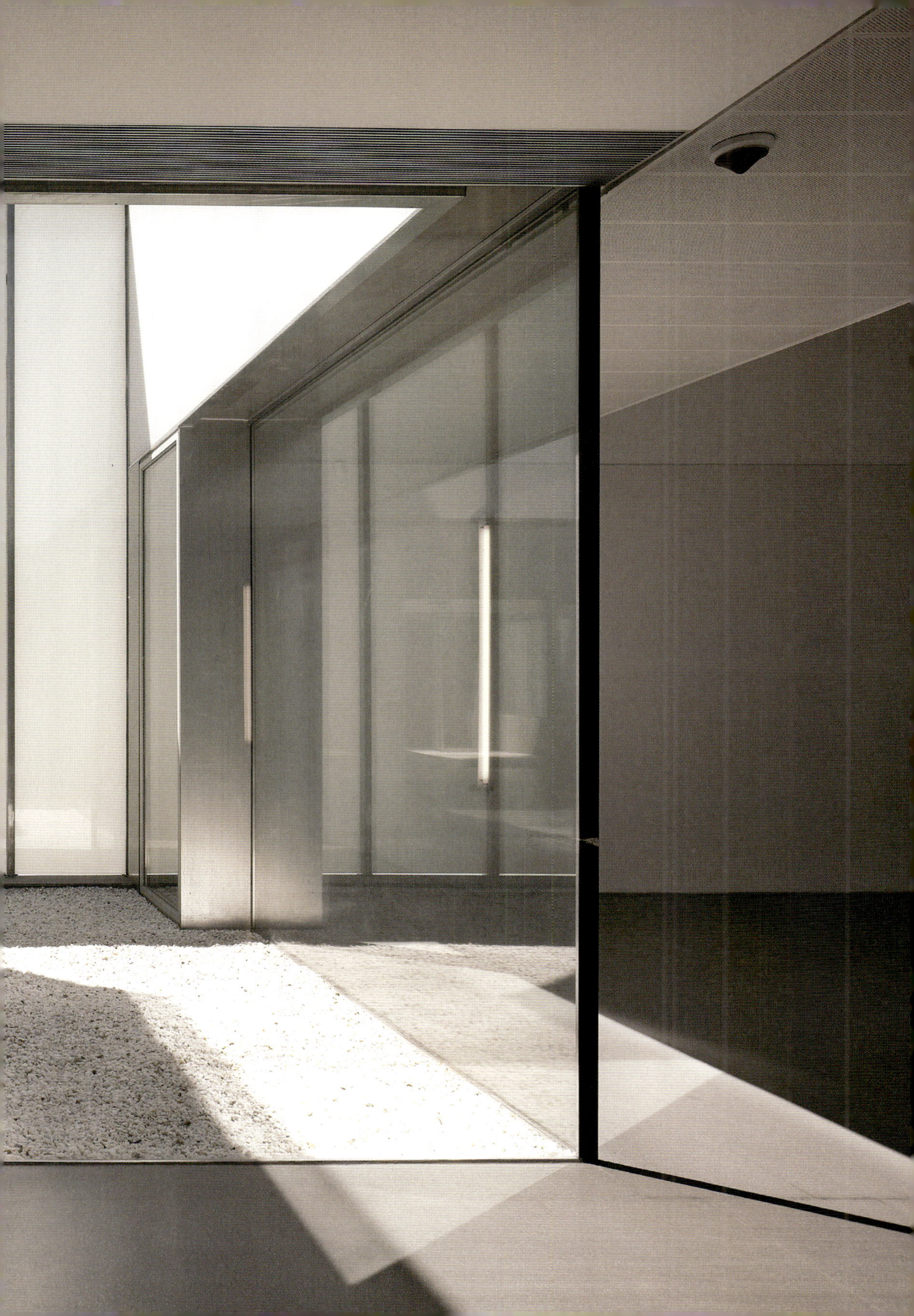

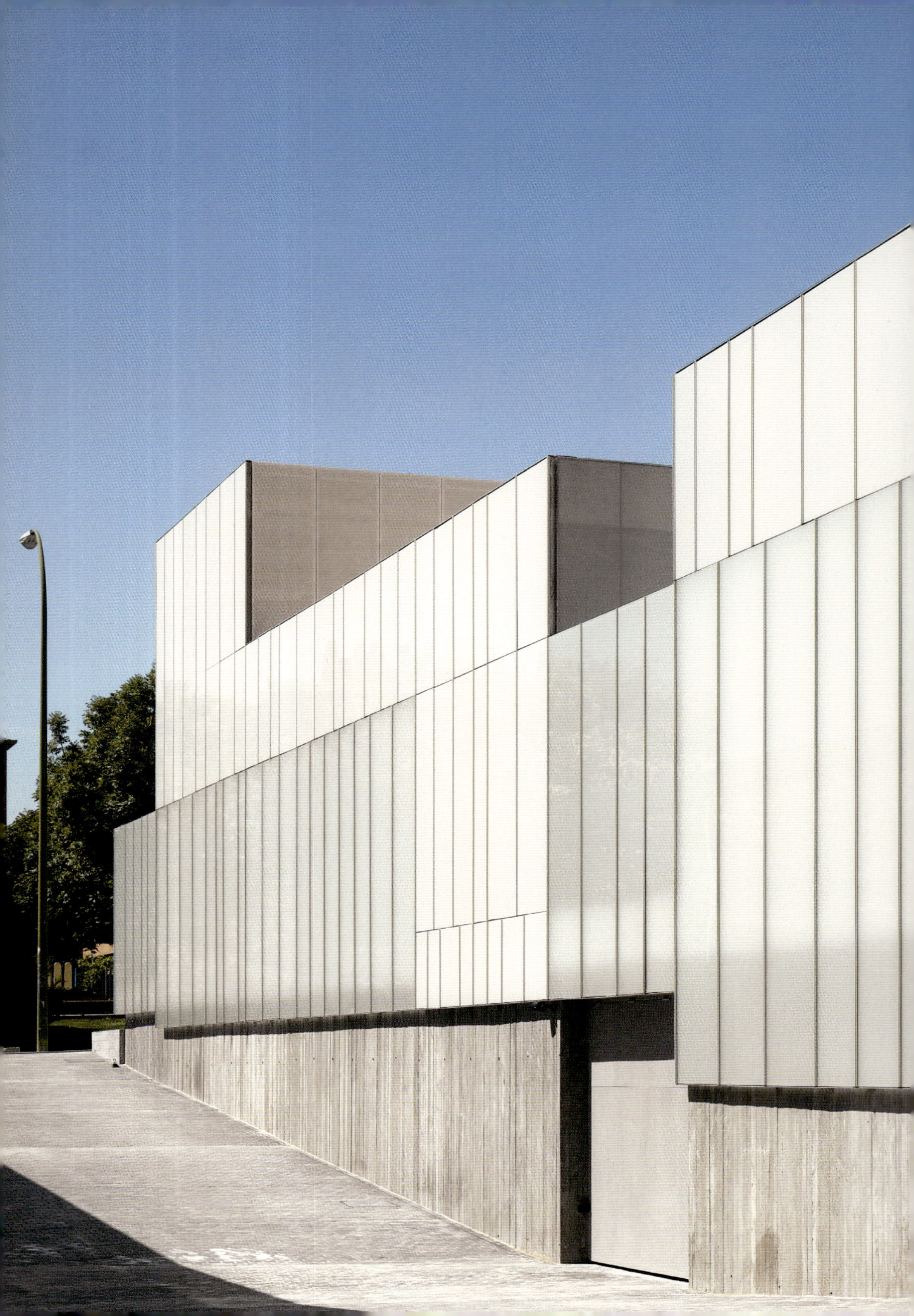

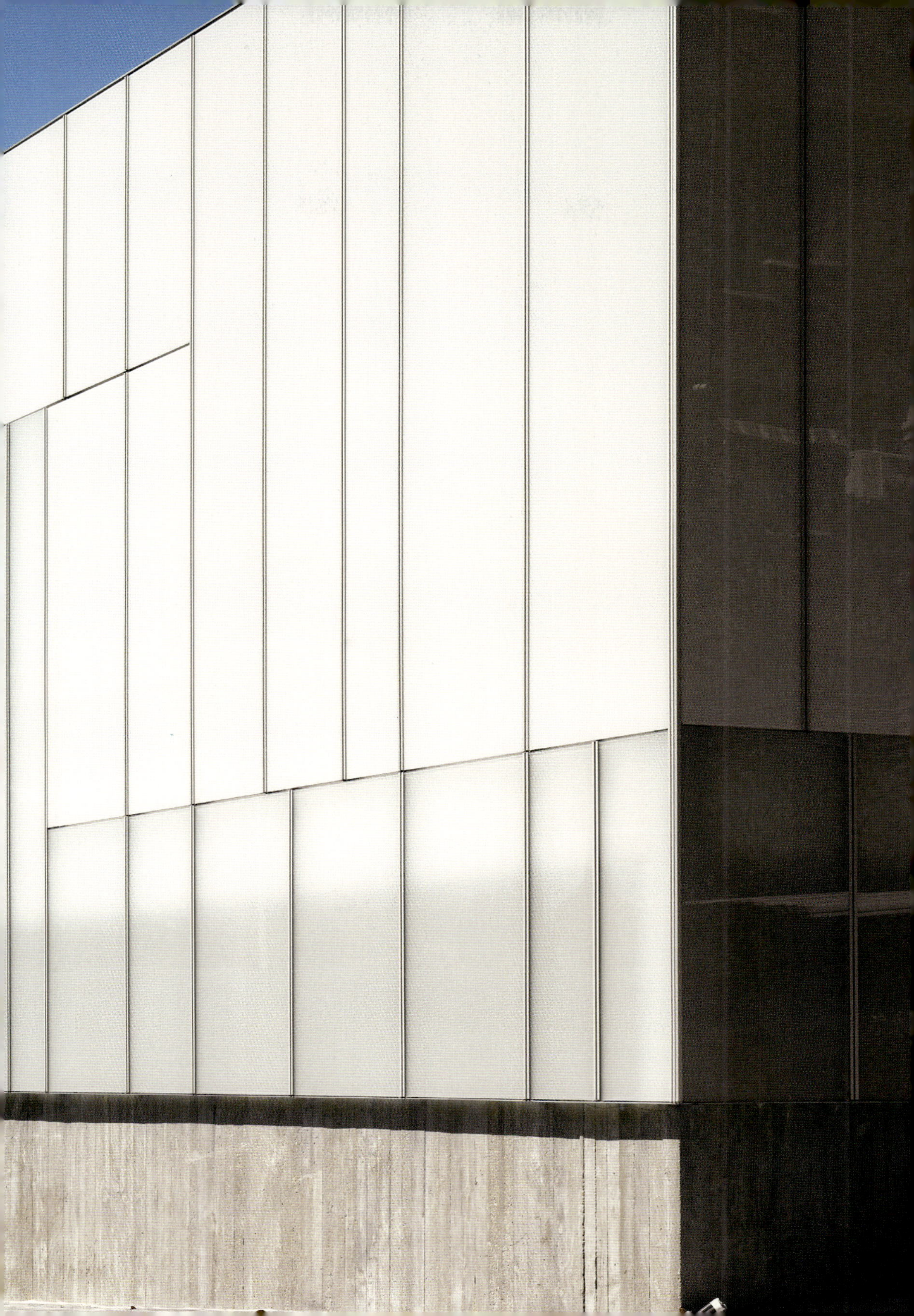

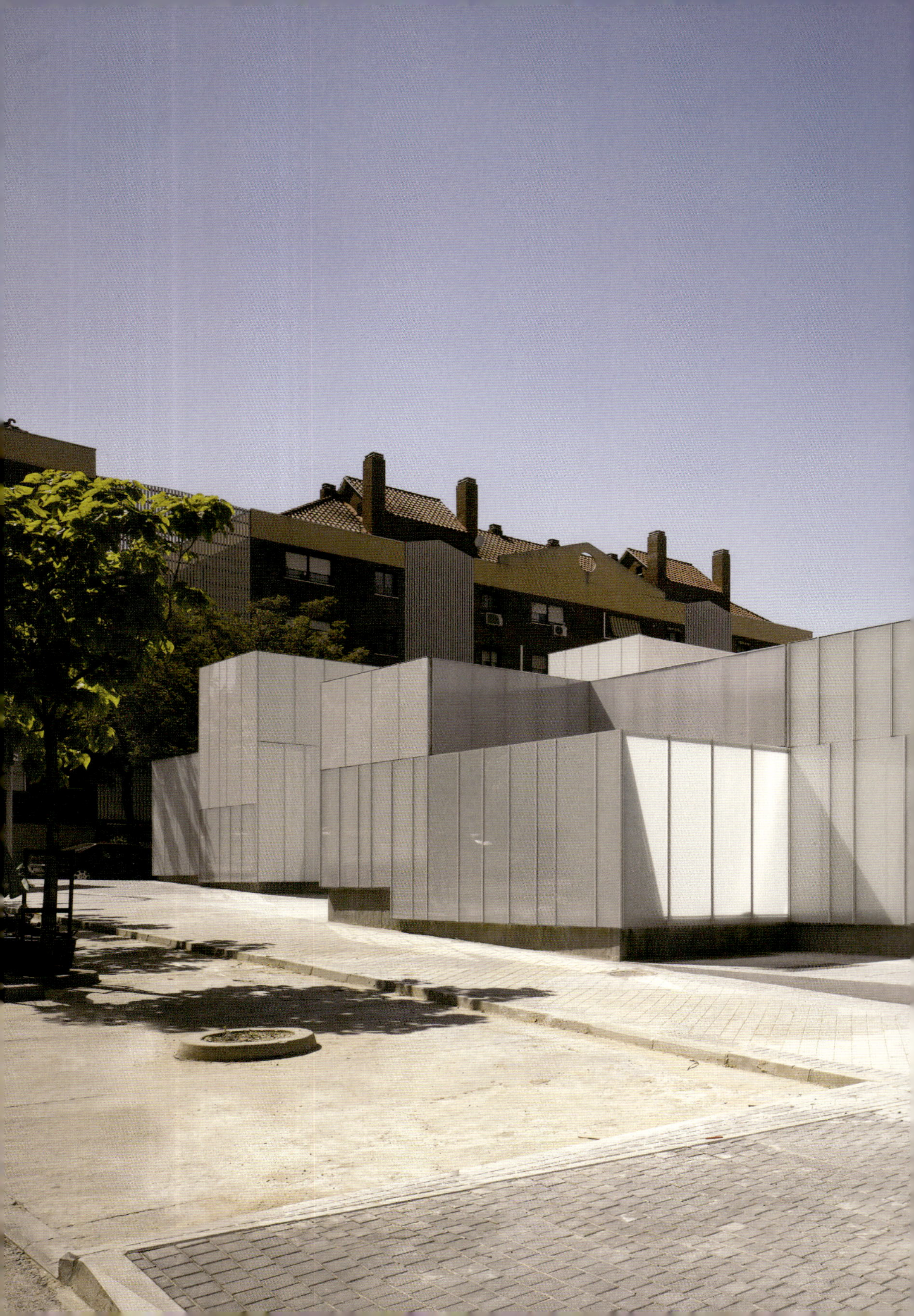

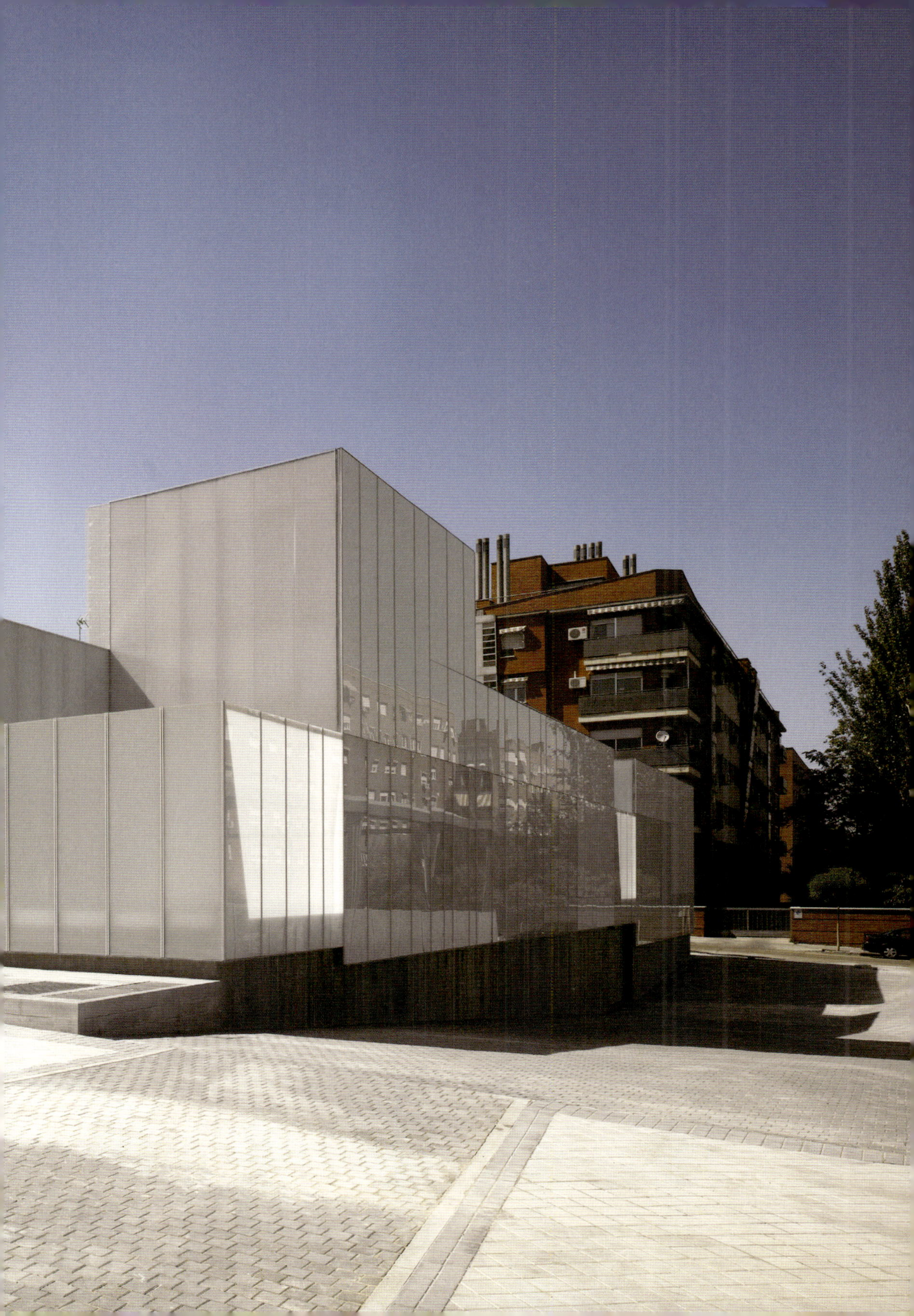

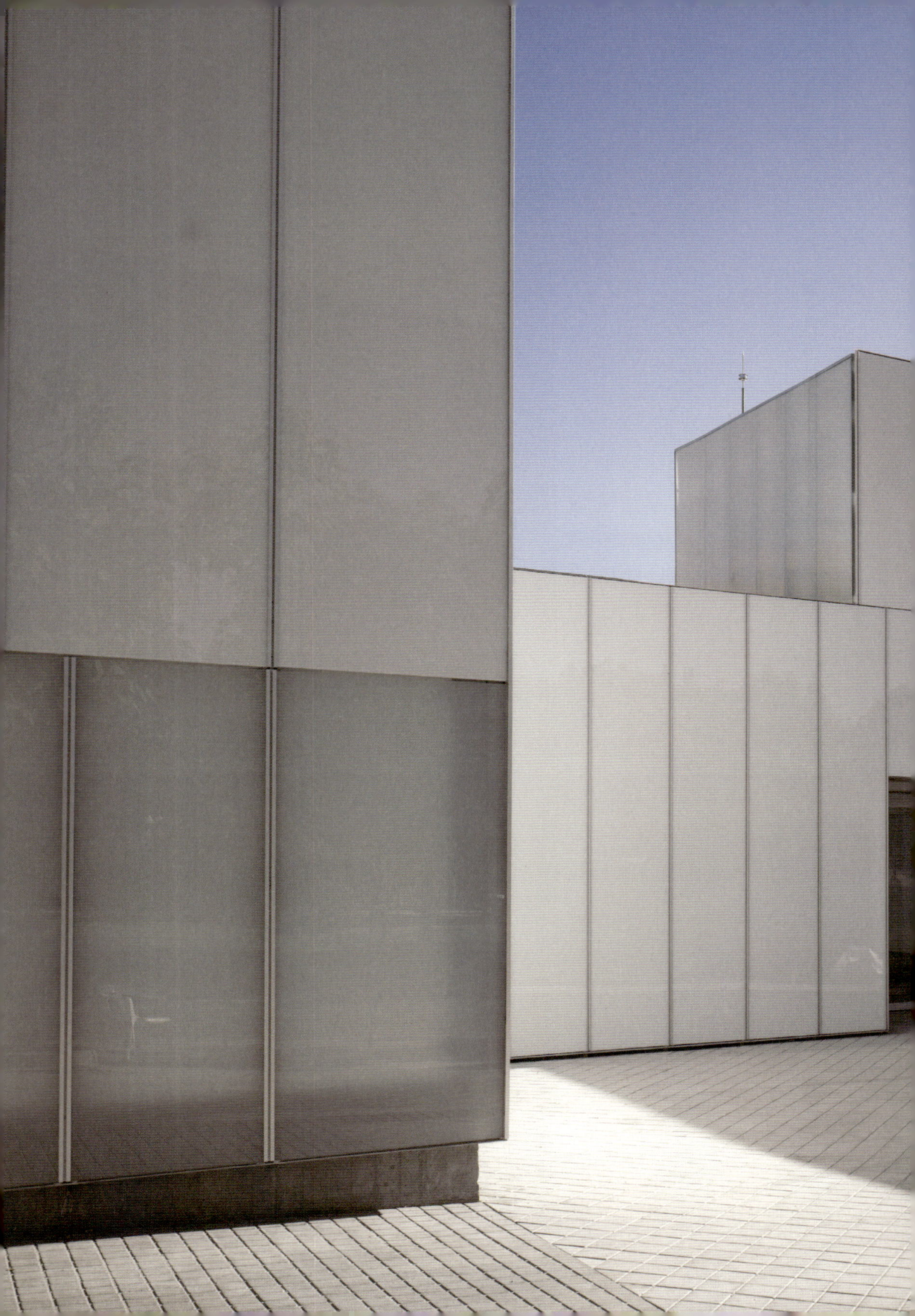

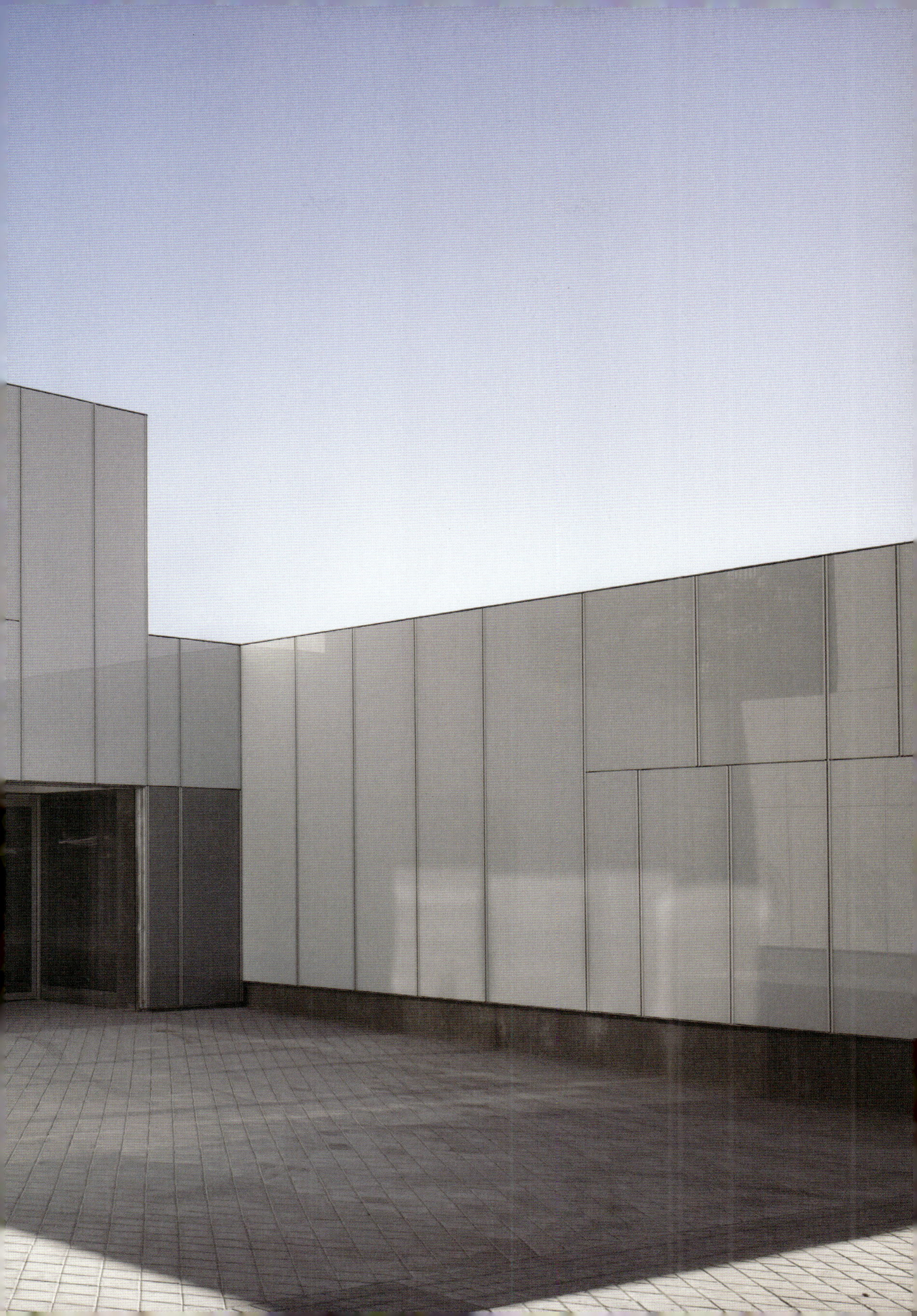

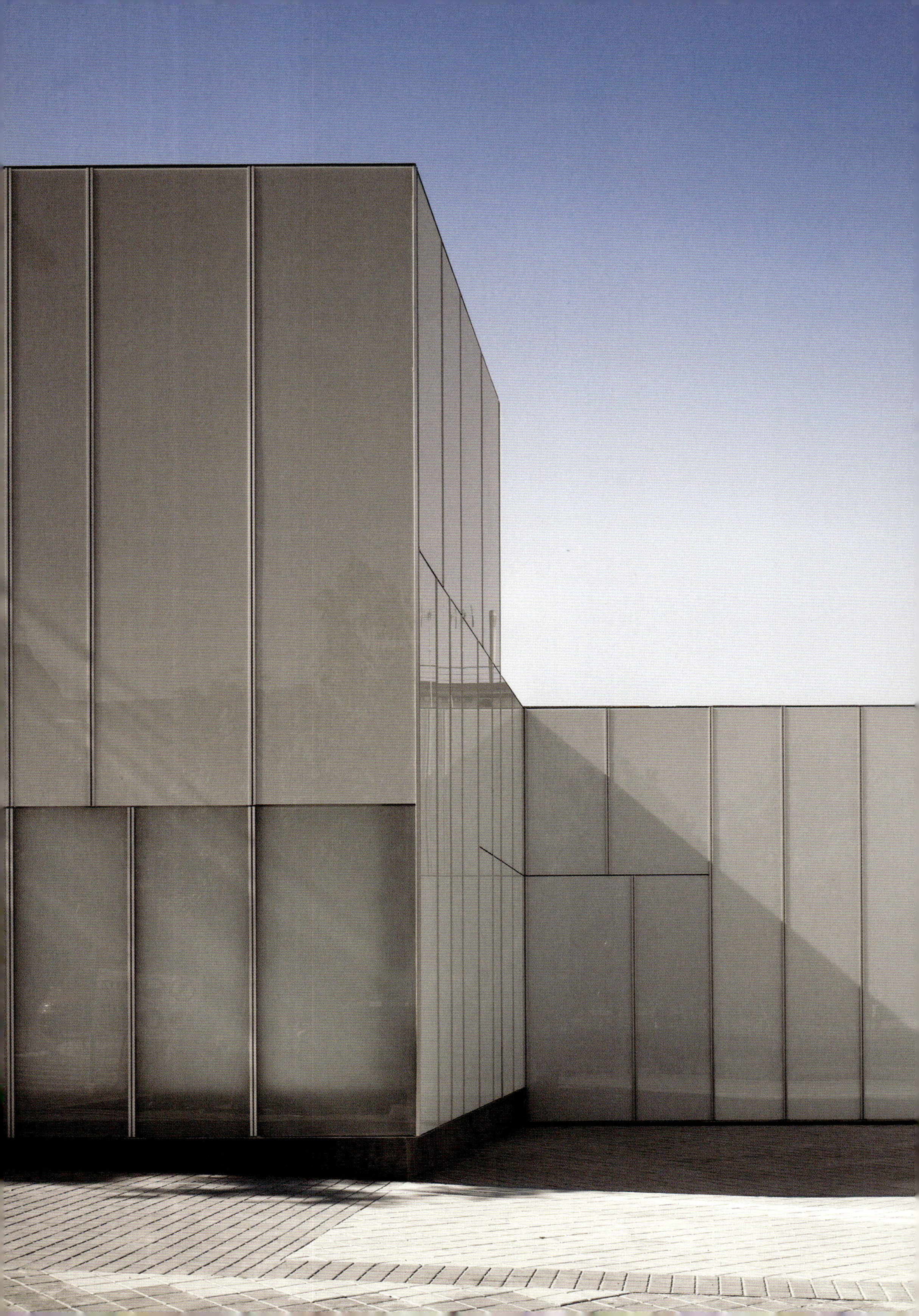

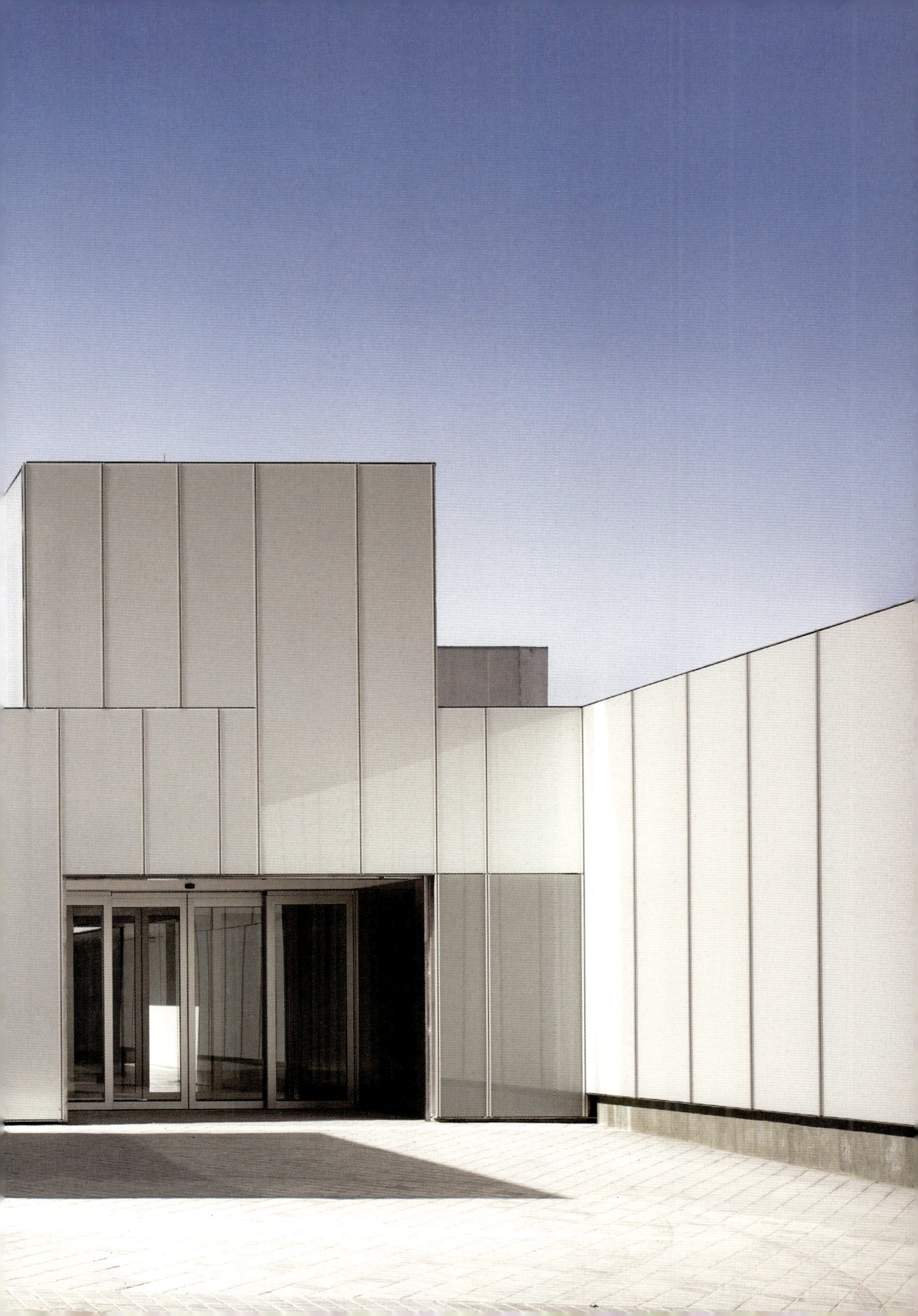

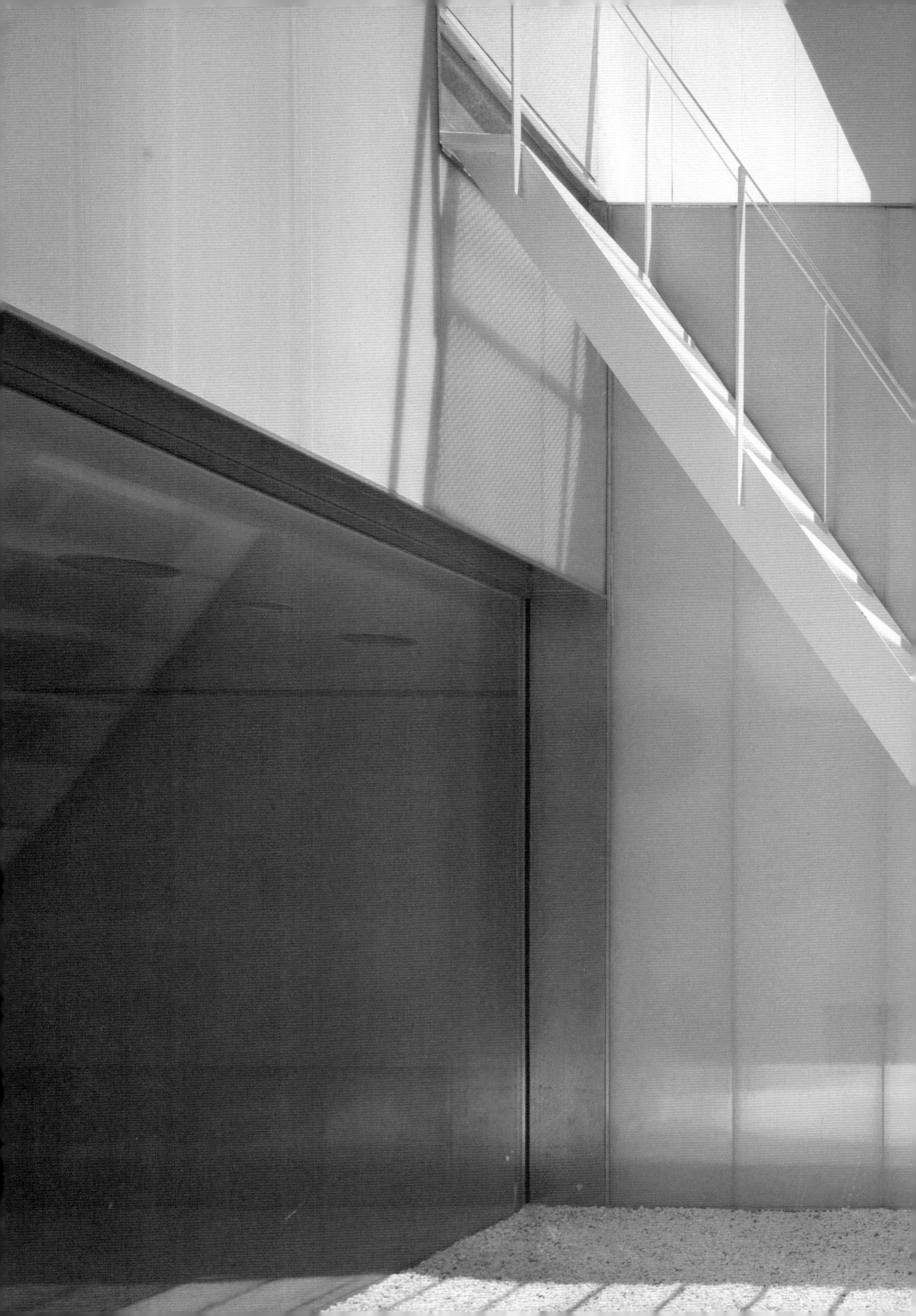

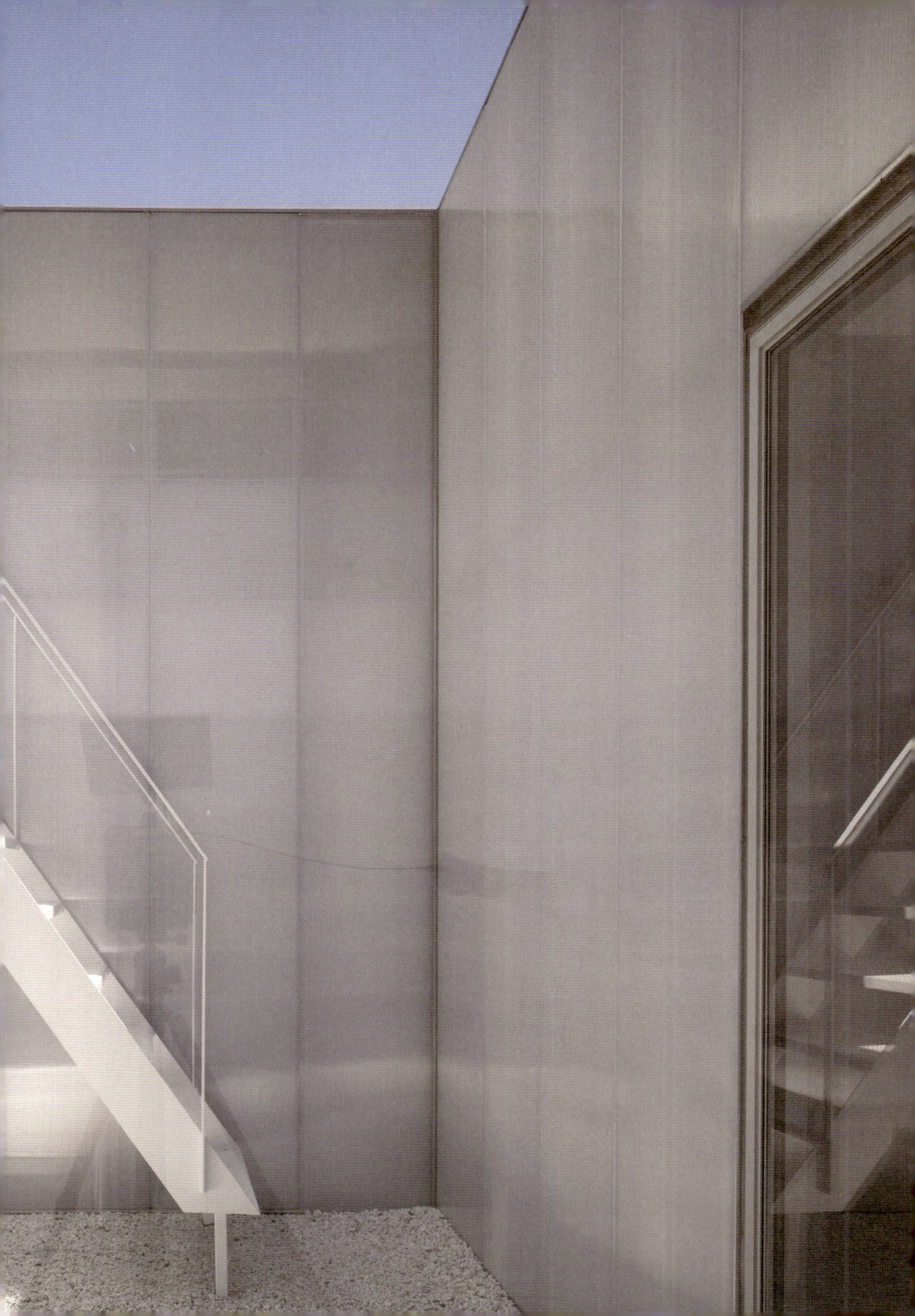

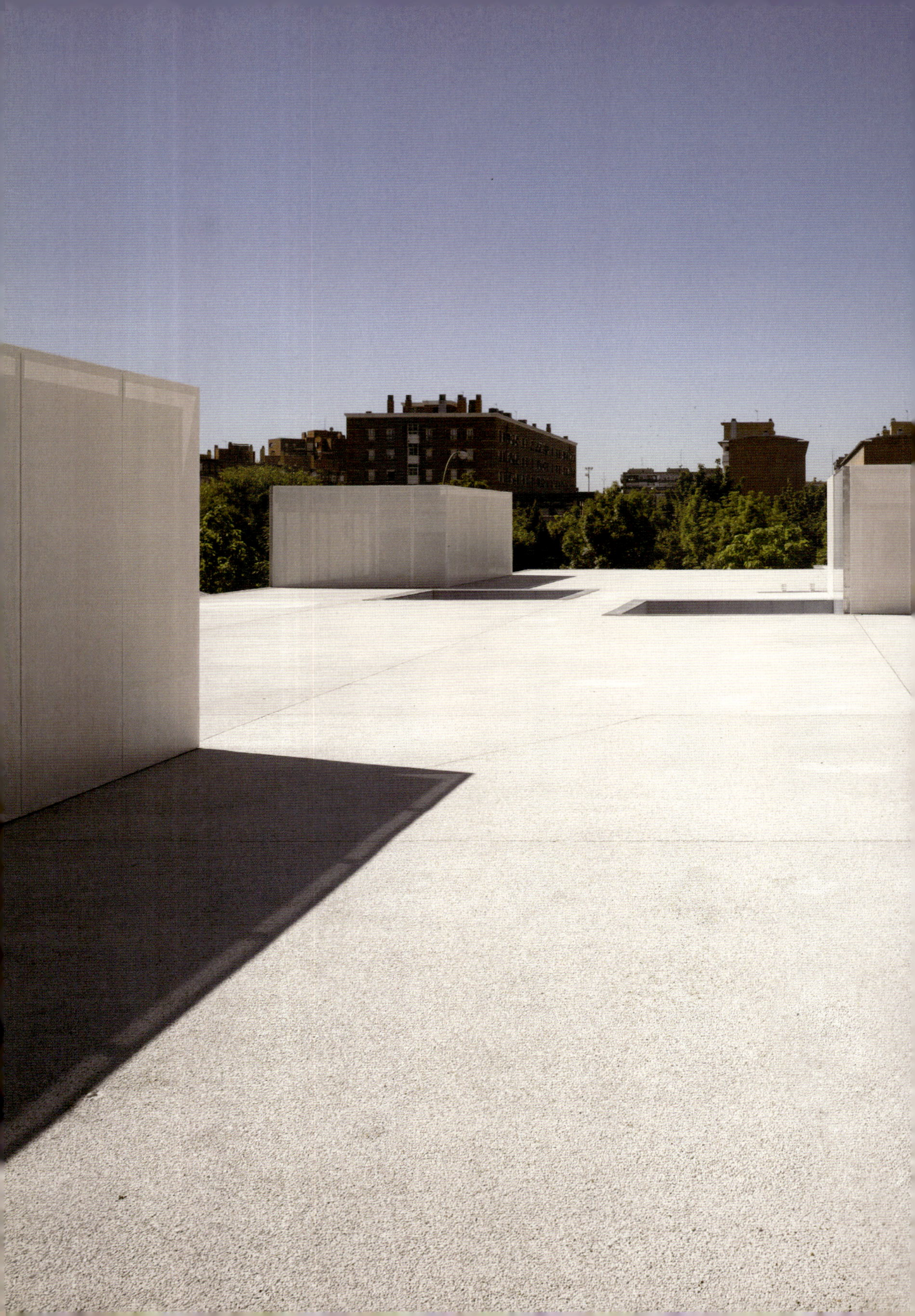

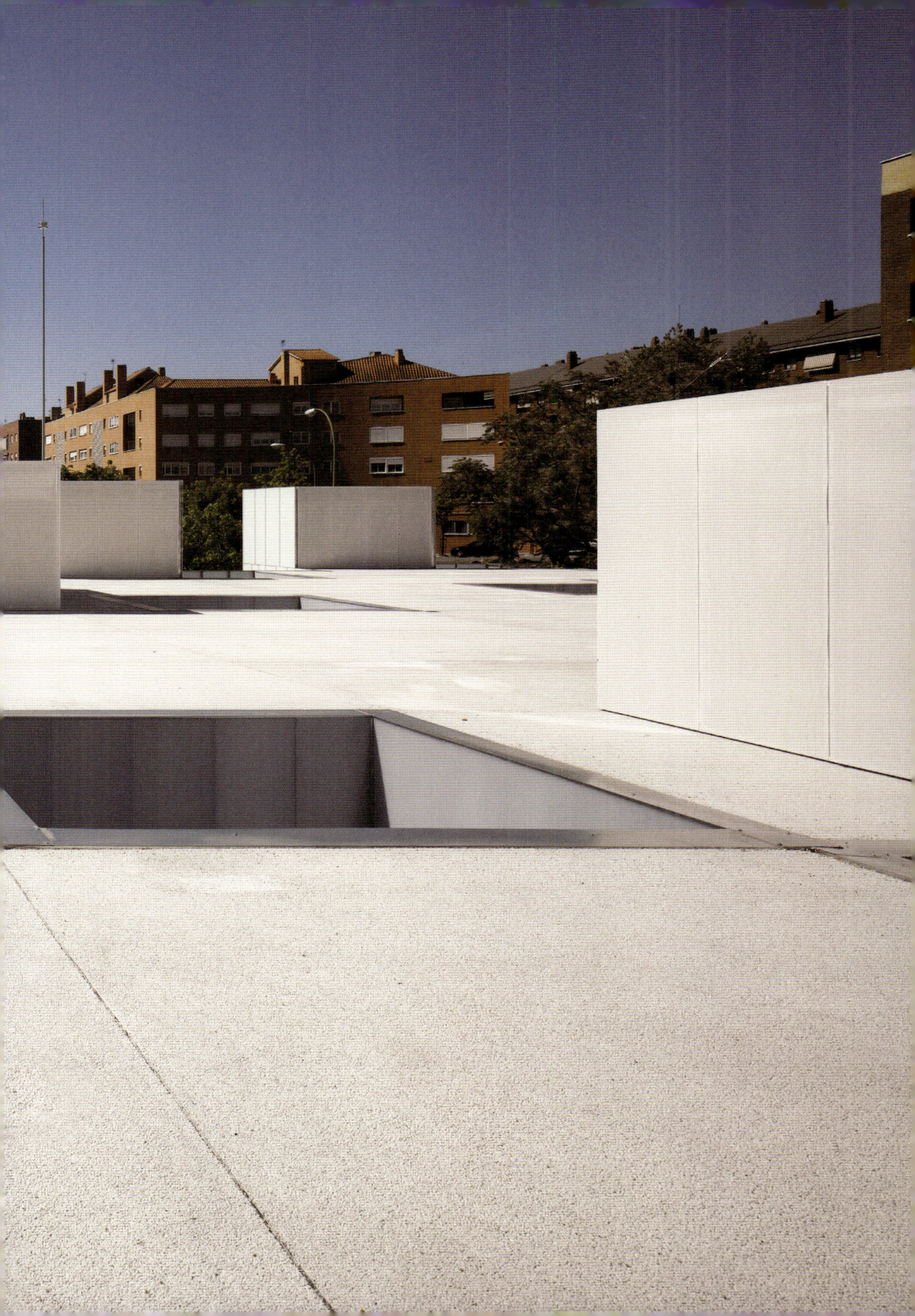

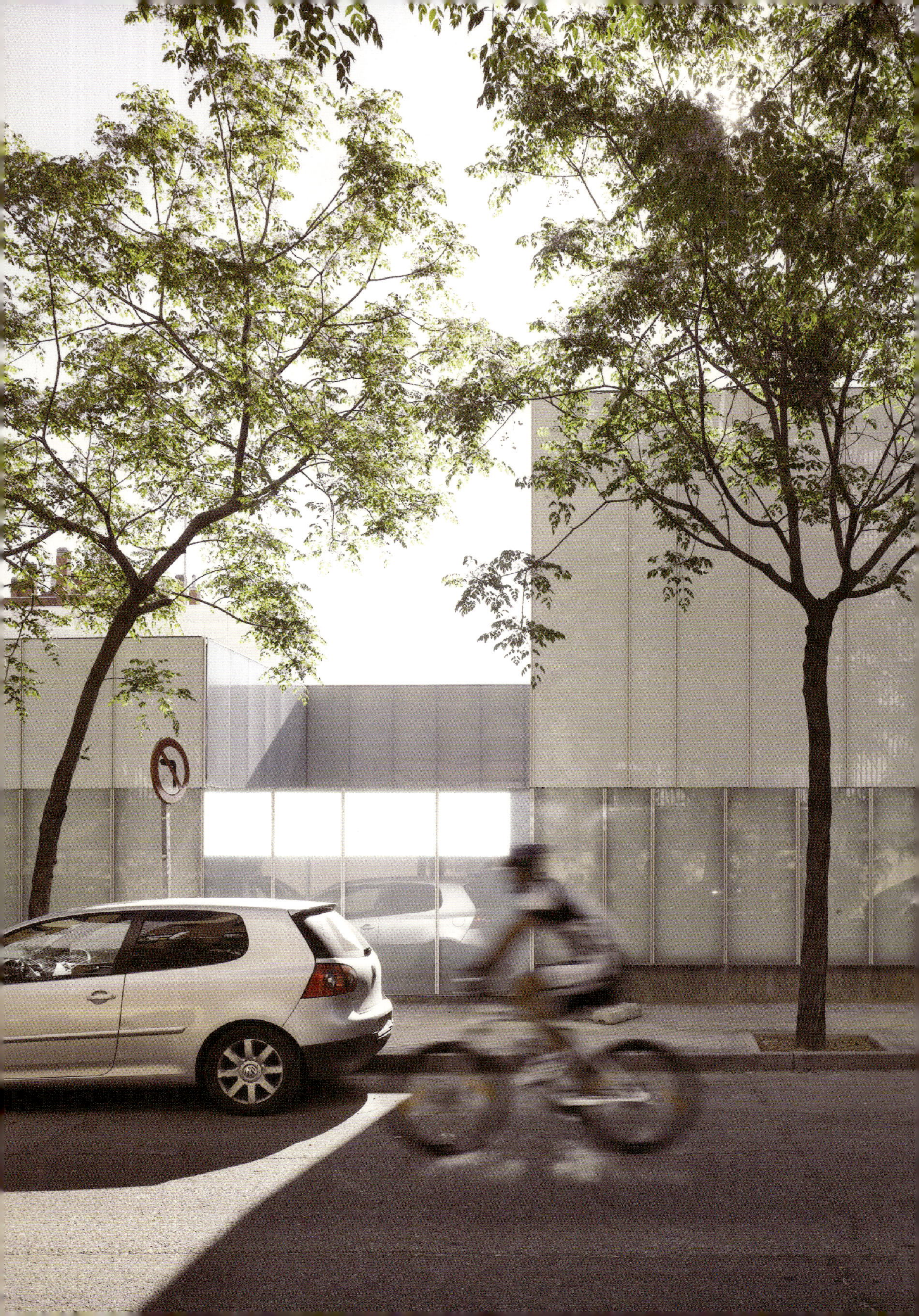

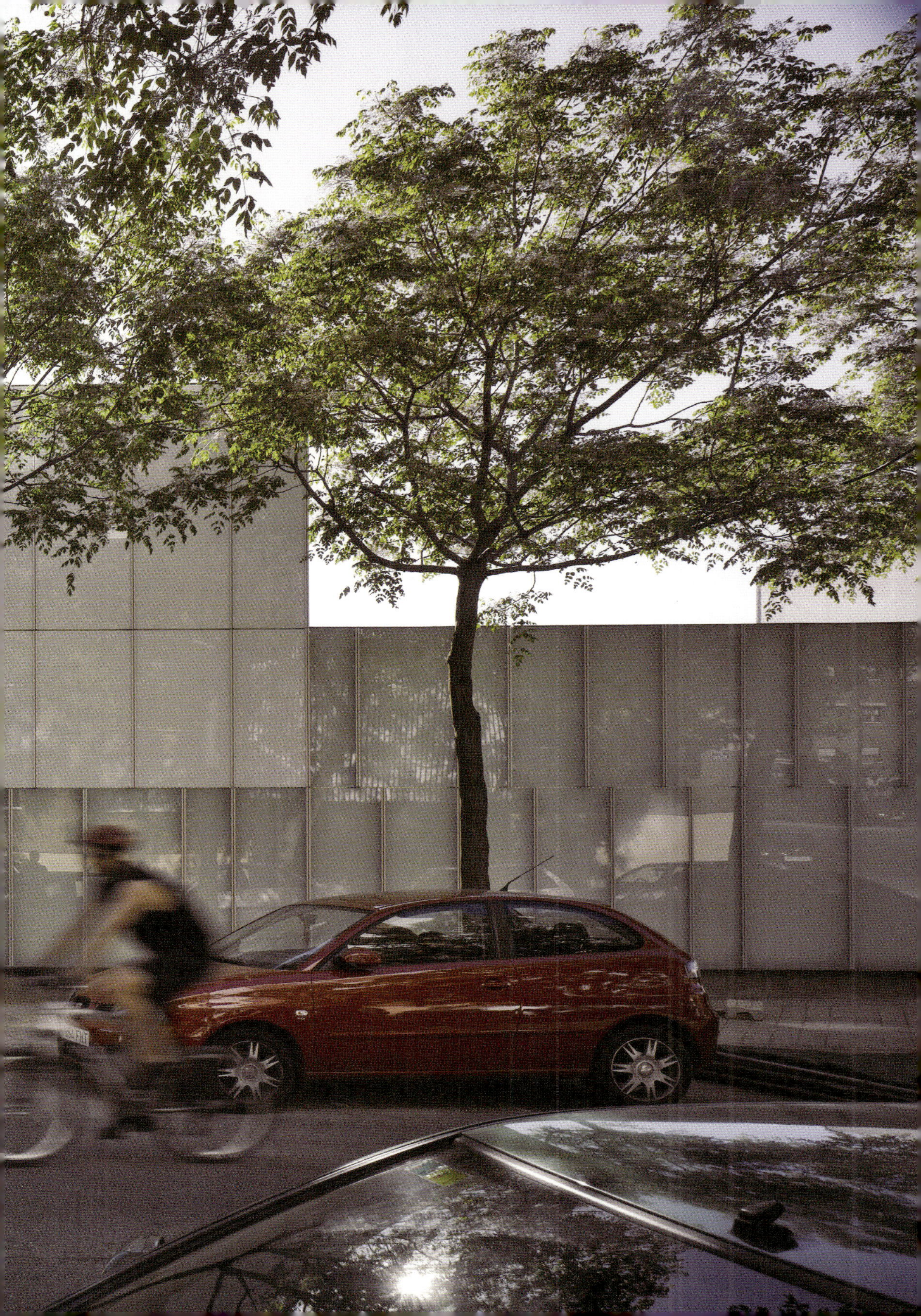

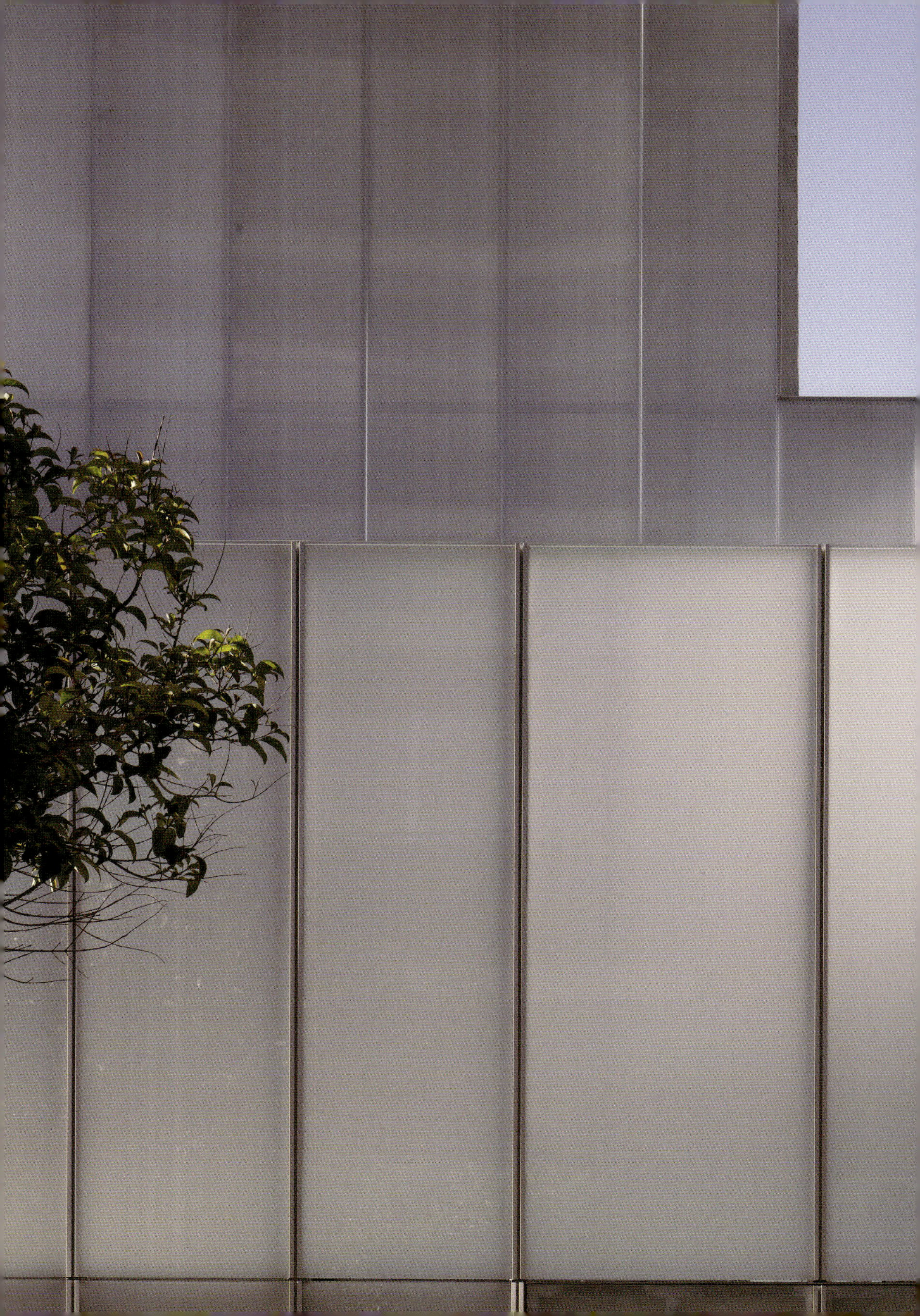

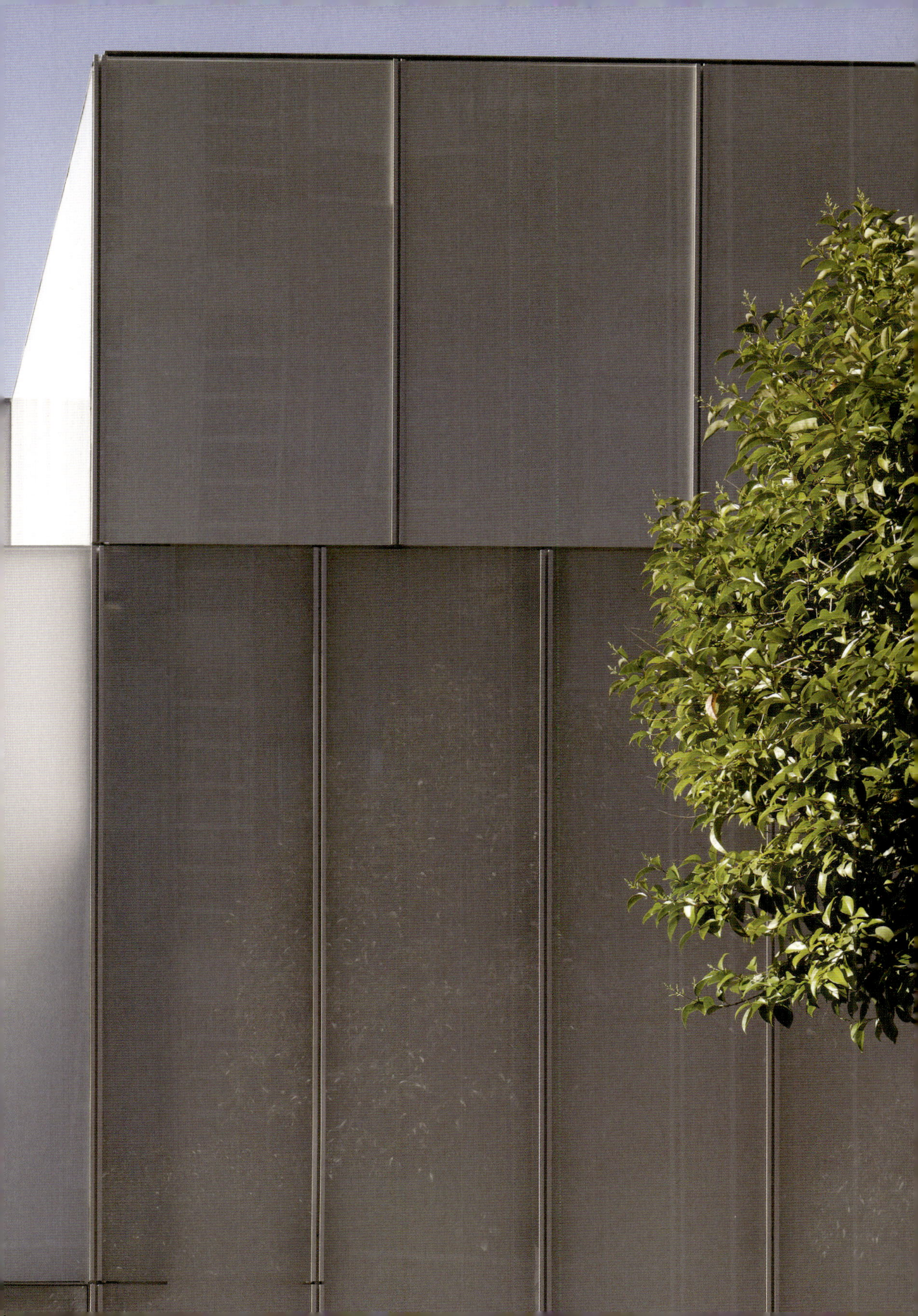

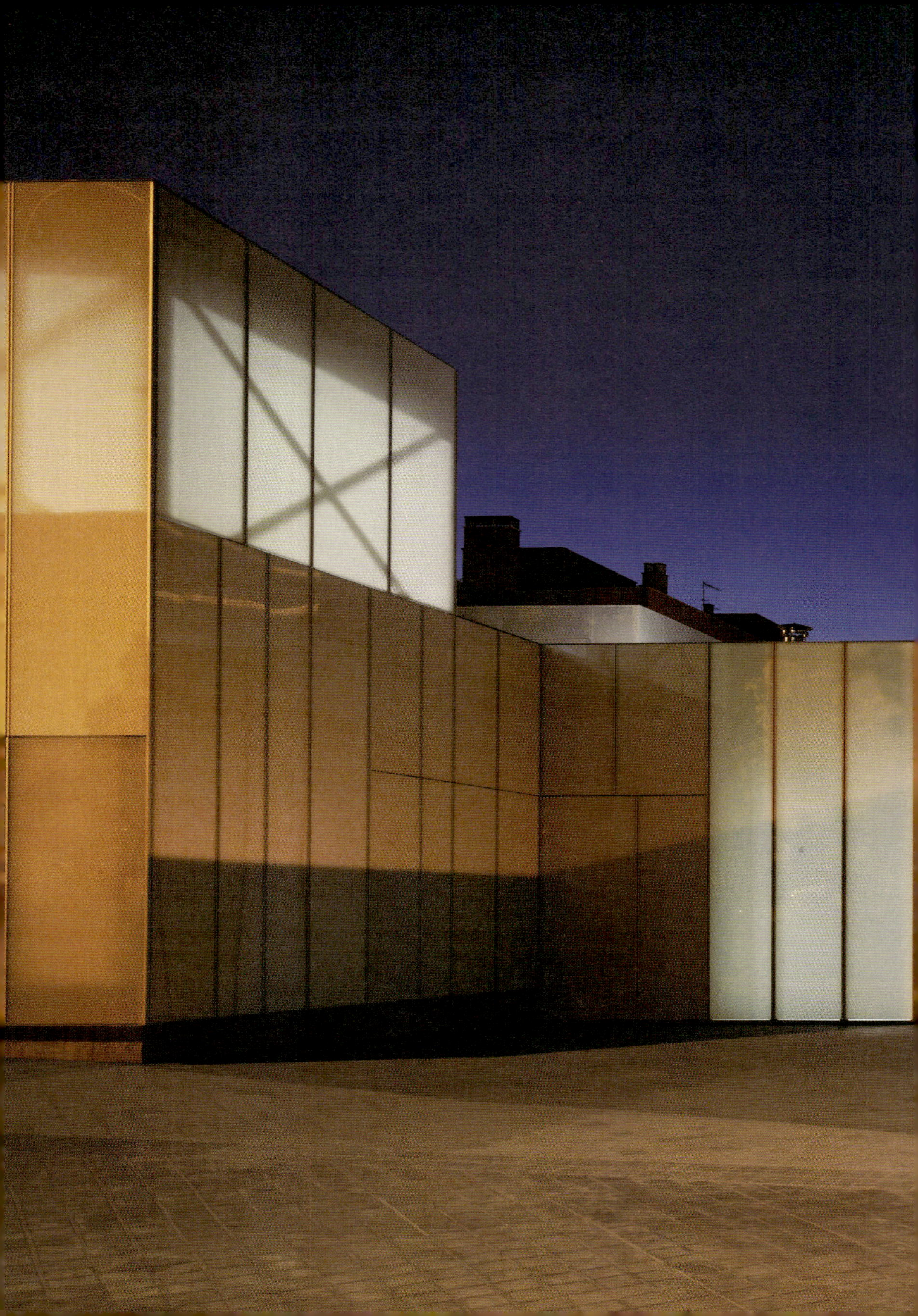

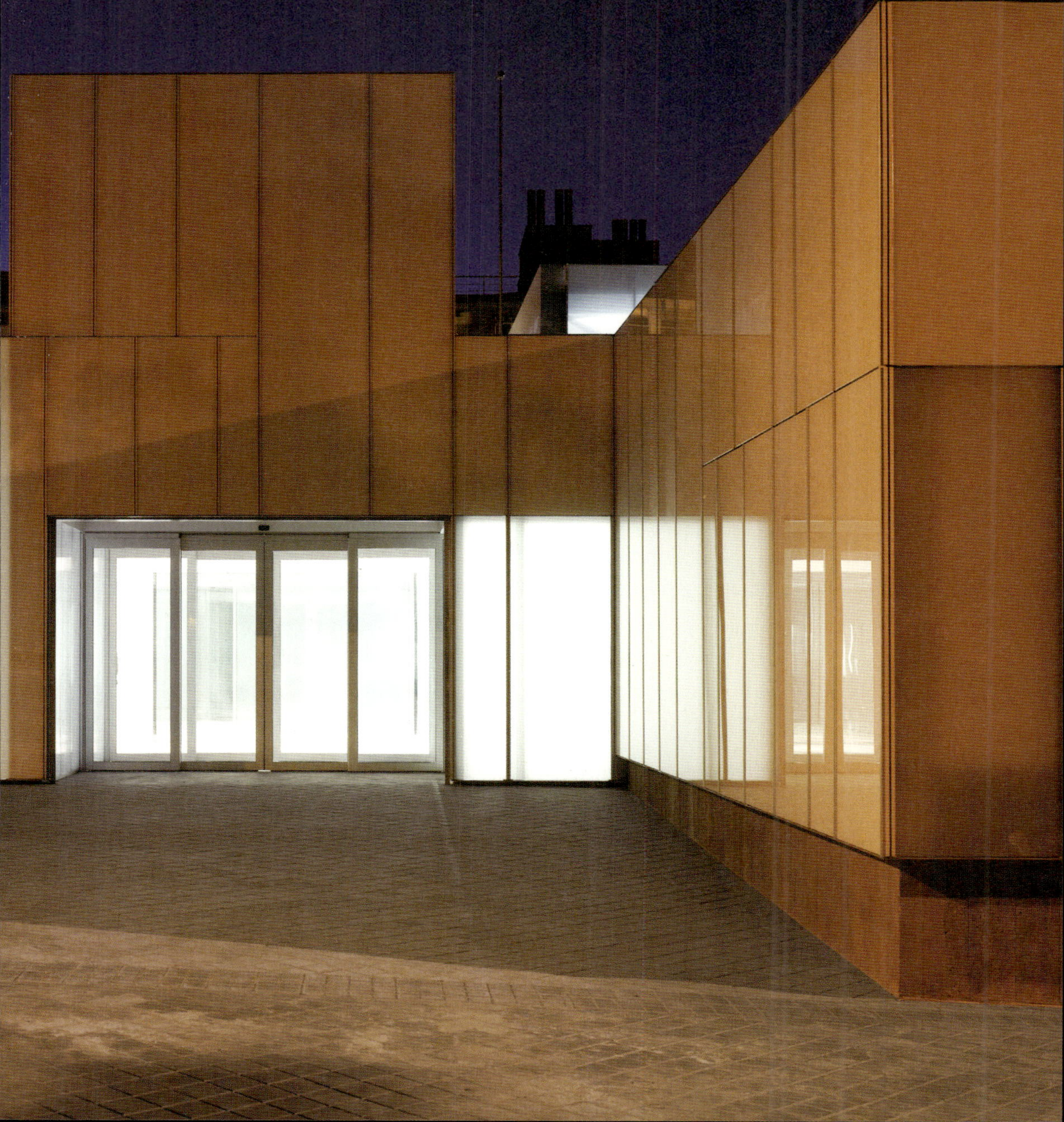

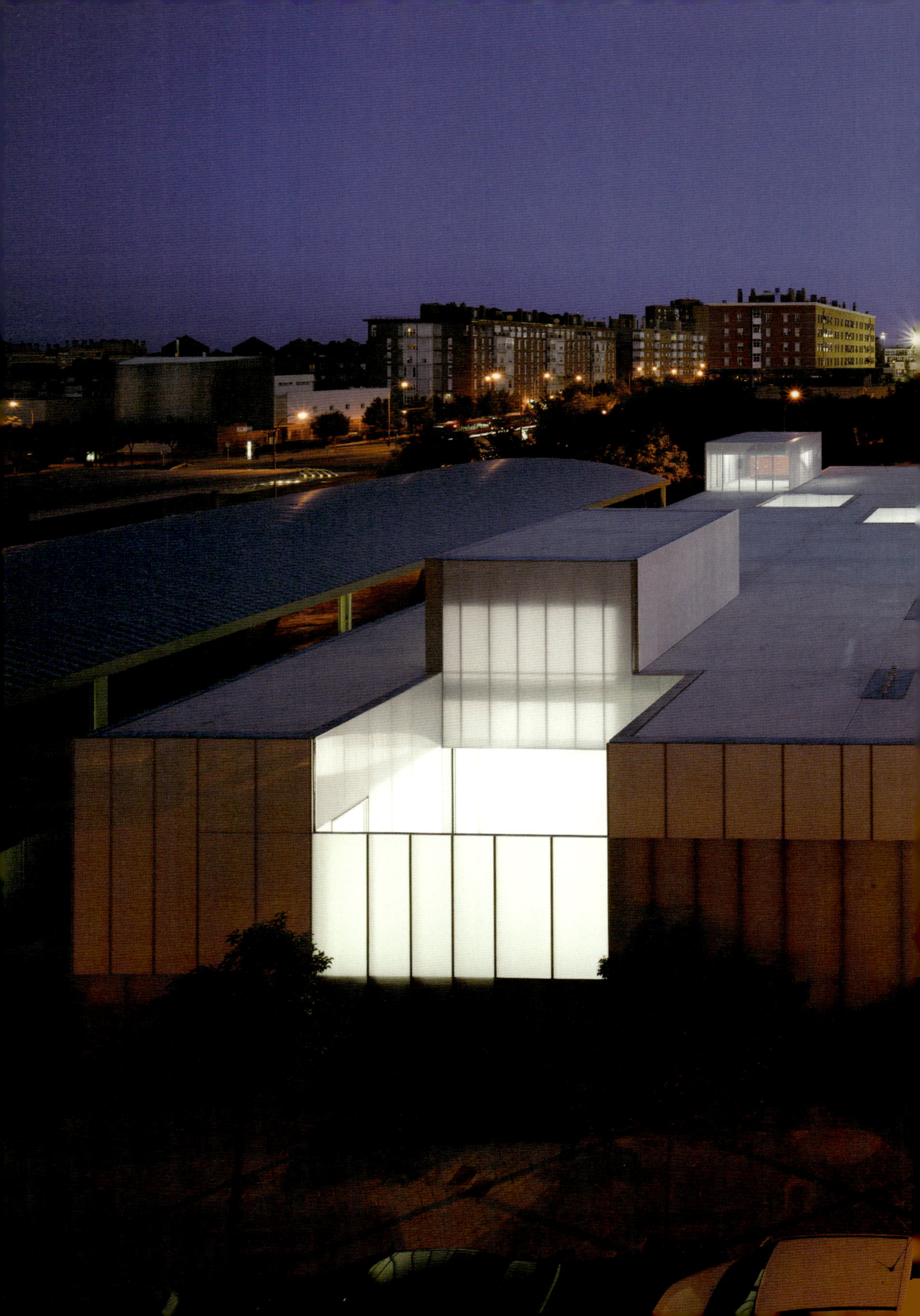

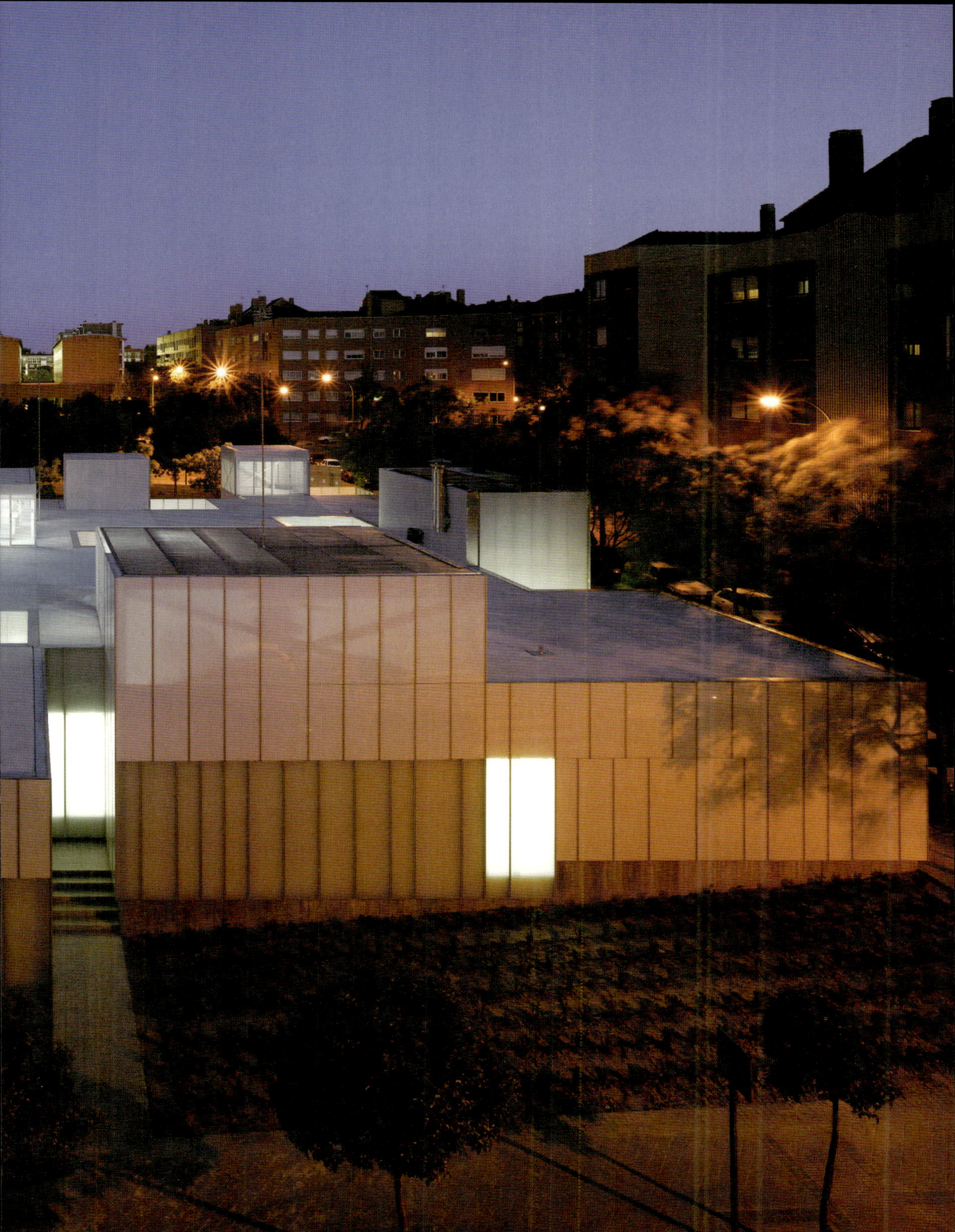

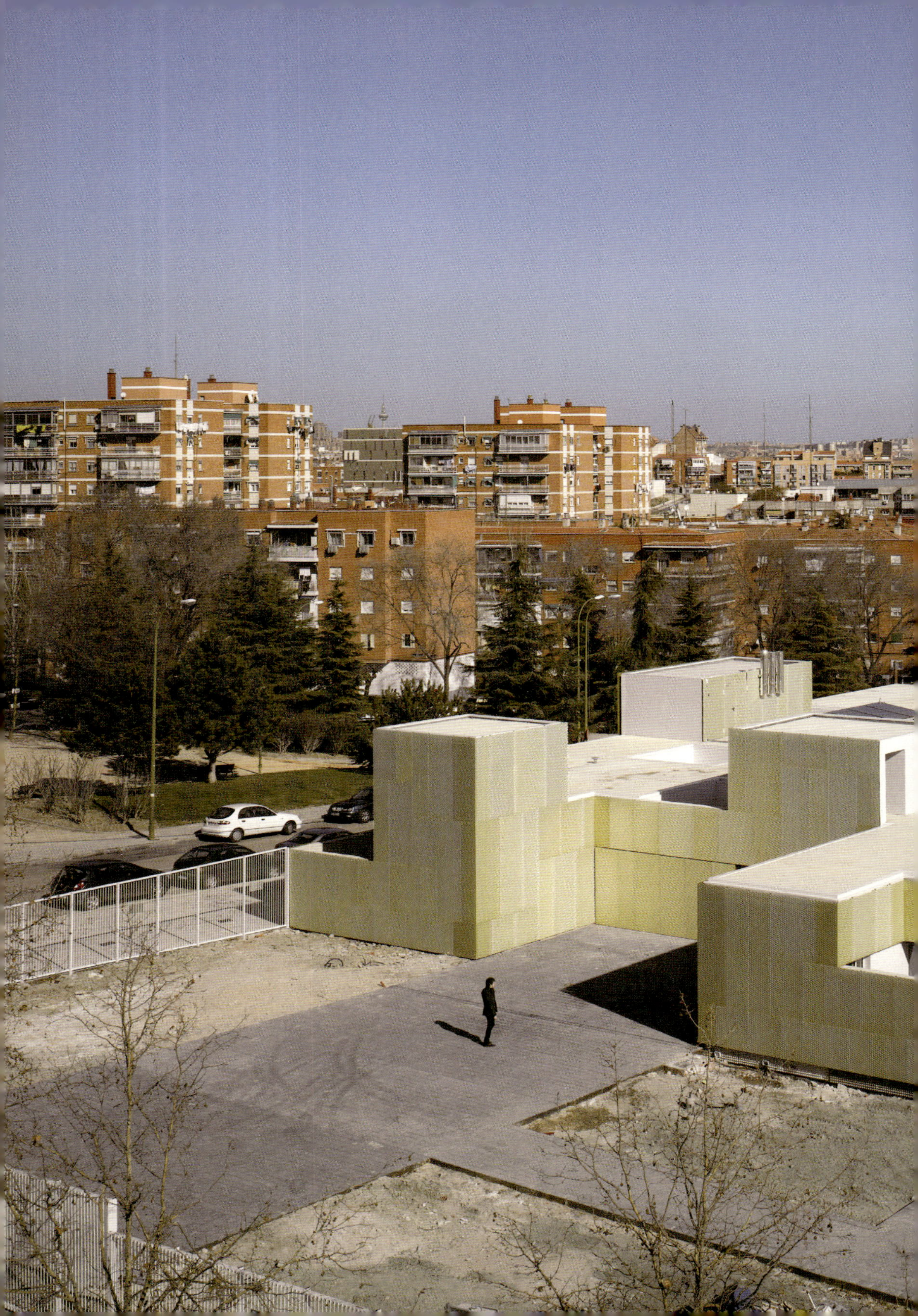

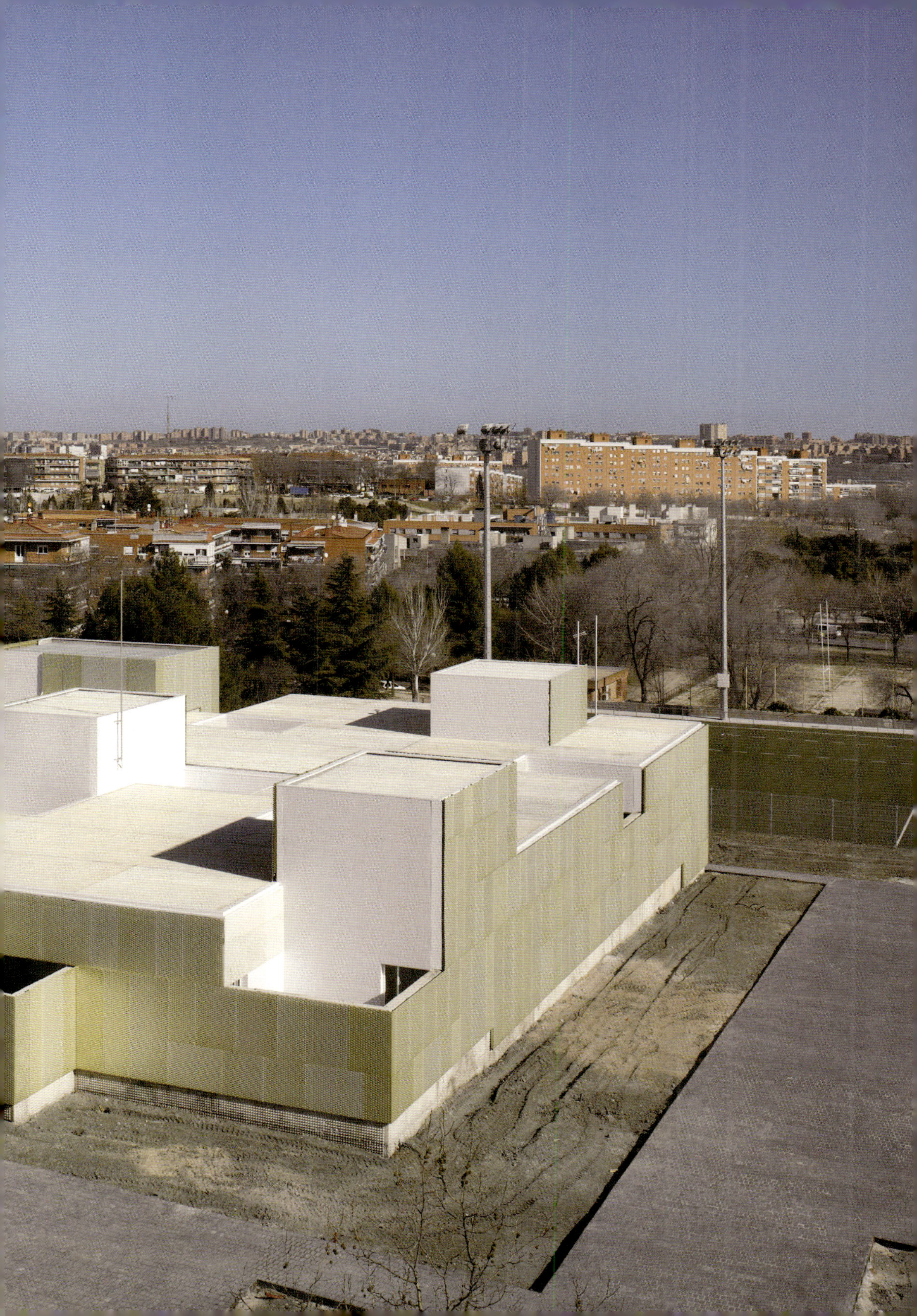

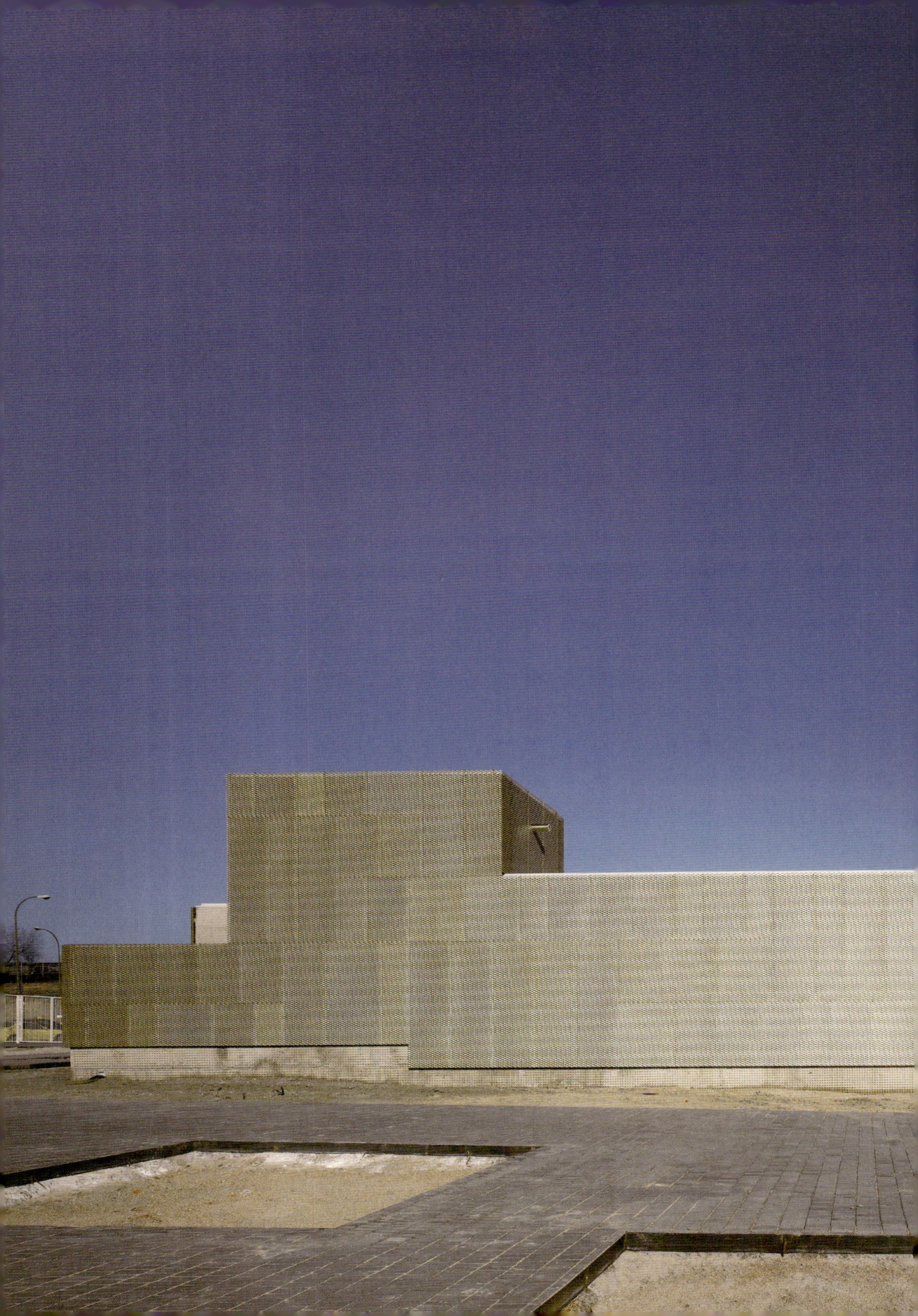

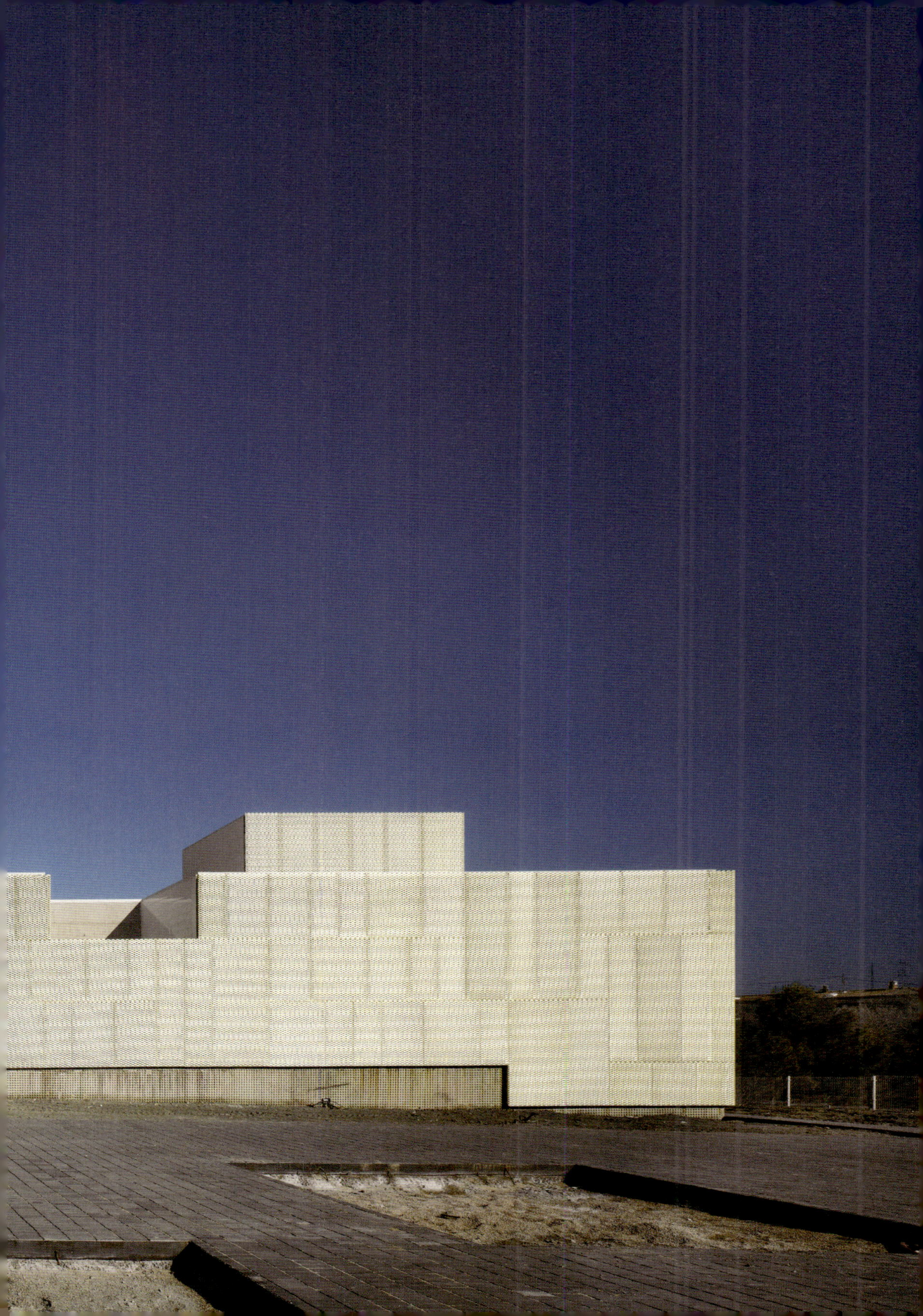

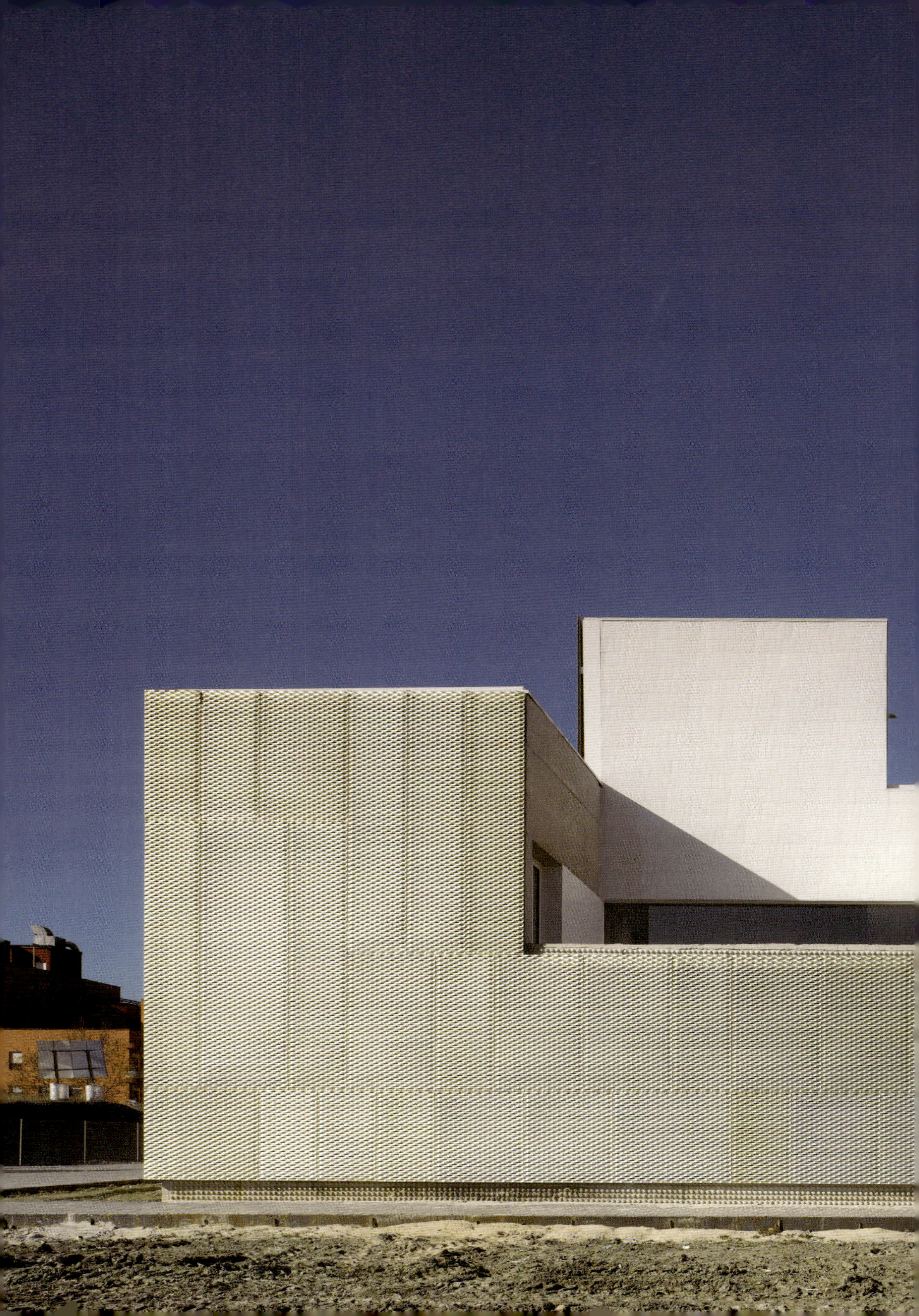

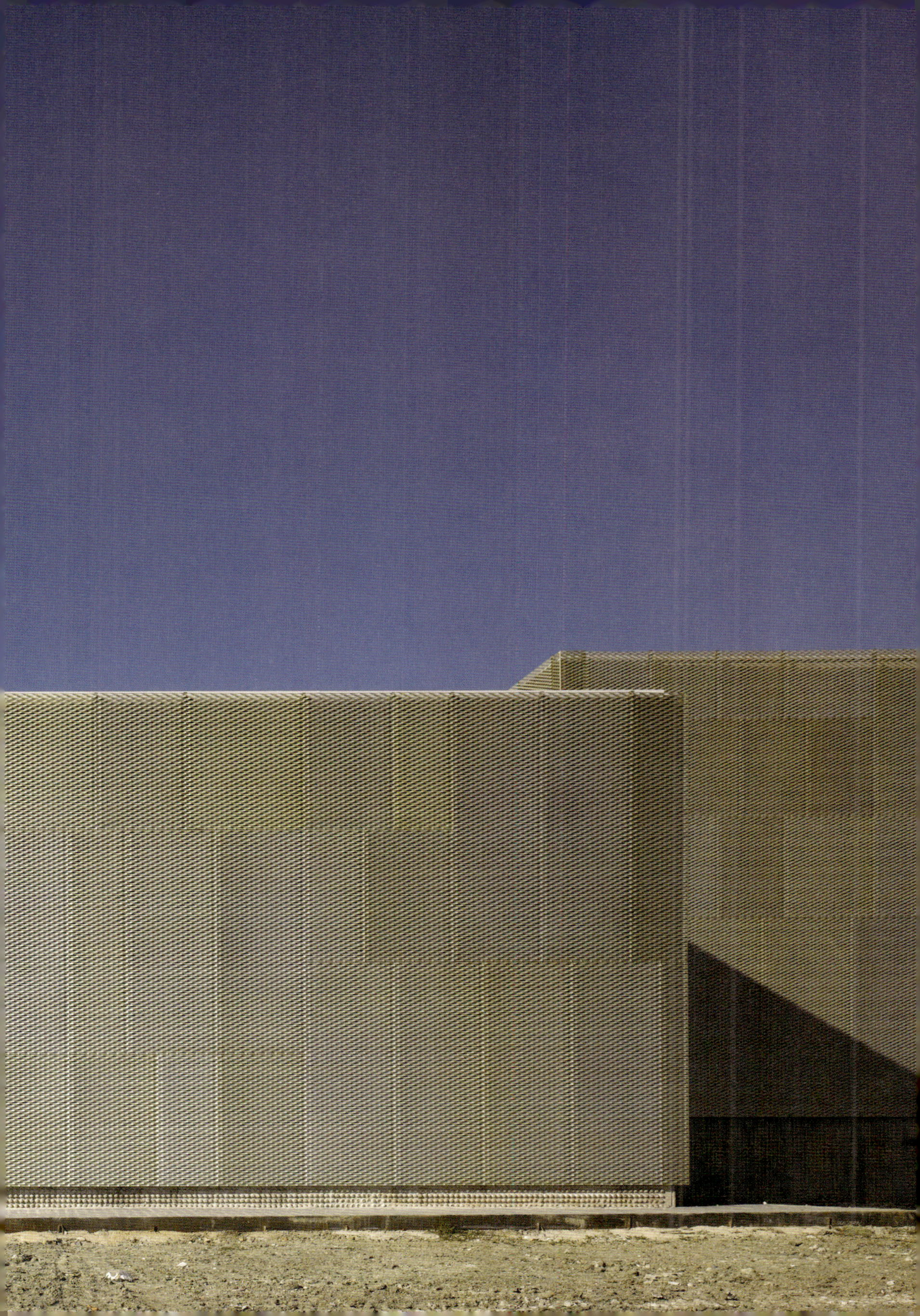

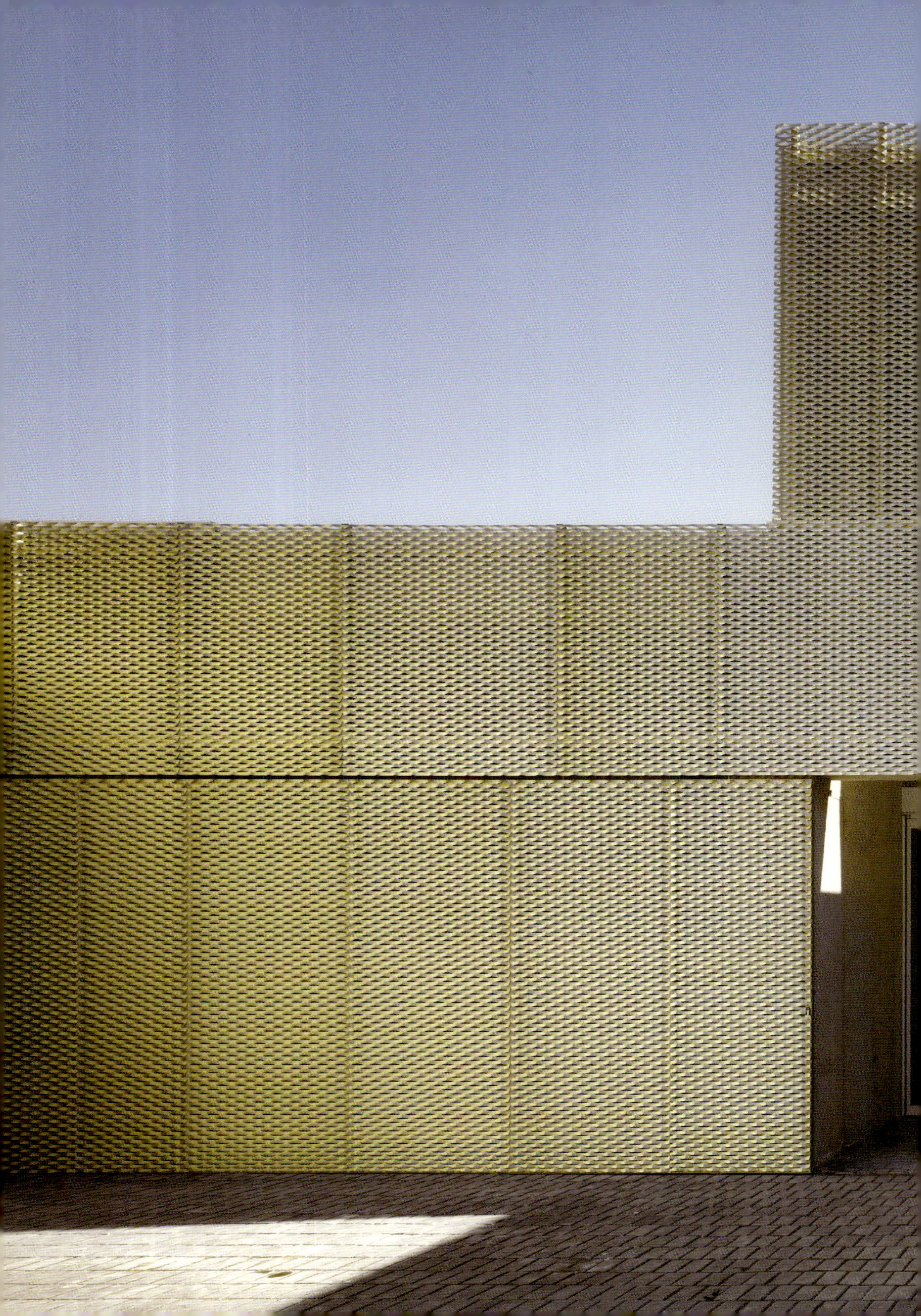

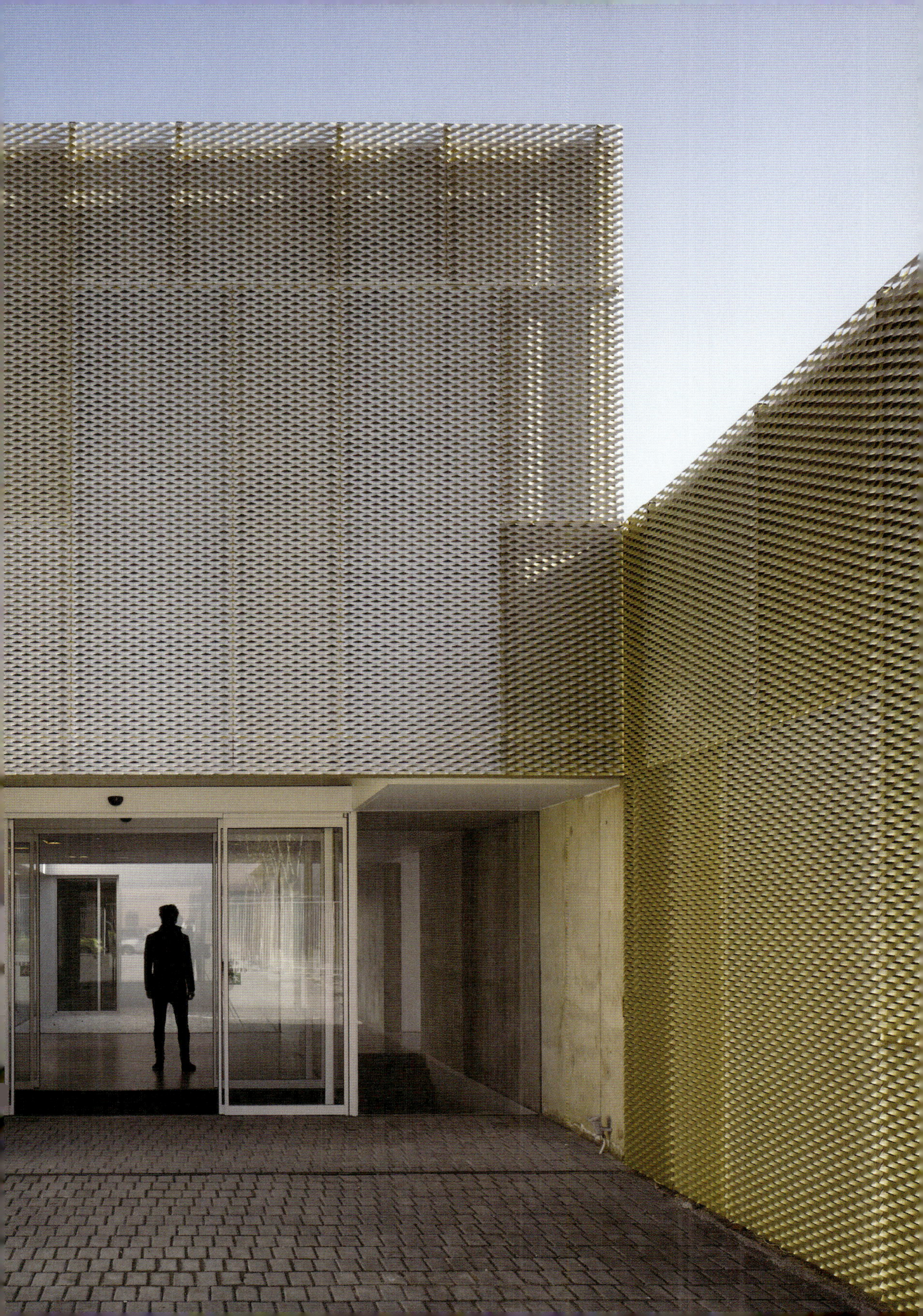

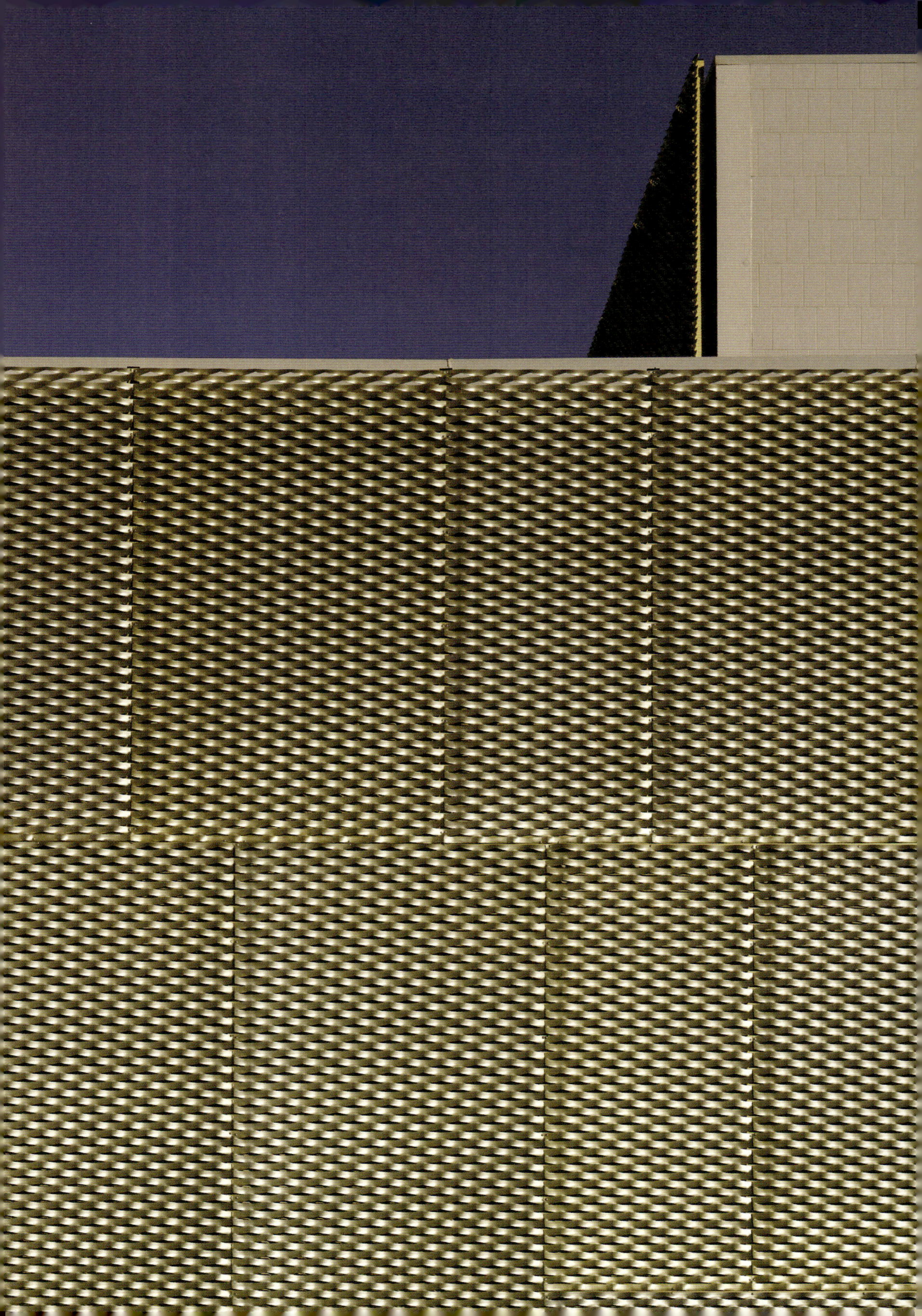

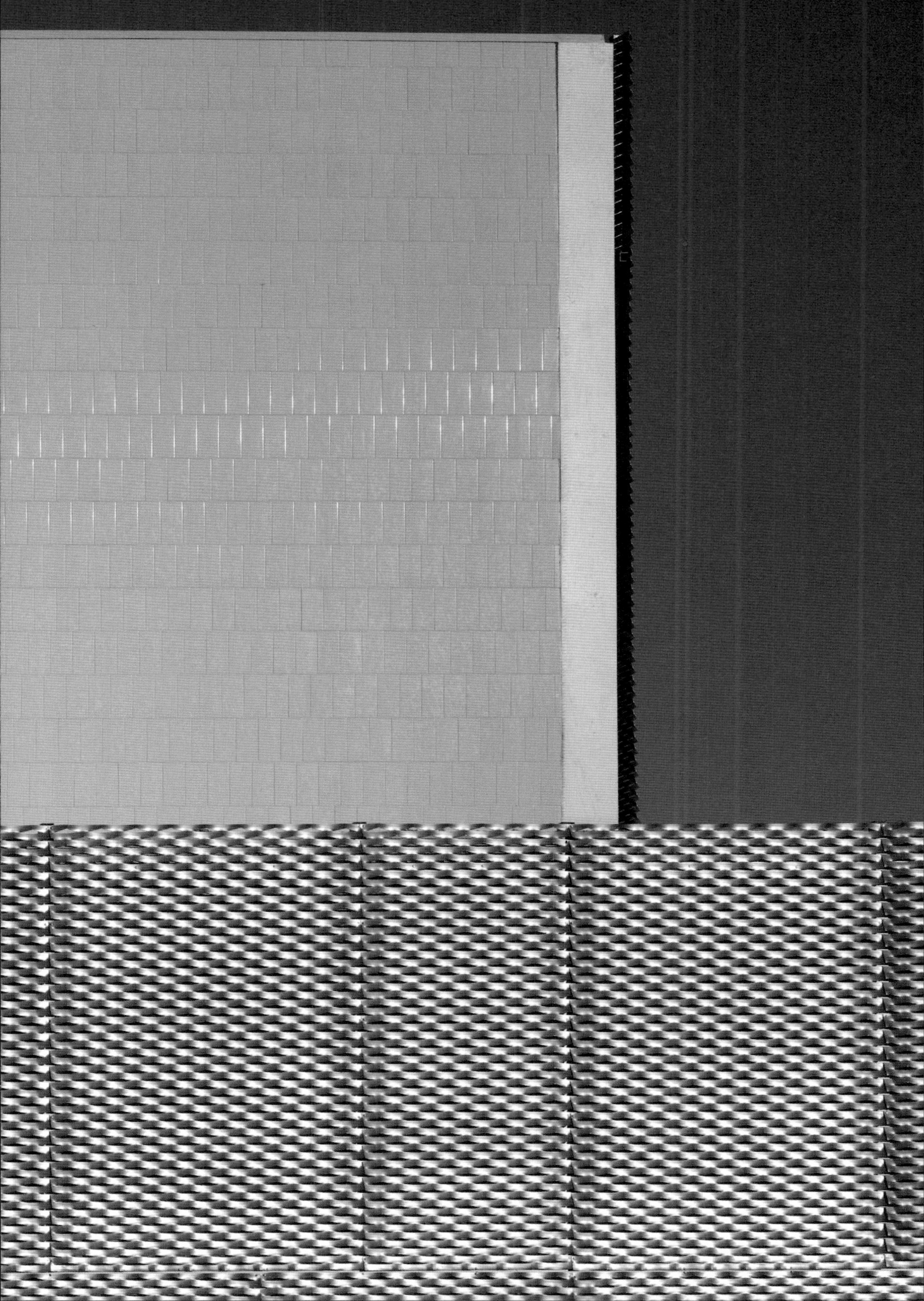

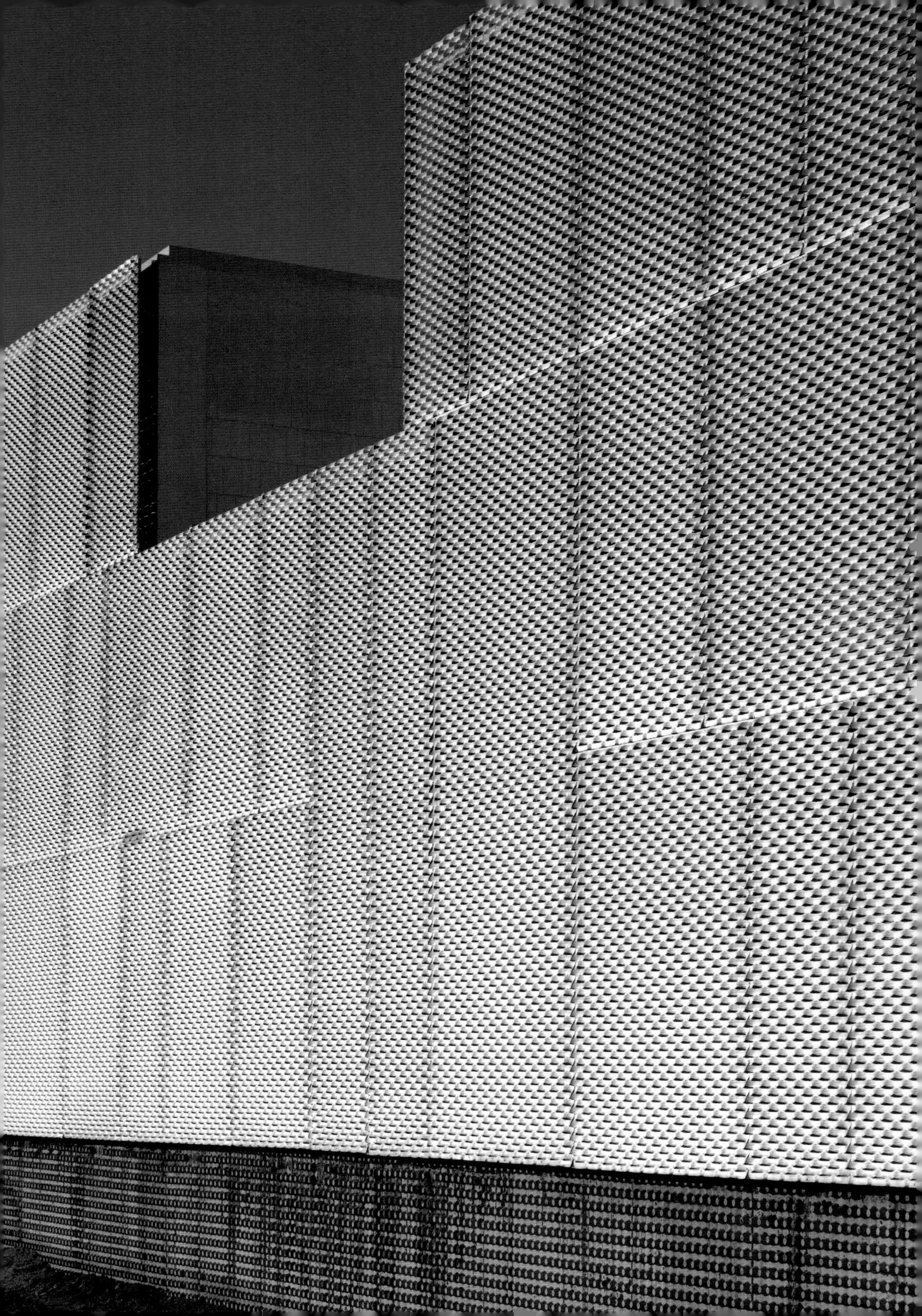

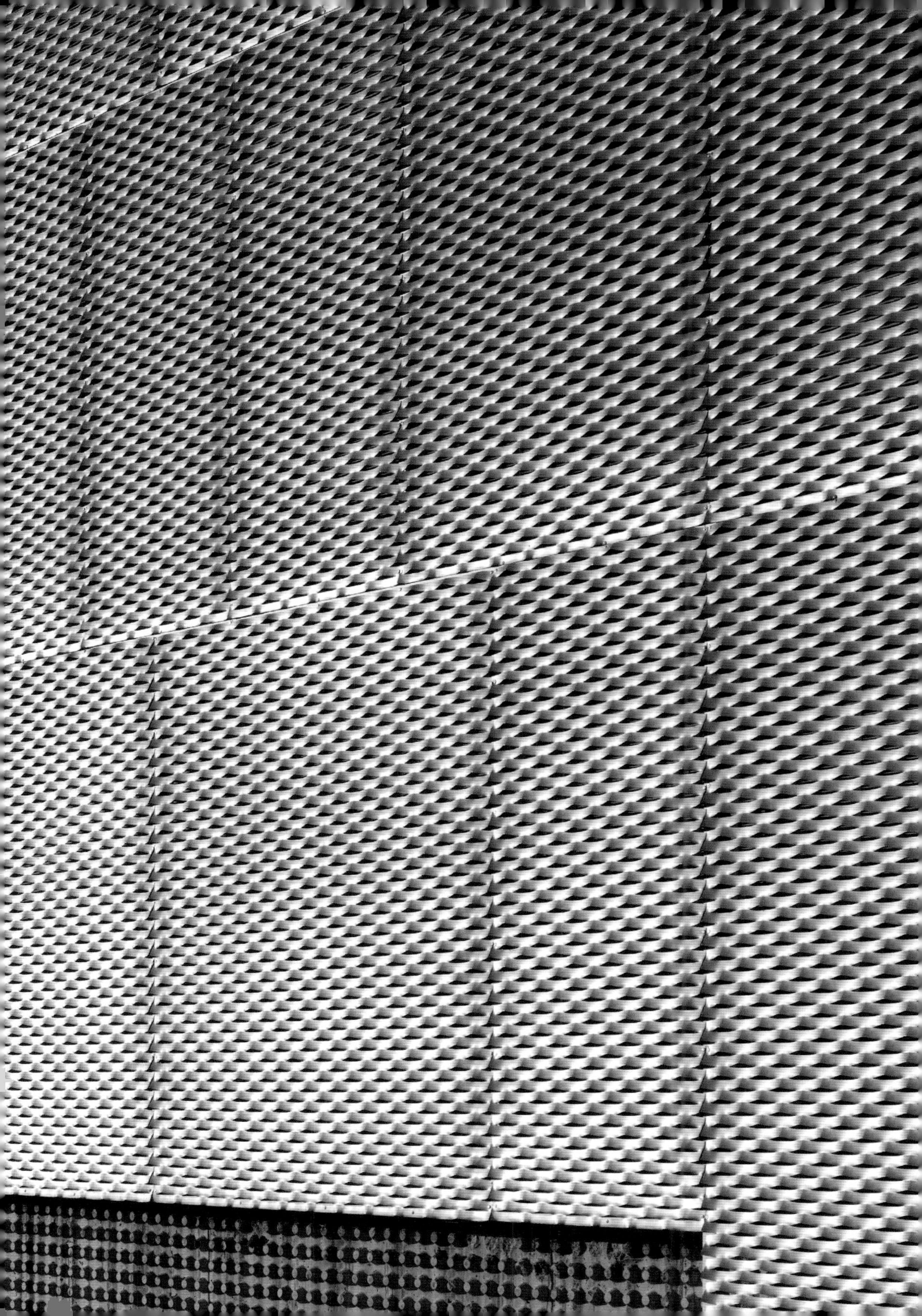

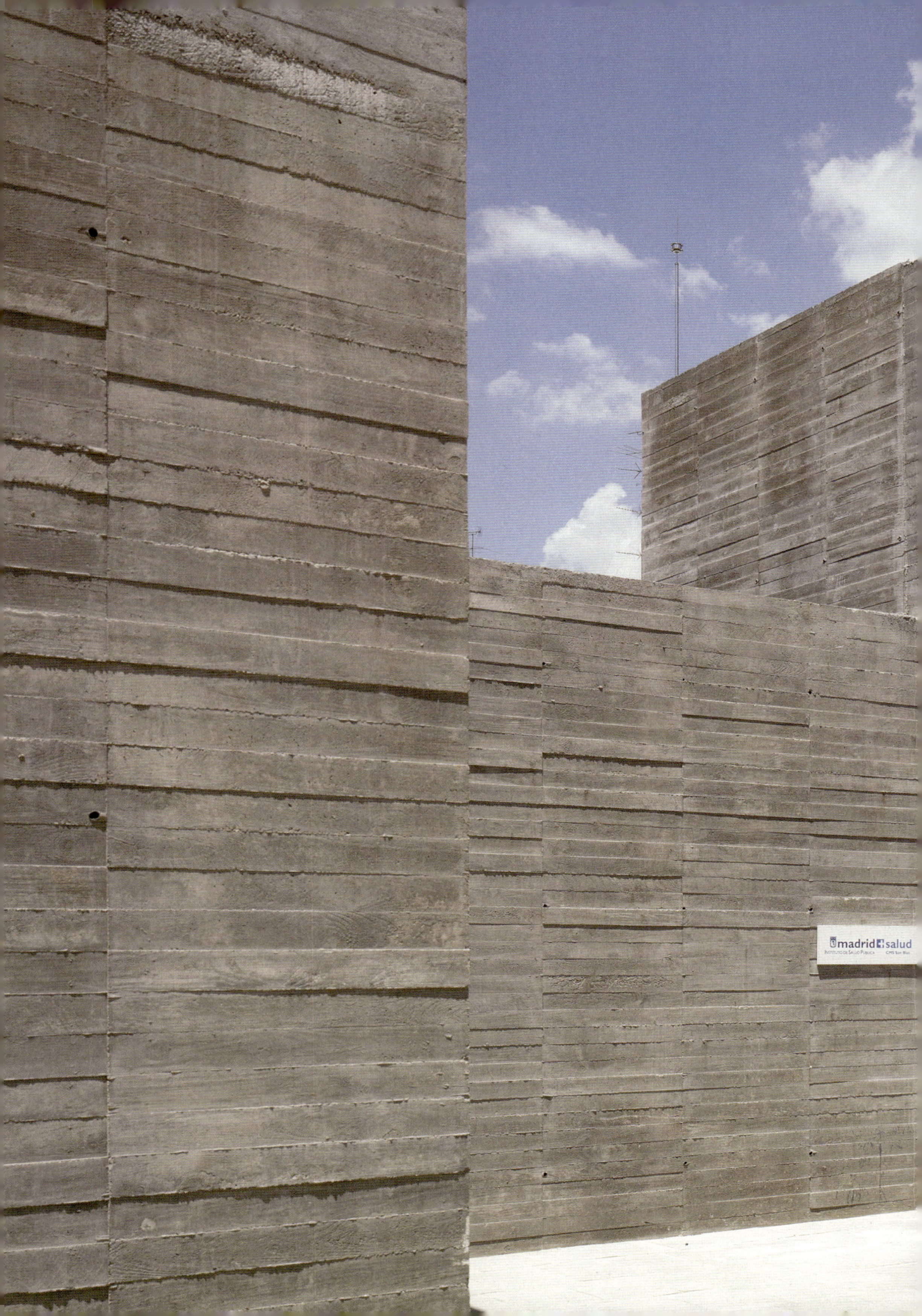
madrid salud
INSTITUTO DE SALUD PUBLICA
CMS San Blas

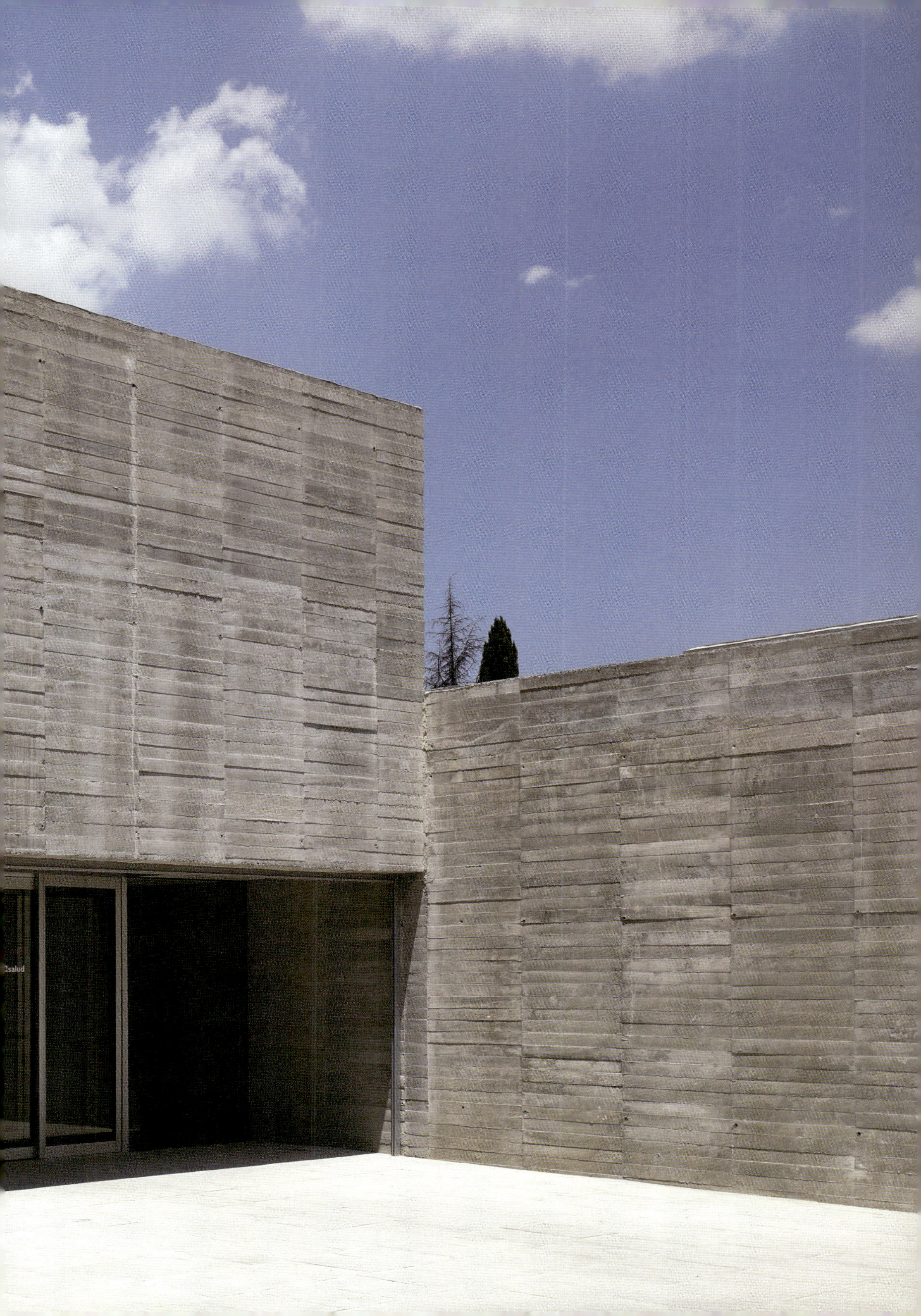

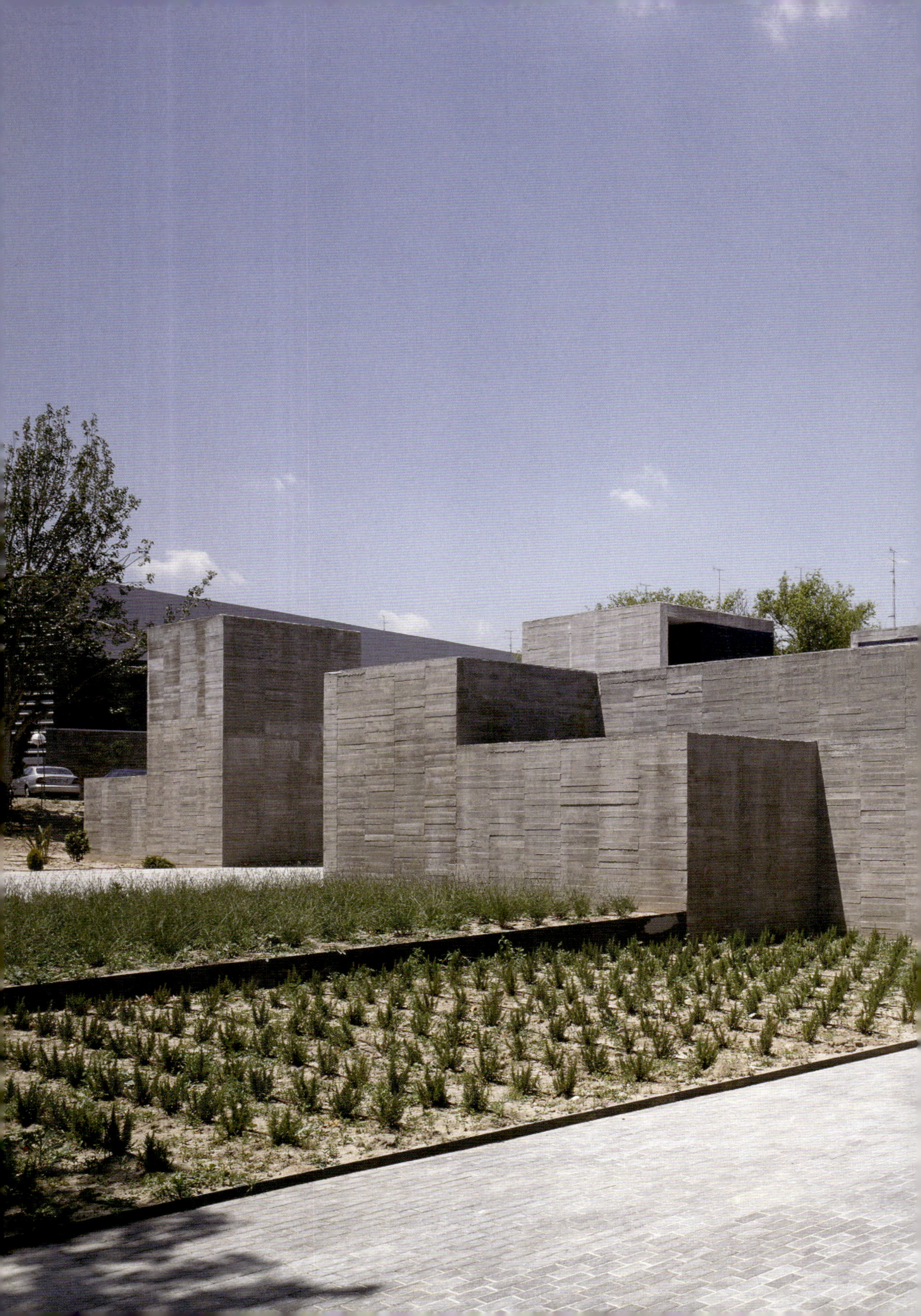

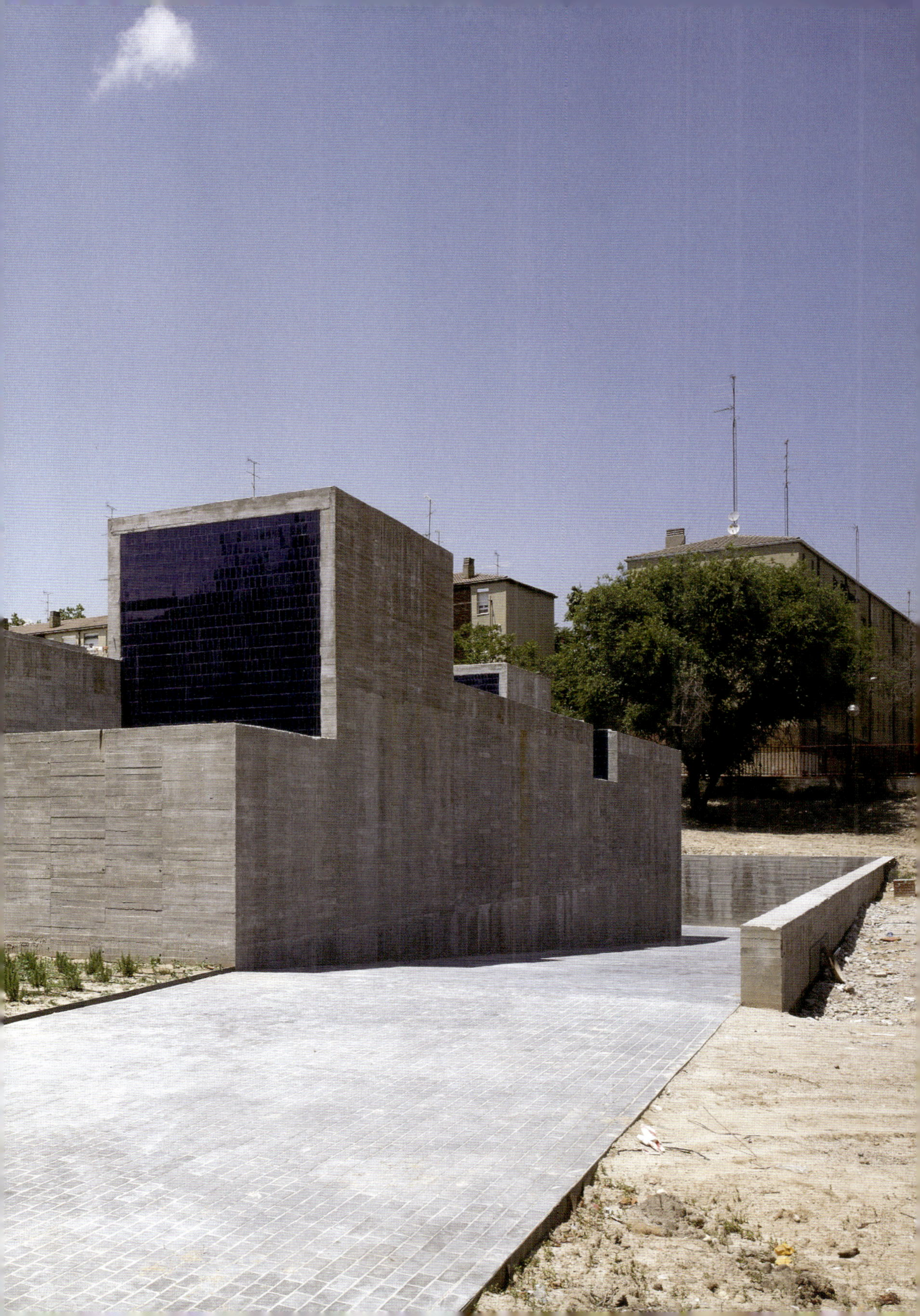

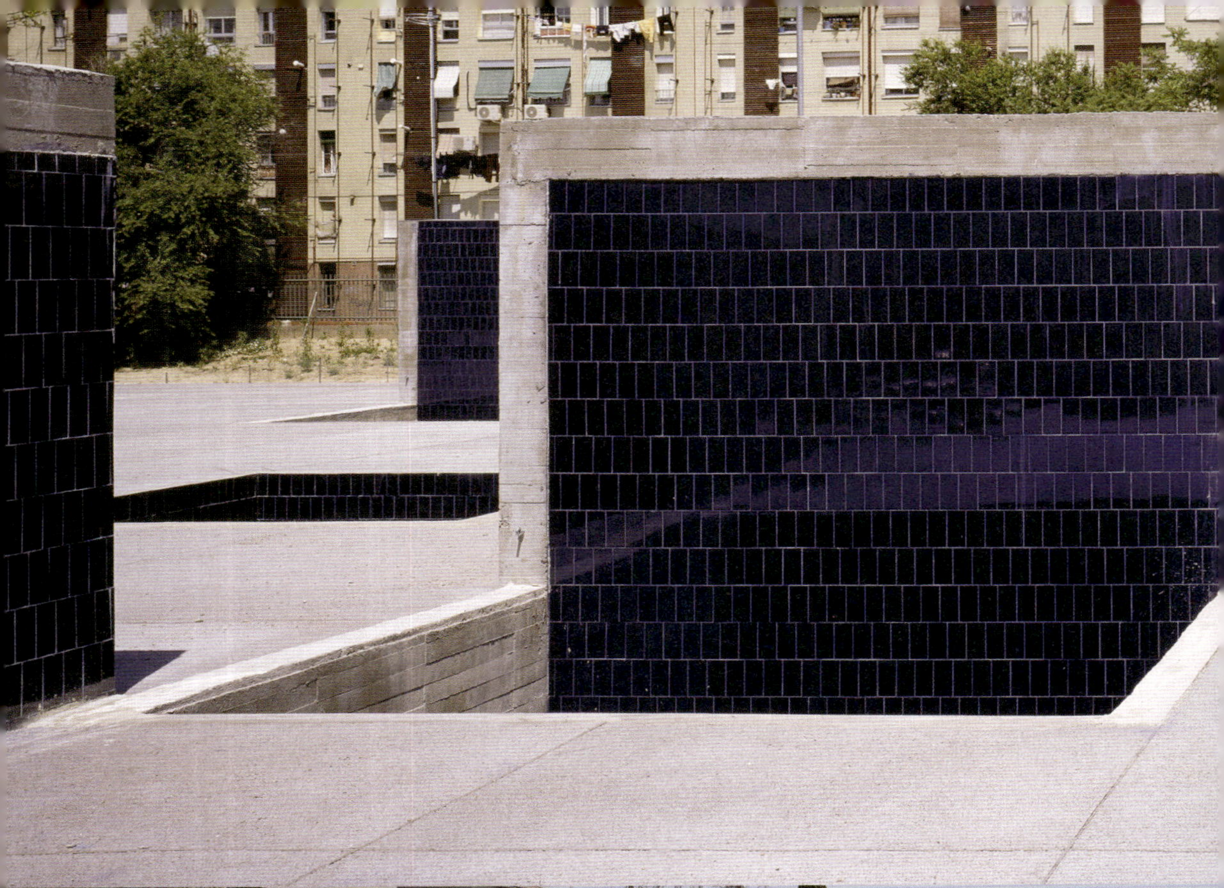
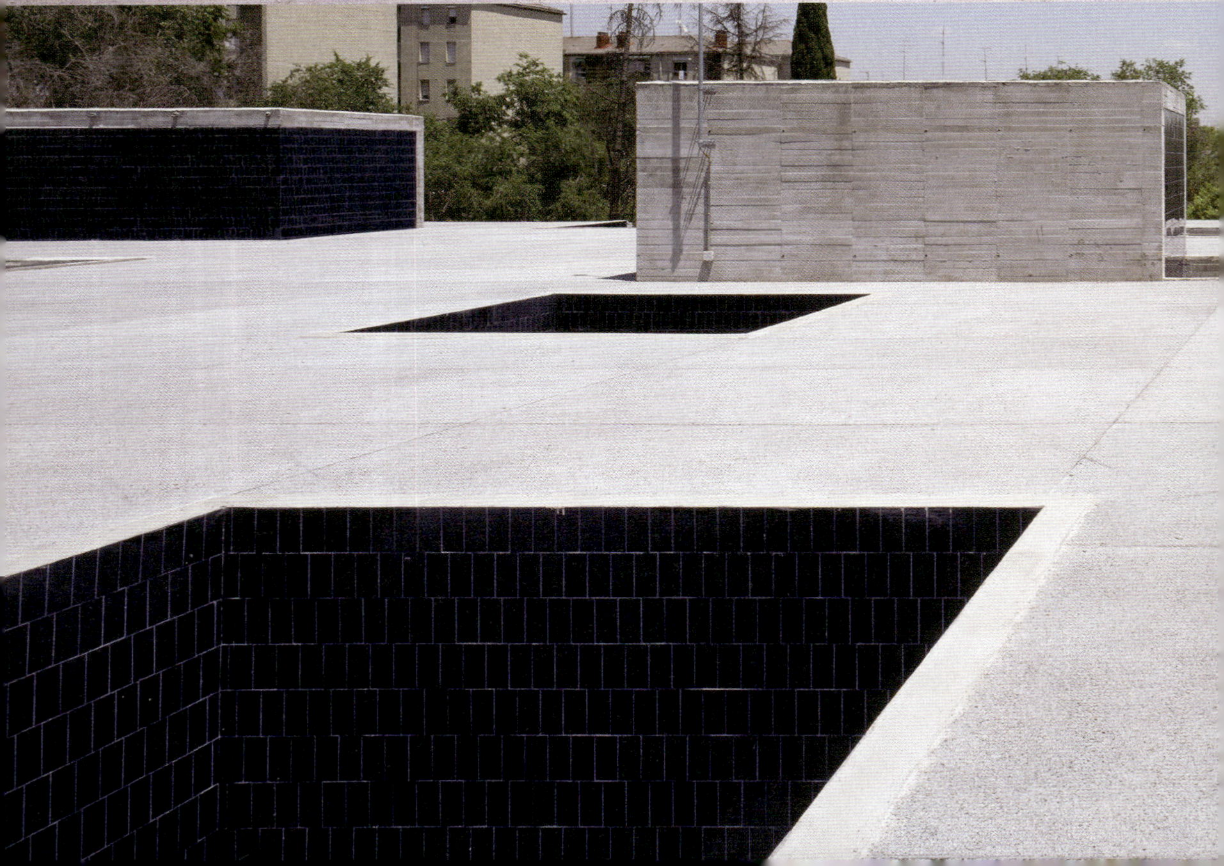

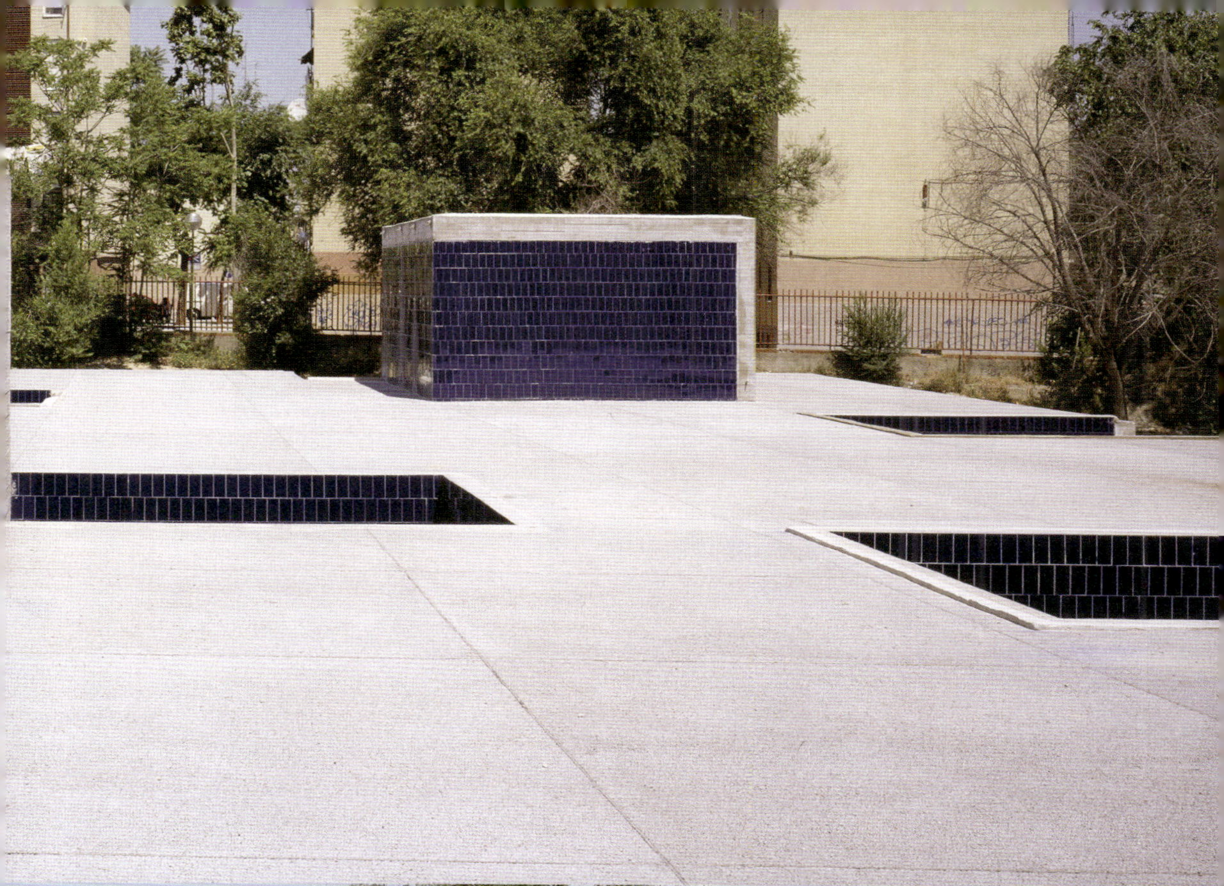

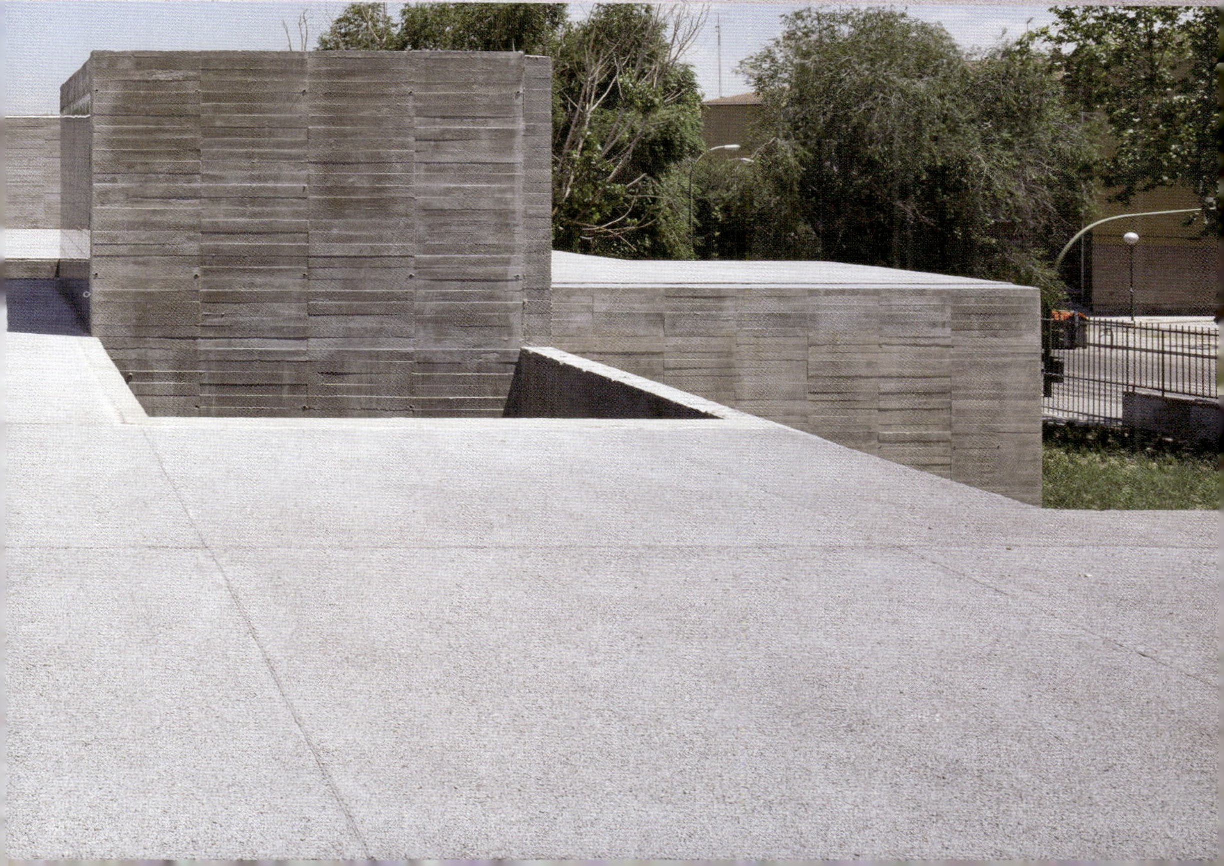

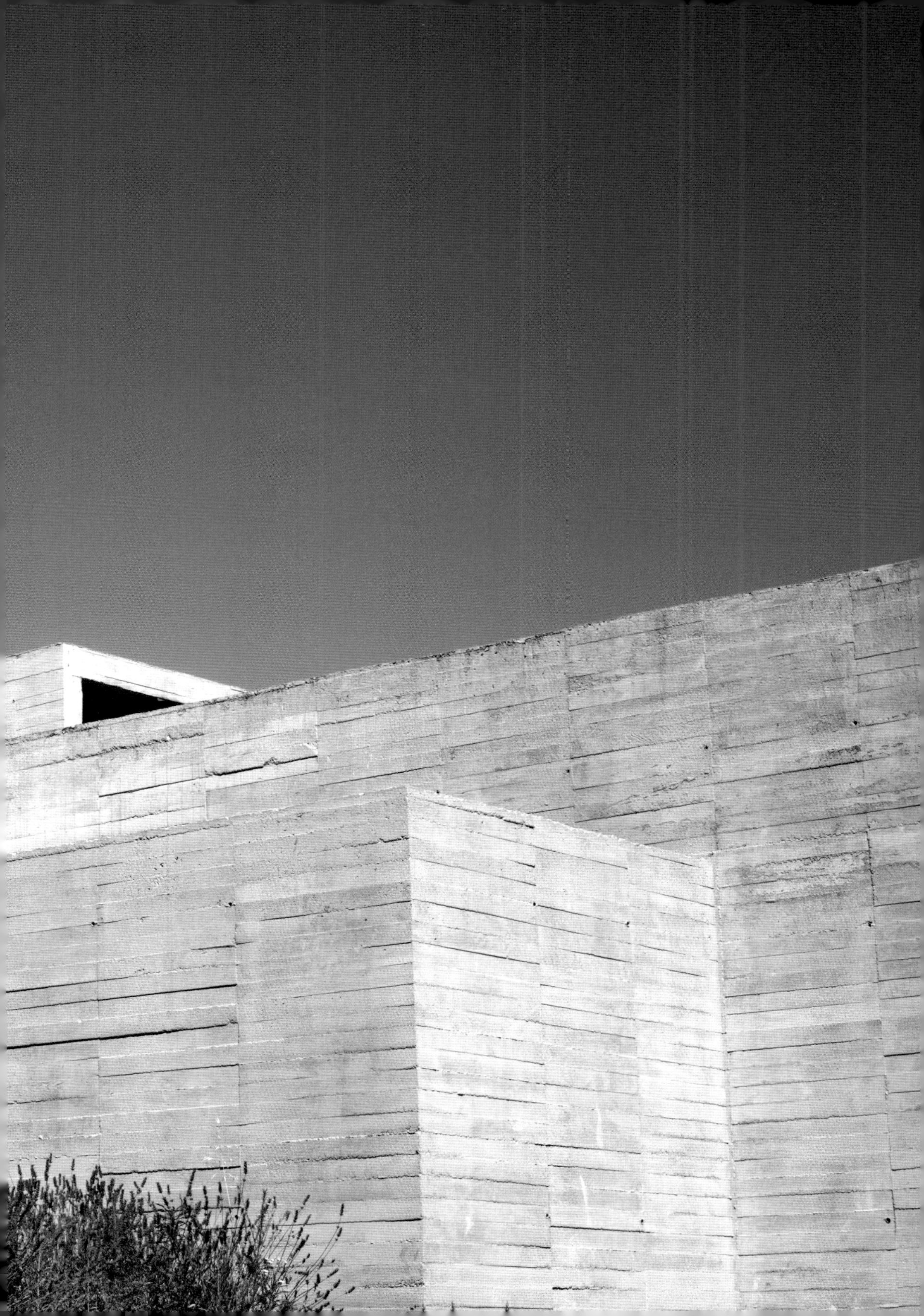

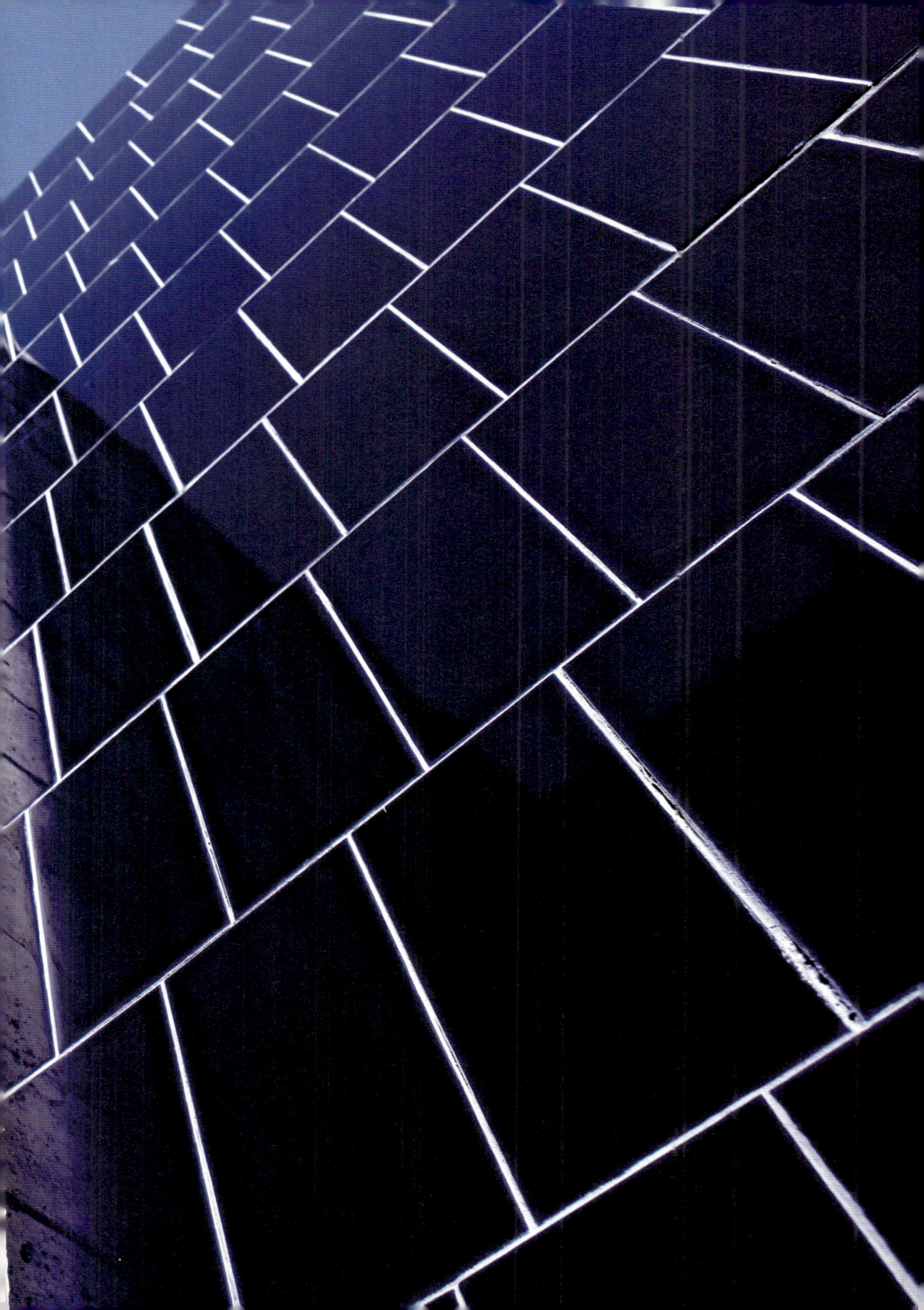

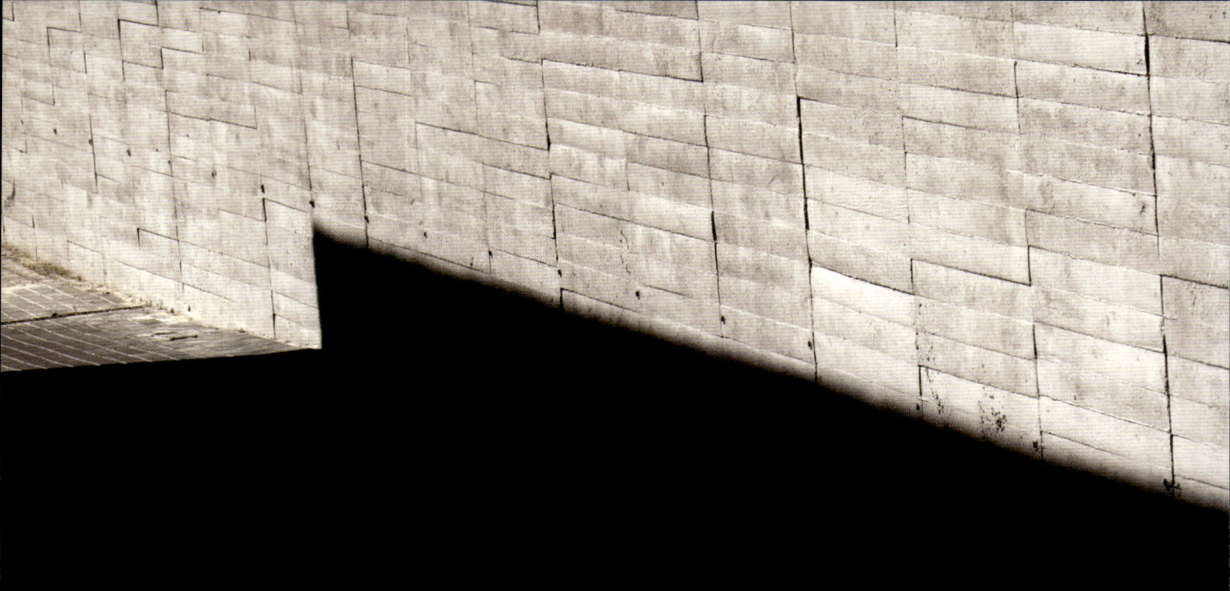

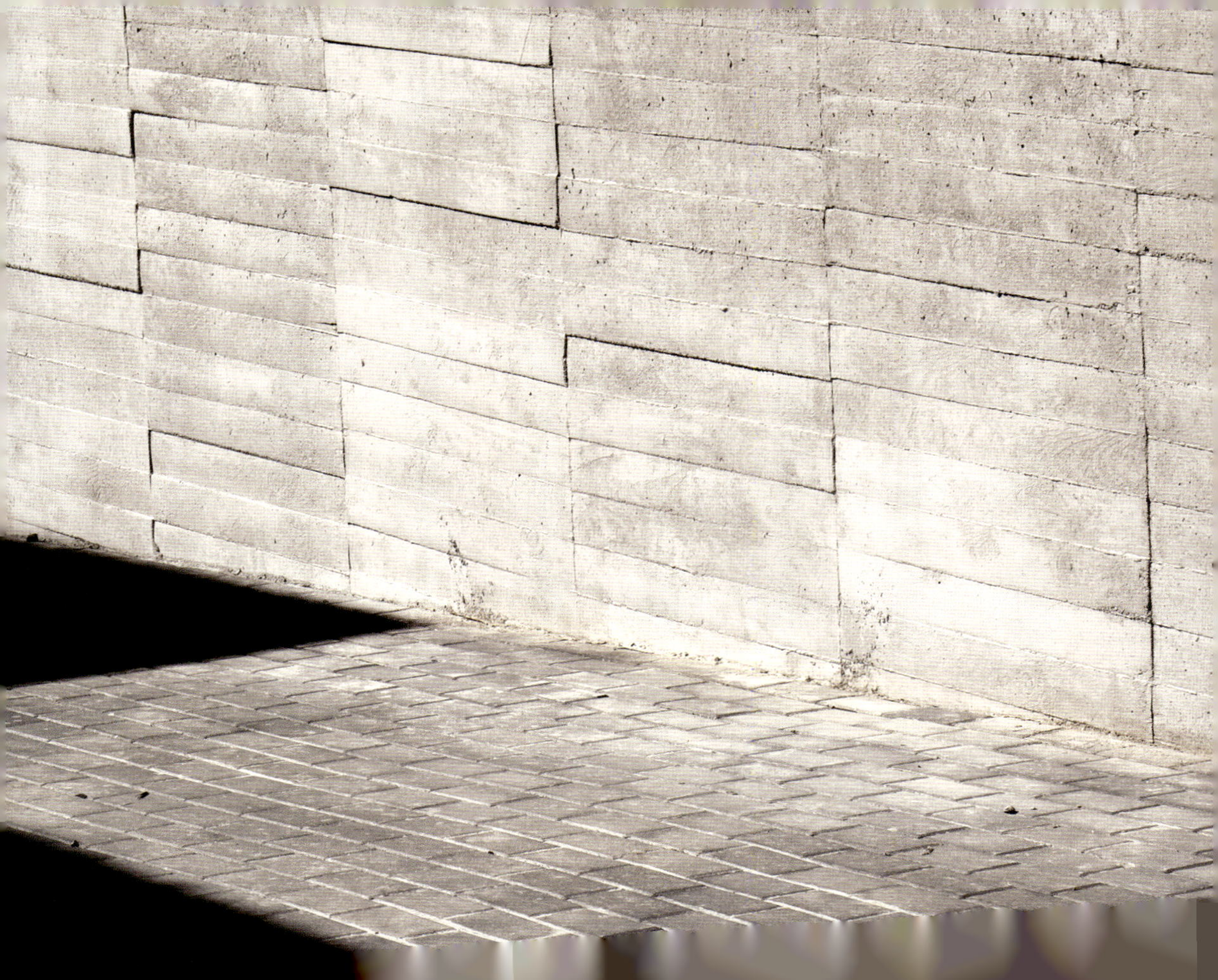

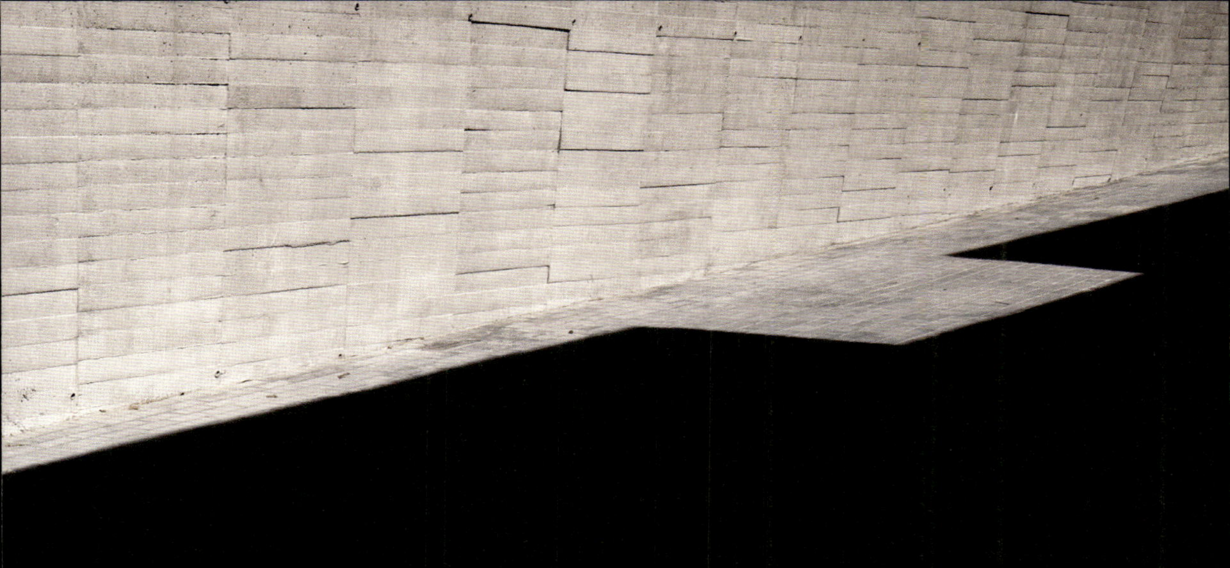

*__Scale of the drawings__: 1/4500 page 17; 1/2000 pages 18, 20, 22, 68; 1/1600 pages 50, 52, 53, 72, 73; 1/800 pages 24, 25, 33, 44, 45, 48, 49, 54, 55, 56, 58, 59, 62, 69, 73, 76, 77, 113, 148, 149; 1/600 page 74; 1/550 pages 98, 99, 101; 1/500 pages 30, 31, 35, 36, 37; 1/400 pages 26, 27, 43, 64, 65, 67, 87, 89, 91, 102, 103, 104, 105, 106, 107108, 109110, 111, 114, 153; 1/275 pages 121, 123, 125; 1/250 pages 80, 81, 82, 83, 84, 85, 92, 93, 94, 95, 151, 154, 155; 1/40 pages 135, 137, 139.

			units	m²	units	m²	units	m²
common	entrance hall	44/49	●	44,35	●	44,35	●	48,48
	reception	14/16	●	14,69	●	15,05	●	14,94
	archive and first storage	20/22	●	21,27	●	20,86	●	20,03
	systems control and security	10/11	●	10,46	●	10,46	●	10.69
	conference room	40/44	●	40,60	●	40,60	●	43,70
	multipurpose room	54/57	●	54,52	●	54,52	●	56,94
	public restrooms	4/5	●	4,16	●	4,08	●	4,75
				190,05		**189,92**		**199,53**
administration and personnel	office	15/18	● ● ●	50,58	● ● ●	50,58	● ● ●	52,51
	waiting area	21/22	●	21,47	●	21,47	●	21,58
	personnel room	29/37	●	29,86	●	36,25	●	36,26
	personnel kitchen	12/14	●	12,85	●	12,30	●	13,37
	personnel changing rooms	6/9	● ●	17,40	● ●	13,32	● ●	12,61
				132,16		**133,92**		**136,13**
primary care	exam room (doctor)	18/19	● ● ● ●	75,60	● ● ● ●	75,62	● ● ● ●	73,92
	treatment room (nurse)	16/17	● ●	34,25	● ●	32,25	● ●	32,16
	pediatric exam	20/22	●	20,15	●	20,15	●	21,66
	pediatric treatment	18/20	●	18,37	●	18,22	●	19,12
	tests room	20/21	●	20,26	●	20,26	●	20,38
	obstectrics	26/28	●	26,34	●	26,34	●	27,19
	midwife	18/22	●	18,22	●	18,22	●	21,38
	social worker	19/21	●	20,77	●	20,77	●	19,70
	mental health	14/22	● ● ●	45,49	● ● ●	57,00	● ● ●	59,30
	waiting area	20/25	● ● ● ● ●	111,30	● ● ● ● ●	111,3	● ● ● ● ●	107,23
	public restrooms	4/13	● ● ● ●	35,26	● ●	23,97	● ●	23,09
	personnel restrooms	4/6	● ●	8,82	● ●	11,15	● ●	11,11
	sterilization	4/5	●	4,94	●	4,13	●	4,31
	storage	4/13	●	4,43	●	6,80	●	12,17
	waste	5/6	●	5,37				
	linen	4/6	●	5,27	●	4,2	●	4,99
	cleaning	5/8	●	5,37	●	7,16	●	5,94
				444,20		**457,55**		**463,65**
service	parking		●	473,59			●	487,80
	general storage	16/41	●	16,19	●	40,55	●	20,79
	electric room	7/11	●	10,78	●	7,34	●	7,45
	mechanical room	45/49	●	45,04	●	48,34	●	48,85
	comunications and UPS	9/11	●	9,84	●	10,12	●	10,05
	garbage room	4/9	●	7,59	●	4,95	●	8,54
				563,03		**111,30**		**583,48**
net area				**1329,44**		**892,54**		**1382,79**

estudio.entresitio is an international award winning practice with bases in Madrid and New York.

Maria Hurtado de Mendoza and Cesar Jimenez de Tejada are founding partners and have worked together since the beginning of their professional careers in 1993. Jose Maria Hurtado de Mendoza joined the office in 2003, after working for Rafael Moneo for four years, and Alvar Ruiz has been part of the team since 2007.

estudio.entresitio is invested in the material actualization of the architectural concept. The practice has extensive building experience with an emphasis on public work that utilizes novel solutions to the functional and necessary without sacrificing the creative or exploratory.

estudio.entresitio has enjoyed much attention. In 2007, Architectural Record selected the firm as Design Vanguard, helping their work to be published and seen in many countries. Their built work has received more than 42 awards and honorable mentions. The firm participated in the 10th, 11th and 13th (2016) BEAU Spanish Biennial of Architecture and Urbanism, the 7th BIAU Iberoamerican Biennial of Architecture and Urbanism, the 7th, 10th and 15th (2016) Venice Biennale, and received the ACSA design faculty award, and the 2014 WAN House of the year award for the #house#1.130. Their latest success is the 1st Prize in the international competition for the National Museum of Memory to be built in Bogotá, Colombia together with MGP.

Awards and recognitions for the the trilogy of clinics San Blas, Usera and Villaverde:
- Prize, health care architecture, ARCHDAILY Building of the YEAR 2012. February 2013.
- First prize, health care category, AIT AWARD 2012, CMS Usera, Frankfurt. April 2012.
- Finalist, health care category, AIT AWARD 2012, CMS Villaverde, Frankfurt. April 2012.
- First prize, ASPRIMA-SIMA 2012, best non-residential building 2012, CMS Villaverde. April 2012.
- First prize, International Biennal "Barbara Cappochin" 2011, CMS Villaverde. July 2011.
- Honorable Mention, International Biennal "Barbara Cappochin" 2011, CMS Usera. July 2011.
- Pre-finalist, XI BEAU (Bienal Española) 2011, CMS San Blas. April 2011.
- Selected, VII BIAU (Bienal Iberoamericana), CMS San Blas. April 2010.
- Madrid's prize, IV Premio de Arquitectura Enor, CMS San Blas. November 2009.
- Third prize, III Premio BigMat de Arquitectura, CMS San Blas. June 2009.
- Honorable Mention, Young architecture award, X BEAU 2009, CMS San Blas. March 2009.
- First prize, XXII Madrid's City Hall awards (best non residential building), CMS San Blas. December 2008.
- First prize, VI Ascer awards (interior design), CMS San Blas. December 2007.

estudio.entresitio
www.entresitio.com
estudio@entresitio.com

María Hurtado de Mendoza
mhm@entresitio.com

César Jiménez de Tejada
cjtb@entresitio.com

José María Hurtado de Mendoza
jmhm@entresitio.com

Álvar Ruíz Villanueva
ar@entresitio.com

Madrid
Gran Via 33, 7I. 28013 Madrid, Spain
T +34 91 701 03 30

New York
134 West 86th st. #4A. NY 10024 USA
T +1 917 870 1092

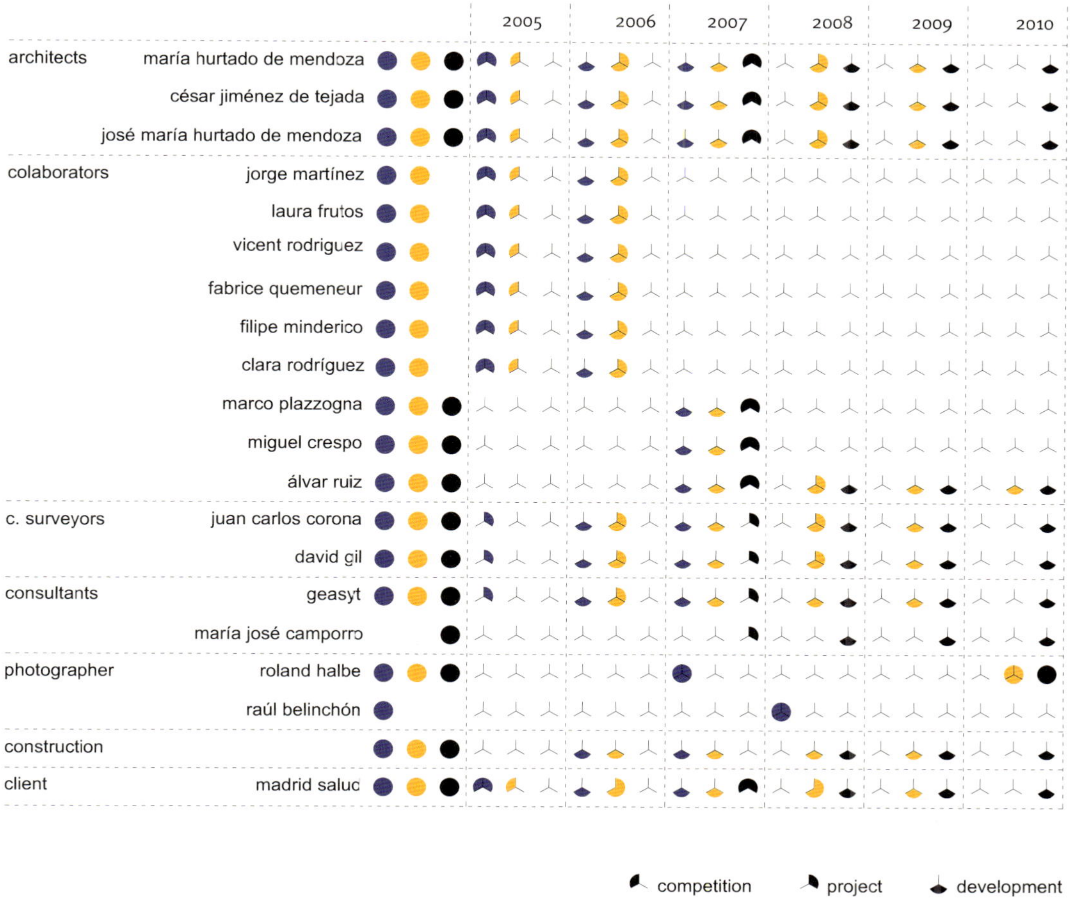
2005
2006
2007
2008
2009
2010
architects
maría hurtado de mendoza
césar jiménez de tejada
josé maría hurtado de mendoza
colaborators
jorge martínez
laura frutos
vicent rodriguez
fabrice quemeneur
filipe minderico
clara rodríguez
marco plazzogna
miguel crespo
álvar ruiz
c. surveyors
juan carlos corona
david gil
consultants
geasyt
maría josé camporro
photographer
roland halbe
raúl belinchón
construction
client
madrid salud
competition
project
development

clinical
an architecture of variation
with repetition

Maria Hurtado de Mendoza
estudio.entresitio

Published by
Actar Publishers
New York, Barcelona

Graphic Design
Ramon Prat Homs

Copy editing
Angela Kay Bunning

Drawings by
estudio.entresitio

Photography by
Pages 158–245: Roland Halbe
Pages 246–251: Raúl Belinchón

Distributed by
Actar Distribution Inc.
440 Park Avenue South, 17th Floor
New York, NY 10016
T +1 212 966 2207
F +1 212 966 2214
salesnewyork@actar-d.com

Barcelona
Roca i Batlle 2-4
08023 Barcelona
T +34 933 282 183
salesbarcelona@actar-d.com
eurosales@actar-d.com

ISBN 978-1-945150-48-7
Library of Congress Control Number:
2017940716
A CIP catalogue record for this book is available from the Library of Congress, Washington D.C., USA.

This publication was supported with funds from the New Jersey Institute of Technology.

ACTAR

NJIT New Jersey Institute of Technology